THE POLITICS OF CHEMICAL RISK: SCENARIOS FOR A REGULATORY FUTURE

# THE POLITICS OF CHEMICAL RISK:
## SCENARIOS FOR A REGULATORY FUTURE

Edited by

Roland Bal

*Leyden Institute for Law & Public Policy,*
*University of Leiden, Leiden, The Netherlands*

and

Willem Halffman

*Department of Science & Technology Dynamics,*
*University of Amsterdam, Amsterdam, The Netherlands*

KLUWER ACADEMIC PUBLISHERS
DORDRECHT / BOSTON / LONDON

A C.I.P. Catalogue record for this book is available from the Library of Congress.

ISBN 0-7923-4891-5

Published by Kluwer Academic Publishers,
P.O. Box 17, 3300 AA Dordrecht, The Netherlands.

Sold and distributed in North, Central and South America
by Kluwer Academic Publishers,
101 Philip Drive, Norwell, MA 02061, U.S.A.

In all other countries, sold and distributed
by Kluwer Academic Publishers,
P.O. Box 322, 3300 AH Dordrecht, The Netherlands.



*Printed on acid-free paper*

Layout and camera-ready copy:
Anne-Marie Krens – Oegstgeest – The Netherlands

Cover design:
Merian Plaat, Plaatwerk – Delft



Printed in the Netherlands

CONTENTS

# PREFACE

This is an unusual book. What is not unusual is its theme. Indeed, many hundreds of books and probably tens of thousands of articles have been written on the subject of chemical risk. Most of these works discuss the possible harm done by specific chemicals, or the way chemicals in general should be regulated. Some of them analyse the way chemical risk is measured or regulated. These works stem from such different disciplines as human or ecotoxicology, pathology, epidemiology, policy science and the study of science and technology, to name just a few.

Neither are the origins of this volume very unusual. Indeed, the sentence "this book is the product of a workshop..." will not sound very unfamiliar to most readers.

Two things make the book unusual. The first is that it brings together authors who seldom meet. A very sharp division seems to run through the field of chemical risk, separating on the one hand people who are actually assessing and managing chemical risk, from people who are studying this activity on the other. These people seem to live in different worlds, speak different languages, have different problems and different answers to these problems. There are several reasons for this divide, of which the most important probably has to do with the boundary between science and non-science. From the 1970s onwards, the separation of scientific from non-scientific issues on chemical risk, i.e. the separation of risk assessment from risk management, has become increasingly important for the legitimation of the regulation of chemicals. Such a separation is moreover, though difficult to reach in practice, deemed possible by actors in the world of chemical risk. That possibility, however, is questioned within social analyses of risk regulations. Scientific assessments of risk are viewed on this side of the divide as social constructions, no different in essence from extra-scientific assessments.

Moreover, the separation between science and non-science itself is, as these analysts express, part of a 'politics of chemical risk'. Not surprising, then, that the two worlds hardly ever meet.

We believe this situation to be detrimental to both sides of the divide, and that there are many things to learn from a confrontation. Since we ourselves are social students of risk regulation, we know that we can learn a lot from actors in the world of chemical risk. But we also believe that we have something to tell them that can solve some of their problems, or at least point in new directions where answers may be found. The divide then need not be as wide as it may seem from an epistemological point of view. The workshop, as well as the present volume, puts this hypotheses to the test, of course.

The second reason why the book is unusual is the way it ends. There are in fact two endings, the first being substantial and the second reflexive. Substantially, instead of ending with a proclamation of some sort, specifying what the problems are and where action should be undertaken, it ends with *scenarios*. That is, instead of narrowing down possible courses of action, it tries to create space to debate different ones. As such it can be seen as an agenda, setting out some of the issues that we, as well as the participants in the workshop, think are important. It further provides a frame, or rather different frames, in which these issues might be discussed. The second ending is a reflection upon 'the workshop as an experiment'. Did we – that is organisers and participants – succeed in analysing and bridging the divide described above?

Needless to say, the organisation of a workshop and the publication of a book cannot proceed without the help of a great many persons and organisations. We would like to thank the following organisations that provided for financial support to the workshop: the European Commission, Directorates General XI and V, the European Association for the Study of Science and Technology (EASST), the Dutch Research School on Science, Technology, Modern Culture, the Leyden Institute for Law & Public Policy, the Health Council of The Netherlands and the Dutch Organisation for Scientific Research.

Arjan Spit did a very good job at making minutes of the tapes that were recorded during the discussions. Wiebe Bijker proved to be an invaluable intermediary between the 'two worlds'. His chairing abilities furthermore go unquestioned. Anne-marie Krens not only proved to be a great help in negotiating with hotels and restaurants and trying to keep us to our time-schedule, but also did a wonderful job at the layout of the book, as did Merian Plaat for the cover.

The editors,
Amsterdam & Maastricht, 10 December 1997

*Willem Halffman & Roland Bal*

# GENERAL INTRODUCTION

This book is the product of a workshop. The workshop *The Politics of Chemical Risk* was organised with a double agenda in mind. One set of goals was related to the future of chemical hazard regulation in Europe. The other was concerned with an attempt to create communication between natural and social scientists working on or in risk regulation. In this general introduction we first discuss the goals that informed the workshop, as well as this volume. After that, we give a short description of the workshop and the book itself. We do not discuss the chapters: these are discussed in separate introductions, preceding each part of the book.

The first and substantial goal was to clarify and elaborate some of the tensions in the regulation of chemical substances in both the workplace and the environment. All industrial countries have developed regulatory systems to assess and manage the risk of chemical substances. While these were at first national initiatives, international organisations, such as the OECD and the EU, are becoming more important actors in this field of policy, taking international harmonisation ever further. These projects run counter to important differences in national regulatory systems. Such differences are not only due to political structures and styles (Vogel 1986), but also to different styles and approaches in regulatory science and assessment, and are even a matter of differences in the way the boundaries between the two are drawn, organised, and maintained.

Some countries tend to rely mainly on expert advice in their regulations, usually in the form of highly discrete expert committees. Others have set

In: R. Bal & W. Halffman (eds.), *The Politics of Chemical Risk*, Kluwer Academic Publishers, Dordrecht 1998: p. 1-6.

up extensive negotiation procedures, in which a wide range of groups participate, even in rather technical discussions (Brickman et al. 1985). International initiatives, such as the North Sea Conference or the EU's setting of Occupational Exposure Limits, continue to put these national mechanisms of science/policy coordination under pressure. As these initiatives intensify, they increasingly raise important questions of how these tensions will work out and about new alternatives for accommodating local differences with translocal integration. How will national consultation procedures relate to international decision making on chemical risks? What are the possibilities for democratic participation in risk regulation on an international level? How will differences in national risk assessment procedures be accommodated? How will the international regulatory system be integrated with different national styles of regulation and government?

The second goal was to stimulate the communication between natural and social scientists in order to mobilise interdisciplinary experiences for this agenda. The regulation of chemical risk is a domain of policy that involves a wide range of actors. People in regulatory agencies, scientists such as toxicologists, epidemiologists, or ecologists, industrial researchers, trade unions and environmental organisations: all have a high degree of first hand experience with the operation of regulatory systems. In particular, the natural scientists involved in regulatory research (and policy), form a rather close-knit community that has ample opportunities to meet and exchange views. Policy analysts and social scientists interact with this community to a much lesser degree, despite an impressive body of research on risk regulation. It is precisely the widely differing forms of integration and distinction of science and policy between different regulatory systems that have been a central topic for the researchers in science studies (cf. Gillespie 1979; Gillespie et al. 1982; Jasanoff 1990; 1992; Wynne 1992; Landy et al. 1990; Limoges et al. 1992; Cambrosio et al. 1992).

The social science approach to risk differs from that of the natural scientists, as is very prominent in a 1992 report of the British Royal Society, *Risk: Analysis, Perception and Management*. The first section of this report is entirely devoted to quantitative approaches that interpret risk analysis as a purely scientific problem, whereas the second section points to the close interconnection between culture, policy and risk and the impossibility of a 'purely scientific' approach (Royal Society 1992; cf. Health Council of the Netherlands 1995). No attempt is made, however, to discuss the differences and tensions between these two positions, let alone to begin to integrate them (Levidow 1994). Our idea was to get beyond this gap, to combine the advantages of practical experience and detailed technical knowledge with the power of social scientists' reflexive contributions, in order to think about possible regulatory futures. The intention was, then, not to reformulate the different agendas of natural and social scientists into one common agenda, but rather to open up the respective positions in order to stimulate debate on what kind of futures can be envisaged for the politics of chemical risk.

In order to do this, we selected three themes about which we saw opportunities for discussion. The three themes are the workings and organisation of the boundary between chemical risk assessment and risk management, the mutual influence of the national and the international arenas of chemicals regulation, and the standardisation and protocolisation of toxicity tests. Far from being the only possible themes, these three provide ample opportunity to discuss the natural and social scientists' contributions.

## The workshop

We wrote all of this in a long starting document, specifying that we wanted one session on the risk management – risk assessment boundary, one on internationalisation, and one on standardisation. For each of these, specific questions were formulated and topics suggested. We sent out this document for comment, and invitations, contributions, and sponsors snowballed. Because we foresaw communication difficulties, we decided to send out a reader containing basic texts from both the regulation of chemicals and the study thereof. We thought it important to keep a close grip on the program in order to keep the project on its intended track, e.g. by asking speakers to talk on specific subjects, specifying the questions we would like them to go into. We sent out abstracts of all talks to the participants beforehand, in order to keep presentations as short and discussions as long a possible. On the basis of the literature and the abstracts, we wrote four 'scenarios for a regulatory future', which were handed down to the participants at the start of the workshop. We included much time for informal gatherings, plenty of food and drinks, and even fitted in the obligatory canal tour in order to maximise informal contacts. On 7 and 8 December 1995, the participants met in Amsterdam, delicately chaired by Wiebe Bijker.

## THE BOOK

The book is made up of four parts. The first three contain discussions of the respective themes: the risk assessment – risk management boundary, internationalisation and standardisation. They are each briefly introduced, specifying the theme and the questions that go with it and summarising the respective chapters, and are concluded with a 'discussions' section, containing the discussions at the workshop. In the last part the two underlying goals of the workshop are brought together: the substantive goal is elaborated in the scenarios, while the communication goal is evaluated in a postscript on 'the workshop as an experiment'.

## References

Brickman, R., S. Jasanoff & T. Ilgen (1985) *Controlling Chemicals: The Politics of Regulation in Europe and the United States*, Ithaca: Cornell UP.

Cambrosio, A., C. Limoges & E. Hoffman (1992) 'Expertise as a Network: A Case Study of the Controversies over the Environmental Release of Genetically Modified Organisms', in: N. Stehr and R.V. Ericson (eds.), *The Culture and Power of Knowledge: Inquiries into Contemporary Societies*, Berlin: De Gruyter; 341-61.

Gillespie, B. (1979) 'British "Safety Policy" and Pesticides', in: R. Johnston & P. Gummett (eds.) *Directing Technology: Policies for Promotion and Control*, London: Croom Helm; 202-24.

Gillespie, B., D. Eva & R. Johnston (1982) 'Carcinogenic Risk Assessment in the USA and UK: The Case of Aldrin/Dieldrin', in: B. Barnes & D. Edge (eds.) *Science in Context: Readings in the Sociology of Science*, Milton Keynes: Open University Press; 303-335.

Health Council of the Netherlands: Committee on Risk measures and risk assessment (1995), *Not All Risks Are Equal*, The Hague: Health Council of the Netherlands, publ. no. 1995/06.

Jasanoff, S. (1990). *The Fifth Branch: Science Advisers as Policy Makers*, Cambridge, MA: Harvard UP.

Jasanoff, S. (1992) 'Science, Politics, and the Negotiation of Expertise at EPA', *Osiris*, 2nd series 7: 195-217.

Landy, M.K., M.J. Roberts & S. Thomas (1990) *The Environmental Protection Agency: Asking the Wrong Questions*, New York: Oxford UP.

Levidow, L. (1994) 'De-reifying Risk', *Science as Culture* 4: 440-56.

Limoges, C., A. Cambrosio, D. Charron & B. Longpré (1992), 'From ecotoxicology to risk assessment in biotechnology: the standardization of microcosms', paper for the Society for the History of Technology conference, Uppsala, Sweden, August 1992.

Royal Society (1992) *Risk: Analysis, Perception and Management. Report of a Royal Society Study Group*, London: Royal Society.

Vogel, D. (1986) *National Styles of Regulation: Environmental Policy in Great Britain and the United States*, Ithaca: Cornell UP.

Wynne, B. (1992) 'Carving Out Science (and Politics) in the Regulatory Jungle', *Social Studies of Science* 22: 745-758.

# PART I

THE RISK ASESSEMENT

–

RISK MANAGEMENT BOUNDARY

# INTRODUCTION

Starting with innovations in the second half of the 1970s, the risk assessment – risk management distinction has become a central organising scheme in regulatory systems. Under the heading *risk assessment* the effects of chemicals in the environment are assessed scientifically, while the political and economic considerations are a matter of *risk management*. The distinction has been institutionalised in regulatory agencies and procedures and has often helped to limit policy conflict by attempting to seal off the scientific parts of the debates from the political ones. If this process is successful, then political conflict is only possible within the confines of the possible, as indicated by the scientific assessment of risk (Jasanoff 1990, 1992). This approach to decision making has strong proponents, especially in the regulatory world, but also among policy analysts, the main advantage being an increase in both the legitimacy and the productivity of the decision making process. However, critics claim that behind the screens of risk assessment, decisions are being made that are essentially political in character and should therefore not be left to scientific experts (cf. Fischer 1990).

Fortunately, there is much undiscovered terrain in between these extremes. Where and how the boundary between assessment and management is drawn turns out to vary between different regulatory contexts and between different points in time. For example, Flip Noordam, of the Dutch Ministry of Social Affairs and Employment, gave a short presentation at the workshop on the different demarcations between risk assessment and management in procedures for occupational standard setting in some European countries. In a comparison between Scandinavian countries and The Netherlands in particular, he showed how the determination of adequate safety factors is considered a matter of politics in the former and a matter of science in the latter.

Furthermore, there is now some evidence that one of the sources of counterproductive policy controversies is precisely the insufficient negotiation between policy actors about where the boundary needs to be drawn. Examples of such disagreement can be found in conflicts over the participation of interest groups in regulatory committees (cf. Castleman & Ziem 1988) or the access of these groups to the information used in assessments (cf. Wynne & Mayer 1993).

The three chapters that follow explore some of the grounds of the risk assessment – risk management boundary. What is this boundary made of? What role does it play in risk regulation? What are the problems it runs into, or creates, and in what ways can these be overcome?

We start this volume with Sue Mayer's and Gillian Glegg's paper on the role of ecotoxicology in standard setting for UK water pollution prevention policies. Although the scientists involved in this process claim that there is a strict boundary between risk assessment and risk management, Mayer and Glegg argue, the practice of standard setting shows that this is a myth. The uncertainties in current risk assessment procedures constantly require scientists to make judgements without a firm scientific basis. Although the existence of these judgements is acknowledged by the regulatory world, this is seen as a mere technical problem, to be resolved with ever more research. Mayer and Glegg claim that regulators and scientists fail to see the fundamentally political presuppositions underlying the way regulatory concepts such as the 'precautionary principle' or 'assimilative capacity' are applied. They argue for a broader political debate on the evaluations that are made in the risk assessment process as a way to improve the quality of decision making as well as environmental protection.

Like Mayer and Glegg, Mark Piney is concerned with the political aspects of risk assessment. His analysis of the setting of Threshold Limit Values by the American Conference of Governmental Industrial Hygienists (ACGIH) shows that they are based on assumptions, resembling the ones underlying the assimilative capacity of the environment. Piney tracks the origins of this paradigm – leading him to the professionalisation of industrial hygienists in the first half of this century – as well as its spread. The 'diffusion' of the paradigm went hand in hand with the adoption of TLVs by nations all over the world in the post-war period. While the TLV-committee of the ACGIH proclaimed in public that TLVs were only health based, Piney shows that all along it was known that they were in fact balancing health effects and economic feasibility. Furthermore, Piney shows that there is an 'anchoring effect' in standard setting, which not only works between committees in different countries, but also in relation to actual exposure, especially in high-exposure workplaces. To overcome this, he suggests that standards should not refer to single exposure limits, but to zones of exposure.

In his contribution on Dutch Maximum Accepted Concentrations, Roland Bal traces the dynamics of boundaries between risk assessment and risk management on three different levels. Firstly, he shows that in the organisational setting, the boundary between risk management and risk assessment has become thicker in the course of time. This has been accompanied with a tighter emphasis on the boundaries between what he calls 'domains of discretion' in the standard setting mandate. In the practice of standard setting, however, no such strict boundaries exist: what is to be called 'assessment' and what 'management' has to be ordered out in the process of standard setting itself. He argues that in order to be productive, the heterogeneity of practice has to be translated in the orderly world of the mandate. Drawing upon work in Science and Technology Studies, he identifies three 'boundary ordering devices' that enable actors within the MAC procedure to make such a translation. Furthermore, he argues that while the boundary between assessment and management generally tends to be emphasised during controversies, this might be counterproductive. In these cases, according to him, more room should be given for negotiating the boundary.

## References

Castleman, B.I. & G.E. Ziem (1988) 'Corporate Influence on Threshold Limit Values', *American Journal of Industrial Medicine* 13: 531-59.

Fischer, F. (1990) *Technocracy and the Politics of Expertise*, London; Sage.

Jasanoff, S.S. (1990) *The Fifth Branch: Science Advisers as Policymakers*, Cambridge, MA: Harvard UP.

Jasanoff, S. (1992) 'Science, Politics, and the Renegotiation of Expertise at EPA', *Osiris 2nd Series* 7: 195-217.

Wynne, B. & S. Mayer (1993) 'How Science Fails the Environment', *The New Scientist* 138, June 5 1993: 32-35.

# 1

*Sue Mayer & Gillian Glegg*

# THE RISK ASSESSMENT / RISK MANAGEMENT BOUNDARY MYTH MAKING AND ITS IMPLICATIONS IN THE UNITED KINGDOM

## INTRODUCTION

In this paper, taking chemical regulation and environmental decision making as an example, we explore the grey area that is the boundary between risk assessment and risk management. In particular, we consider how the lack of clarity in this area reinforces a certain approach to pollution control and how it gives this approach the influential label 'scientific', but at the same time limits alternative approaches to pollution control by an implicit (and sometimes explicit) assertion that they are 'non-scientific'. We also look at how this is integrated into the changing political situation in the UK, where there is a growing lack of trust in institutions, as well as a cynicism about democratic processes.

The aim of the work reported here was to determine how scientists involved in the regulatory process approach the issue of science and its use as a management tool. The paper draws on interviews with water pollution scientists in the Department of the Environment (DoE), the Water Research Centre (WRc), the National Rivers Authority (NRA) and Her Majesty's Inspectorate of Pollution (HMIP) and elsewhere, conducted during 1994 (the NRA and HMIP have since been amalgamated to form the Environment Agency). In these interviews the respondents were asked their opinion of current approaches to pollution regulation in the UK, how they thought this would change in the future and what sort of role they see for science

In: R. Bal & W. Halffman (eds.), *The Politics of Chemical Risk*, Kluwer Academic Publishers, Dordrecht 1998: p. 13-26.

in this operation. Around 20 interviews were carried out each lasting upwards of an hour.

## Risk management: Water pollution regulations in the UK

The UK operates its risk management through a regulatory system which assesses chemical pollutants on an individual, chemical by chemical basis (see ENDS, 1992). The concentrations of individual chemicals are classified as safe or not depending on the use class of a river – for fishing or water abstraction, for example. In many respects, this amounts to determining the Assimilative Capacity of the receiving environment – that is the amount of a pollutant a particular environment can accommodate without causing more harm than is deemed acceptable. Therefore, licences are issued detailing specific chemicals and the maximum concentrations or loads which may be discharged. Many effluents will contain many different constituents but only very few will be consistently named and therefore specifically controlled via the licence.

Based on the determination of safe levels, consents are given to industries to release a given amount of a certain chemical or chemicals in their waste effluents. To define this 'safe' level there has to be an understanding of the toxicity, distribution and fate of the chemical in the environment, in addition to information on amounts and locations of releases. Thus, to describe an acceptable discharge from a particular site, information is needed to predict how the chemical will behave once released. This is considered the domain of risk analysis. It is portrayed as a purely technical endeavour, providing information for risk management which also draws on the economic and political criteria.

## Risk assessment: Ecotoxicology

To assess the risk associated with the release of a chemical into the environment it is necessary to know what sort of effect that chemical may have on the receiving waters. To do this the science of ecotoxicology is applied and its information used in an attempt to draw cause and effect relationships which define the risks posed by the pollutants. The role of ecotoxicology is seen as providing the scientific input to risk management which is then combined with the social, economic and political factors.

Ecotoxicology includes establishing the normal status of ecosystems, investigating predictive tests of toxicity, developing models to extrapolate from laboratory effects to effects on ecosystems and monitoring those effects in the field (Barlow et al. 1992). Ecotoxicology can also involve assessment of the quality of the environment exposed. In the aquatic environment specifically, this assessment generally depends upon chemical measures of environment quality, such as the levels of particular pollutants in the water, sediments or biota, or assessment of generic parameters such as biological oxygen demand.

In this way, ecotoxicology can be seen as an applied, 'regulatory' science. Its purpose is to supply scientific data for use in decision making about the control of polluting chemicals by, for example, defining the amount of a chemical which may be discharged without causing detriment to the receiving waters. However, despite an apparent precision implicit in the lists of features of ecotoxicology, a considerable amount of uncertainty exists. In particular, there are seldom sufficient data to carry out a complete assessment of a chemical and its receiving environment, as shown by the study by Mathiesson et al. (1992) of estuaries around the UK.

While it is acknowledged that flexibility is necessary in the interpretation of research for regulatory purposes, the ways in which such uncertainty is interpreted are not known. This contributes to the situation where the boundary between risk assessment and risk management becomes opaque and often impenetrable.

## REGULATORY DECISION MAKING: BRITISH REGULATORY SCIENTISTS' ACCOUNTS

Over the last thirty years there has been substantial investment in the development of chemical standards and methods of monitoring. We asked scientists whether they considered the current system was satisfactory.

Most of the interviewees pointed to inadequacies of the current system. While chemical tests for the presence and absence of chemicals are widely used at present because they are practical and the techniques are relatively well developed, these were not considered adequate for the future. Even those who were quite sceptical about the severity of the problem caused by chemical discharges to rivers, accepted that some improvements to the current approach were needed. The main reason given for this was that they did not relate easily to evidence of environmental harm, i.e. it was seen to be difficult to link cause and effect. Thus, although the regulations as they currently stand depend on being able to establish safe levels of chemicals in the environment, define harm, and monitor environmental quality, there seemed to be an acceptance that this was not being achieved.

*Developing environmentally relevant standards*

A number of shortcomings have been identified which are undermining confidence in the ability of single chemical toxicity testing to protect the environment. These include the large number of chemicals that have to be regulated, the fact that they are usually present in mixtures and the inability of such tests to identify the subtle, chronic effects that these chemicals may have (Matthiessen et. al. 1992; Dethlefsen 1986). This has led to an interest in the monitoring of environmental effects of chemicals in biological terms, and a concomitant move to defining standards in this way. The literature shows that real optimism exists in the UK science policy community that it is possible to realise environmental protection using these methods. This has fuelled a drive towards the development of biological monitoring techniques, although concerns about practical problems have been raised (e.g. Whitehouse et al. 1996). The majority of scientists interviewed, whatever their institutional affiliation, saw biological effects monitoring and whole effluent toxicity testing as the best way forward.

However, there was still dispute over the relevance of the biological responses seen and their link to the chemicals in the environment. While endorsing a more biological approach, there was widespread caution about utilising tests whose significance was not understood. In general, scientists felt that this approach had to be linked to chemical monitoring data so that a cause-effect link could be established. Clear, 'scientific' evidence of harm was perceived to be necessary before action to regulate a chemical or discharge could be justified. In other words, it was seen as necessary to identify that a biological effect was "... something that [was] genuinely going wrong" rather than simply a response. The biologically based tests were viewed as a solution to the problem of establishing environmental relevance, but in turn, they lead to a similar debate over cause and effect.

In addition, one of the striking features of the interviews was the tendency of interviewers to portray evidence from biological tests as over-emphasising the risks. For example, one senior Government scientist said about a new biological enzyme test, EROD:

> All it is, really, is a response of the animal which has led it to trigger a means of dealing with the environmental challenge it has faced in just the same way that if you met a tiger or something as you walked up the street. Your adrenalin level would shoot up and you would be able to run a heck of a lot faster than you would otherwise be able to do. That would be a good thing! So it isn't necessarily bad at all.

And, in relation to biological tests demonstrating the effects of oestrogenic compounds, one scientist from the WRC noted:

> The oestrogenic effect ... it's an interesting and difficult area and one where ... in some ways, certain people are overreacting because the science is not there yet.

Many similar statements were made by others, although they gave no scientific justification for balancing the risks in this optimistic way.

The relevance of biological indicators to environmental effects of a chemical or a mixture of chemicals was not the only problem identified by interviewees. They also highlighted the difficulties of establishing standard, reproducible methods and the need to identify key ecological characteristics. A further problem which has been identified is a fundamental lack of understanding of ecosystems and their variability, which is essential if it is to be possible to distinguish between natural and anthropogeniciclly induced fluctuations.

*The solution: more research*

Scientists interviewed appeared to consider the problems of establishing environmentally relevant standards as technical ones. The difficulties of extrapolating from laboratory tests to field conditions and of establishing environmentally relevant tests were considered to be resolvable with more research. These were not generally seen as fundamental flaws in the approach, but more as technical hitches which could be remedied with greater resources and more time. For example, when asked what was needed to address the uncertainties and inadequacies in the current system, one senior scientist replied: "a bigger budget". Another commented that there was no reason why we should not be able to define and monitor environmental quality if the resources were available.

It was almost always thought possible to address these difficulties and uncertainties with science if sufficient resources were invested. Only one interviewee really questioned whether 'more science' was a sufficient, or logically feasible, option when he noted:

> Well, there's a basic problem from an analytical chemist's point of view ... there are too many chemicals around to try and measure.

This reservation was not, however, expressed by others. When asked whether, given sufficient resources, ecotoxicology could provide precise and relevant tests, one NRA scientist said: "Yes. Like everything else it is the will." Another, from a research institute, when asked about the ability of science to define environmental quality, was similarly optimistic when he said: "Yes. It would not be that difficult."

Thus, the general message that came across strongly was that although the approach of setting standards was problematic in some ways, and issues of environmental relevance still had to be addressed, this was possible with additional investment in research. Some of the government scientists believed, for example, that a two-year research project already underway into the problem of oestrogenic substances in sewage could yield practical, useful policy answers upon its conclusion.

Some of this research has now been published (Institute of Environment and Health 1995), and has concluded that:

> ... a causal relationship between exposure to environmental oestrogens and adverse effects on human reproductive health has not yet been established. Further information from epidemiological and experimental studies is still needed to allow assessments of risk to be made based on weight of evidence.

However, other research published at the same time (Foundation for Water Research 1995, cited in ENDS Report 1995), and in relation to oestrogenic compounds causing endocrine disruption in wild fish populations, concluded:

> It is possible that conclusive proof ... will never be obtained ... (and that) at some stage environmental managers will have to decide whether to act on the basis of burden of evidence.

Thus the policy answers do not seem quite as easily obtained as was suggested. Furthermore, despite the extent of the need for further information, the scientists interviewed rarely mentioned the problem of the practical achievability of new and vast testing programmes for thousands of new and existing chemicals. None of the UK scientists raised the issue of the time delay of waiting for results from scientific data or the problem that, in the interim, chemicals are regulated on the basis of debatable methodologies and uncertain extrapolations.

### *Attitudes to precaution*

Scientists in enforcement agencies (NRA, HMIP) in particular, saw measurable and widely agreed standards and methods as essential to enable them to carry out their duties. In making judgements about what was meaningful, interviewees were also clear that the standards had to be achievable.

These scientists and others often expressed the view that industry should not be 'unduly and unnecessarily burdened'.

Also, in describing what constitutes sufficient evidence of harm, senior scientists in the civil service stated that if laboratory tests alone demonstrated harm, then this was not adequate for chemicals already in the environment. It was noted that industry could be unnecessarily harmed if controls, based on such laboratory tests and without clear evidence of cause and effect, were brought in. As one senior scientist said:

> I'm afraid I don't go much for the idea of turning everything off at the factory; I don't think that's realistic.

Many voiced the need for precaution by saying that while definitive proof of a harmful effect was not necessary, clear evidence was and another commented:

> You have to be careful going into the precautionary principle because you could be having a detrimental effect on an industry or particular discharger for no good reason.

Others echoed these statements, making reference to cost-benefit analyses, social acceptability and financial constraints. They clearly felt that these factors were in some way involved in their deliberations and, although scientists spoke as if they saw the matter as being purely technical and scientific, many of their comments suggest that other considerations were influencing their attitudes. Great importance was given to the perceived need of industry to dispose of its waste in the aquatic environment. This was evident in their feeling that cause and effect had to be demonstrated before scientific approval could be given to action.

Equally striking was the way in which the implications of scientific uncertainty in relation to the significance of biological tests was portrayed. In these cases an optimistic interpretation was given but this was justified, not on scientific grounds, but rather in the interest of fairness to industry. A similar inclination on the part of scientists to give industry the benefit of the doubt in cases of scientific uncertainty has been described by Abraham (1994) in relation to drug safety.

While interviewees professed to be concerned about the interests of industry, avoiding discharges through process modification, or product substitution, was rarely raised in a positive way. When questioned about these options, clean production, closing certain factories, or stopping discharges of whole effluents, was frequently portrayed as being an 'unrealistic' or 'extreme' option. Several of the scientists also mentioned that these features brought the discussion into the realms of politics and economics and away from science. Similarly the precautionary principle was often seen to be extreme, 'unscientific' or unachievable.

In public debates about policies for dealing with chemical waste, the Precautionary Principle is often accused of being used politically (e.g. Stebbing 1992). In contrast, scientific support for the ability of science to determine 'safe' levels of pollutants through use of the Assimilative Capacity approach, gives the impression that the threat of pollutants can be measured and controlled.

The Assimilative Capacity is said to be based on two principles (Portman & Pradvic 1992). Firstly, there is a definable quantity of a substance that can be released into the environment without causing pollution and, secondly, there is a certain level of environmental change which is non-harmful. However, there is also a third, yet rarely stated, principle or assumption which holds that the system is closed and unaffected by any other chemicals or stress factors. While scientists like Portman and Pradvic (1992) accept that harm is socially defined, what they do not question is the ability of science to actually define the quantity of a substance that will not cause that level of harm in what is, in reality, likely to be an open system. There are also scientific studies that question the practicality of current regulation on a chemical by chemical basis which raise, for example, the problems of effluent complexity (Glegg & Johnston 1993). Therefore, taking a precautionary policy goal, such as eliminating the discharges of all xenobiotics, is also arguably consistent with the scientific evidence to date.

Indeed, paradoxically, the same critics of the political nature of the precautionary principle have used explicit political judgements about economics and social practices to justify the assimilative capacity. For example, Portman and Pradvic (1992), important protagonists in the precautionary debate, talk negatively about the 'economic realities' associated with the application of clean technologies. Similarly, Stebbing (1992) concludes that "It is no longer practicable to accept a strategy for pollution control that fails to recognise environmental capacity as part of an ecological market economy."

Scientists thus appear, at times, to see themselves as better placed than the public or politicians to establish definitions of environmental quality but, when doing that, they make a range of social assumptions about what is possible, desirable and achievable. This is not surprising, yet it is frequently denied in public statements about 'scientific' or 'non-scientific' approaches.

## THE IMPLICATIONS

The underlying issue at this particular risk assessment – risk management boundary, as well as in other environmental policy fields, is how to arrive at a socially acceptable compromise between demands for environmental protection on the one hand, and low economic costs on the other, using the best available scientific understanding. Such a compromise is a matter of political values.

It is accepted that UK scientific advisers have to exercise value judgements in formulating their scientific advice. This process should be open to democratic political procedures. But in practice, given, in part, the size of administrative agendas and workloads, these become administrative decisions, made under a constitutional fiction of accountability for each decision, via the relevant Minister, to Parliament. Thus advisers assume they are following the consensus, or at least the dominant political values, when they judge questions in which scientific and policy dimensions are woven together. For example, most scientists interviewed in this study must assume they follow the consensus in the way they invoke the principle that undue costs and pressures should not be placed on industry. In this way the expert judgement process, often simply called the science of risk assessment by its practitioners, is more like a condensed politics. It assumes itself to be legitimate by representing genuine social values, but does not open itself up to the direct expression and negotiation of these.

One implicit assumption in these processes of privileged expert judgement is that all industry is producing unambiguous social benefit. Yet, for example, social research has shown that consumers have considerable concerns about the social value of different kinds of consumer products. For example, foods produced by intensive farming are starting to be rejected in favour of organic foods (e.g. Goodman & Redclift 1991: 239-256). The ways in which such moral concerns are expressed may be patchy and unsystematic. They may, especially, be uninformed by relevant knowledge about, for example, actual environmental side effects and problems of the products. But there is no doubt that these concerns exist increasingly in the public's mind. Yet allowing expert judgement of these values to take place as part of the process of regulatory science is to impose a particular and contentious set of value prescriptions in the name of science. This is why the risk assessment – risk management boundary is really a myth and one which has disturbing implications.

Although scientists involved in the process of regulatory standard setting believe themselves to be expressing legitimate societal values, particularly those of official institutions, the evidence is that such institutions are losing legitimacy and political purchase. A more broadly based, hitherto alienated and marginalised political culture is beginning to organise its own expressions of value in civil society (Marr 1995). If even flexible and pragmatic parliamentary versions of political representation risk being stranded high and dry by these profound developments, so much the more must it be for those much narrower and more presumptive forms of representation in which scientific advisers honestly strive to represent what they think of as consensus policy values in their expert judgements.

The demand for precaution in environmental protection arose out of wider, legitimate cultural values and experiences, yet this move is in danger of being inadvertently hi-jacked by a restricted idea of the way in which knowledge and values articulate together in policy. Instead of seeing that the indeterminacies of precautionary policy commitments favour a broader debate as to what this means in practice, it is delegated to science on the assumption that scientific knowledge can, as usual, define the boundary conditions, now just more precautionary, to which society can continue to pollute.

This delegation to science obstructs the wider need for the public culture of consumerism, advertising and debate to address, in an informed way, questions about the social benefits of, and needs for, products and services. The direct environmental risks of these may be a matter of uncertainty, but that need not be threatening if we can resolve their effects in other ways. For example, by not being so obsessed with having consumer goods (or so many of them). It would then be in the domain of democratic responsibility to make judgements about how much uncertainty over risks we wish to tolerate in relation to products and processes whose importance to society can at least be questioned.

The 1995 Norwegian Gene Technology Act may be a good example of a modern piece of legislation which expressly sets out to cultivate such a broad societal debate (and the capability for it) on need, as an integral part of the risk assessment regulatory responsibility. Thus the wider cultural debate about need, benefit and alternatives, together with a wider social responsibility for environmental protection and for defining sustainable development, would serve to remove much of the heat from risk debates. It would free institutions from their anxious searching for positive knowledge as opposed to admitting unknowns and unknowability.

*Acknowledgements*: This study was conducted while Sue Mayer was a Visiting Research Fellow at the Centre for the Study of Environmental Change, Lancaster University, funded by the Greenpeace Environmental Trust. We are grateful to Brian Wynne and Robin Grove-White for stimulating discussions and support.

## REFERENCES


Abraham, J. (1994) 'Distributing the Benefit of the Doubt: Scientists, Regulators and Drug Safety', *Science, Technology & Human Values* 19: 493-522.

Barlow, S.M., J.M. Bridges, P. Calow, D.M. Canning, R.N. Curnow, A.D. Dayan, I.F.H. Purchase & C.W. Suckling (1992) 'Toxicity, Toxicology & Nutrition', In: *Risk: Analysis, Perception and Management*, Report of a Royal Society Study Group, London: Royal Society; 35-65.

Dethlefsen, V. (1986) 'Marine Pollution Mismanagement: Toward the Precautionary Principle', *Marine Pollution Bulletin* 17: 54-57.

ENDS (1992) *Dangerous Substances in Water: A Practical Guide*, London: Environmental Data Sevices Ltd.

ENDS (1995) *Fish studies strengthen case for curbs on APE's*, London: Environmental Data Services Limited, ENDS Report 246: 5-6.

Glegg, G. & P. Johnston (1993) 'The Policy Implications of Effluent Complexity', in: B.Nath, L.Candola, L.Hens & J.P.Robinson (eds.) *Environmental Polution, ICEP 2*, London: European Centre for Pollution Research; 121-28.

Goodman, D & M. Redclift (1991) *Refashioning Nature: Food, Ecology and Culture*, London: Routledge.

Institute of Environment and Health (1995) *Environmental Oestrogens: Consequences to Human Health and Wildlife*, Leicester: University of Leicester.

Matthiessen, P., J.E. Thain, R.L. Law & T.W. Fileman (1992) 'Attempts to Assess the Environmental Hazard Posed by Complex Organic Mixtures of Organic Chemicals in UK Estuaries', *Marine Pollution Bulletin* 26: 90-95.

Marr, A. (1995) *Ruling Britannia: The Failure and Future of British Democracy*, London: Michael Joseph.

Portman, J.E. & V. Pradvic (1992) 'The Precautionary Principle – Does it Prevent Marine Pollution?', *Chemistry and Ecology* 7: 135-37.

Stebbing, A.R.D. (1992) 'Environmental Capacity and the Precautionary Principle', *Marine Pollution Bulletin* 24: 287-95.

Whitehouse, P., Crane, M., Redshaw, C.J. & Turner, C. (1996) 'Aquatic toxicity tests for the control of effluent discharges in the UK – the influence of test precision', *Ecotoxicology* 5: 155-168.

# 2

*Mark Piney*

# EXPOSURE LIMITS, PRACTICABILITY AND HEALTH RISKS ARGUMENTS FOR A PARADIGM SHIFT

## INTRODUCTION

We live in a quantitative age in which it is said that if something isn't measured or measurable it hardly exists, has no meaning or it cannot be managed. It is a very pervasive and persuasive creed. Politicians, managers and consumers feel happier and more in control if they have numerical scores to judge success or failure or productivity. In the arena of risk and risk management quantification dominates and when it comes to chemical exposure at work the demand is always for a limit, a number to work to. But what do such numbers mean and where did they come from? Interestingly, they are a relatively recent invention and before they existed governments had other ways of regulating risks from chemical exposure.

To understand what occupational exposure limits (OELs) are, we need to examine where they came from, which professional groups produced and promulgated them and what we buy into when we ask that fateful question: is exposure below the OEL?

This contributions will describe how work processes lead to certain exposures. Specifically, in the first section, it will describe the typical exposures of three work groups exposed to silica dust and how such exposures were regulated in the 19th and early 20th Centuries. The chapter then goes on to examine the development of industrial hygiene (IH) and industrial toxicology (IT), and the OEL paradigm these professions forged. This will involve setting out a *working definition* of the paradigm. The development and mean-

In: R. Bal & W. Halffman (eds), *The Politics of Chemical Risk*, Kluwer Academic Publishers, Dordrecht 1998: p. 27-73.

ing of Threshold Limit Values (TLVs), still the exemplary OEL, will be examined. TLVs are 'reasonably practicable' OELs and this reality will lead to a description of what, 'as far as is reasonably practicable' (AFARP) means in practice and the way 'soft' evidence of health effects comes up against the 'hard' facts of practicability and cost. Having described the boundaries in which OELs setting is constrained, the working definition of the OEL paradigm will be revisited and redefined, leading to a discussion of the range of factors which affect the setting of limits and, conversely, the effects single number OELs have on control of risk from chemical exposure. Out of these discussions come arguments for a paradigm shift. The modified paradigm will probably require the setting of two types of standards and how this might be done is described. Finally, just before the conclusions, we return to the stoneworkers we start with and examine what difference the modified paradigm would make to them and the risk of silicosis.

## PROCESSES, JOBS & EXPOSURE

Before delving into the history, meaning and problems which come with OELs, it is important to put the discussion in a work context and this context is all about the industries people work in and the processes they undertake or work with. We will start with three groups of workers who are exposed to silica dust. Fine (respirable) silica dust causes silicosis, a progressive lung scarring disease. Ever since humans have dug mines and extracted minerals from the earth people have contracted silicosis. The risk is not new. Nowadays, people are still exposed to silica dust and still contract silicosis.

The first group works in a quarry in charge of a primary crusher and is exposed on average to 0.8 milligrams per cubic metre of air ($mg/m^3$) respirable quartz dust. The second group are stonemasons working on high silica architectural stone, using various traditional chisels but also regularly using powered tools. This group is exposed on average to 2.0 $mg/m^3$ respirable quartz dust (see Photographs 1 and 2). The third group are pottery workers pouring china slip into moulds, making cups and vases. This group is exposed on average to 0.2 $mg/m^3$.

*Photo 1*

Before occupational exposure limits (OELS) controls such as exhaust ventilation were specified sometimes together with recommended airflow rates. Controls were specified but control effectiveness in terms of an exposure target was not. Photograph shows ineffective captor hoods at a powder weighing operation.

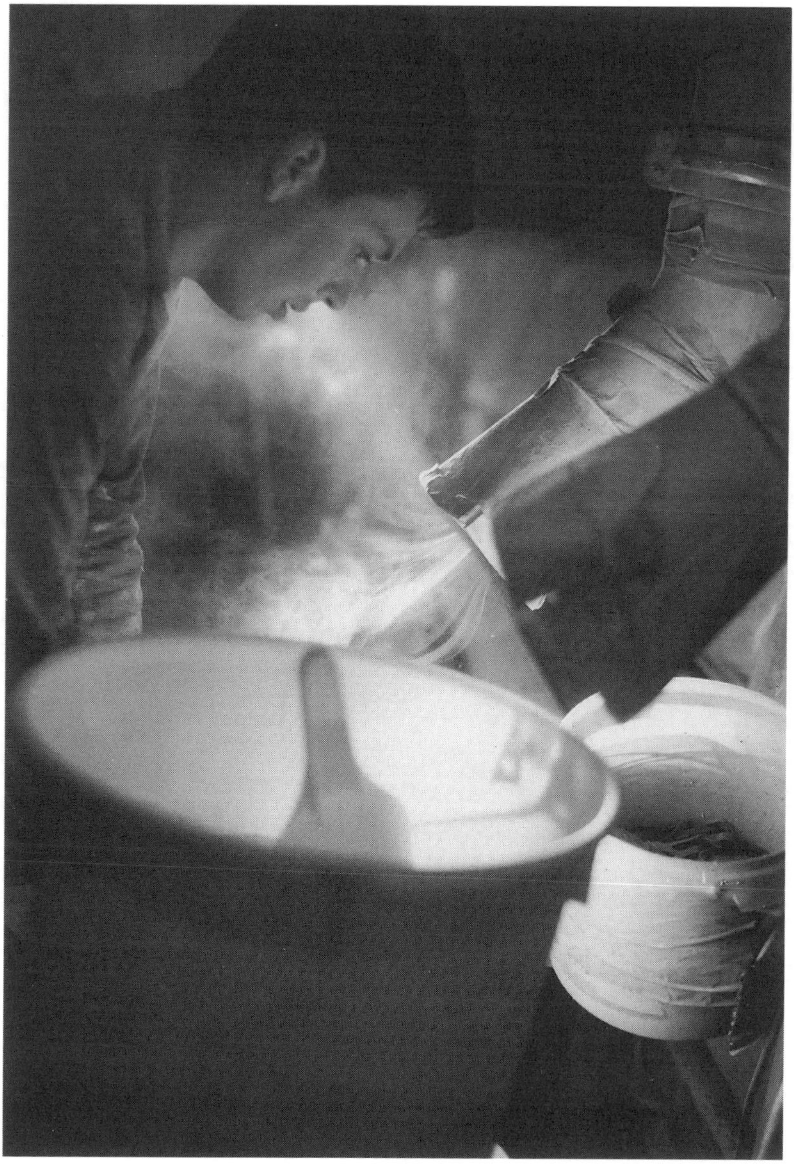

*Photo 2*
Guidance for control of dust as stone masonry operations was all in terms of specification standards. Photograph shows commercially available exhaust ventilation system recommended by the UK Factory Inspectorate in the 1930s. Was the system shown effective enough? For work on high silica stone such as gritstone probably not.

**MILLSTONE DRESSING**

**Dust removal by Localised Exhaust Ventilation**

**(Used at Messrs. Barry, Ostlere & Shepherd Ltd., Kirkcaldy)**

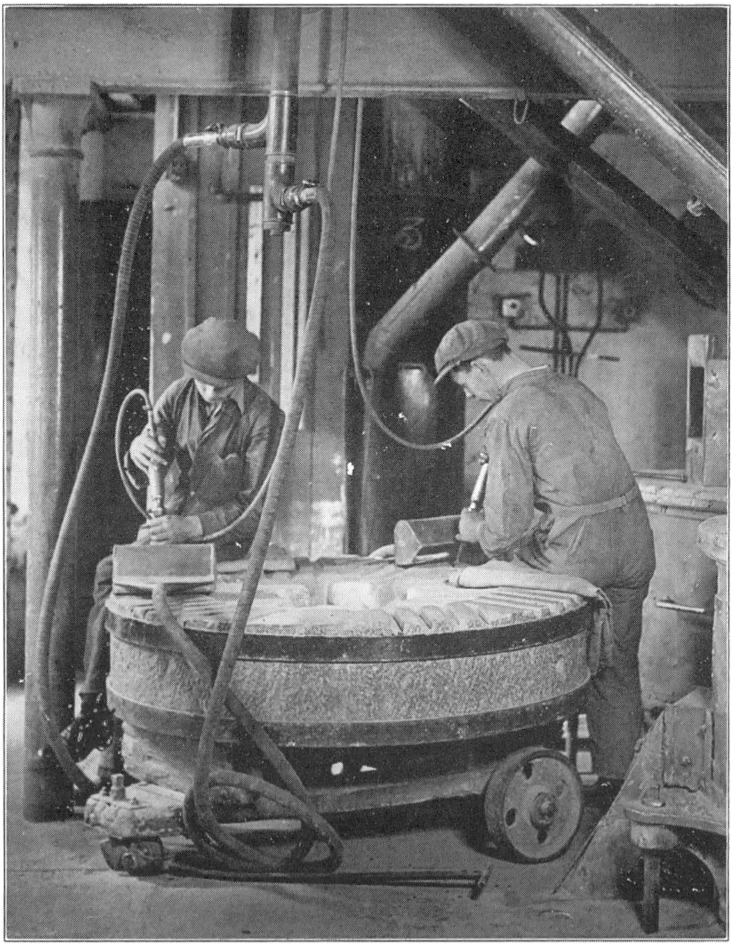

In the United Kingdom (UK) the Maximum Exposure Limit (MEL) for respirable quartz is 0.4 mg/m$^3$ (8 hour Time Weighted Average, or TWA). This standard is judged to be reasonably practicable – defined and discussed later in this chapter – for all processes generating silica dust in the UK. For the quarry work group and the stonemasons the standard clearly tells any assessor that there is a real risk of silicosis if current exposures continue and further indicates that controls need to be applied. The pottery workers' exposures are below the limit and taking the MEL at face value, the pottery owner could be forgiven for thinking that no further controls are needed and that there is no risk of silicosis. For silica dust there is substantial evidence that this conclusion is wrong but the MEL does present a problem to an occupational hygienist or other assessor trying to minimise the risk of silicosis. We will return to these three work groups towards the end of the chapter and see how a different approach to standards might better protect their health.

## PROFESSIONS AND PARADIGMS

> Both normal science and revolutions are ... community-based activities. To discover and analyse them one must first unravel the changing community structure of the sciences over time. A paradigm governs, in the first instance, not a subject matter but rather a group of practitioners. Any study of paradigm-directed or of paradigm-shattering research must begin by locating the responsible group or groups (Kuhn 1970: 179-80).

Single number OELs were developed and promulgated by two science-based professions in the USA in the 1930s and 1940s. Professions can be seen as species evolving to fit societal ecological niches and this is a useful metaphor for plotting and describing the development of professions (Hale et al. 1986). But industrial hygiene and industrial toxicology are also science-based professions. To understand what this means in terms of professional behaviour and belief, the ideas of Thomas Kuhn are useful and form effective additions to simply viewing IH and IT in terms of professional development. Kuhn developed and popularised the paradigm concept. He argued that one could view scientific subjects in terms of pre-scientific periods where no, multiple or dual paradigms exist and paradigmatic periods when schools of science all accept the same paradigm, and at that point one can say that the science of X started proper. Up to this time, various schools put forward fundamentally different explanations for the same phenomena. Only after a certain school's views becomes the generally accepted paradigm can the community of scientists, who accepted the paradigm, settle down to what Kuhn calls 'normal science' and move into a period of post-paradigm productivity. A dominant paradigm has a very dramatic effect on the productivity of a science. Once a paradigm is accepted by a group of practitioners, scientific activity, or 'normal science' consists of puzzle solving and "... a devoted attempt to force nature into the conceptual boxes supplied by professional education" (Kuhn 1970: 5).

Masterman, in her essay 'The nature of a paradigm', counted 21 somewhat different definitions of 'paradigm' in the first edition of Kuhn's book and it is an elusive and elastic idea much abused and misinterpreted since the *Structure of Scientific Revolutions* was first published in 1962. Whatever it is, a paradigm is not 'basic theory' and perhaps Masterman defines the ideas contained within the word 'paradigm' best. She said that:

> A paradigm is a set of scientific habits. By following these, successful problem solving can go on: thus they may be intellectual, verbal, behavioural, technological; any or all of these (Masterman 1970).

In addition, Masterman also clarified how a paradigm works and declared that a paradigm;

> ... is something which can function when the theory is not there... It is an artefact which can be used as a puzzle-solving device and to be used this way it has got to be, in the mind's-eye of the scientist, a concrete 'picture' which is used analogically. It has got to be, in Kuhn's words, 'a way of seeing' (Masterman 1970).

A paradigm is learnt, and a scientific profession reproduces itself by the younger or aspiring members studying the standard texts and exemplary problems and solutions.

While Kuhn was concerned with purer sciences, much of what he says can be read across to applied science-based professions such as industrial hygiene (IH), with some qualifications. The main one being that professions need clients and constituencies who will employ or support them, otherwise they cannot exist. Whereas, in the Kuhnian framework the emphasis is on the theory and practice of professional scientists and the competition which occurs between different groups and between different schools within groups. A client does not exist and employers of scientists, as a group, should have no affect on the science produced by those working to the current paradigm. In pure sciences a strong argument can be made, and is made by Kuhn, that little or no societal influences intrude. In the more applied sciences professional imperatives and the clients' needs are more likely to intrude.

Industrial hygiene, and industrial toxicology (IT) are not, and never have been, pure Kuhnian communities of disinterested scientists. They have always, and will always, feel the tug of two sets of overlapping but incongruent loyalties. For they are, at one and the same time, applied scientific professions trying to behave scientifically and professionally at the same time: they are both professional scientists and scientific professionals (Piney 1989).

## Early process controls, industrial hygiene and exposure limits

### *Public health risks and the 'dangerous trades'*

Certain industrial diseases became reportable in the UK from 1898. The figures reported showed that nearly 2,000 cases of acute poisoning lead cases were recorded in the UK in 1900, and of these a significant percentage died of acute encephalopathy. A similar picture emerged in the USA in those States which had reporting systems amongst what were known there and in the UK as the 'Dangerous Trades'. The factory system concentrated people in one place and the division of labour concentrated people in one job. By this process, the effects of the mechanisation and regimentation of production, certain groups became highly exposed to poisons which before may have been used on occasions by relatively skilled workers as they manufactured a whole product. In addition, by the application of chemistry to production and the creation of new products, new chemical risks were produced. By these various mechanisms, the exposure of particular working groups was dramatically increased in the 19th Century in industrialised countries.

*Specifiying standards for the 'dangerous trades'*

In the last quarter of the 19th Century the concerns of the UK Factory Inspectorate (FI) began to encompass acute occupational health issues such as lead poisoning. In 1878 the Factory Workshop Act, "empowered Inspectors to require mechanical ventilation, whenever they saw fit in workrooms in which dust, gas, vapour or other impurities were generated" (Djang 1942). Towards the end of the 19th Century a series of enquiries were held from which a variety of Regulations were developed with fairly detailed process, work arrangement and ventilation requirements. This approach, whereby controls to be applied to the process are specified in some detail, started at this time in Europe and the USA, and grew in the early part of the 20th Century. In fact, there was a certain amount of interchange and similar specification standards were developed and applied in Germany, France, Great Britain and the USA (photograph 3).

Two people who made a very significant contribution in the UK around this time were Thomas Legge and Elmhurst Duckering, the former being the first Medical Inspector of Factories. Both were involved in detailed studies of lead absorption and poisoning and silica dust exposure and silicosis. Earlier, some use of air measurements was made by the UK FI. Inspectors measured carbon dioxide concentrations to assess the adequacy of general ventilation in factory workshops, starting in the 1880s, but Duckering took measurements much further. Examining a number of dusty processes, mainly involving lead, he measured emissions and exposure and analysed the sources in terms of major contribution to exposure. From his analysis he was able to propose controls based on changes of process and ventilation.

Thomas Legge combined Duckering's exposure measurements with his knowledge of the epidemiology of lead poisoning and symptoms and came to the following conclusion published in 1912:

> Somewhere about 2 milligrams, or 0.002 grams of lead we regard as the lowest daily dose which, inhaled as fumes or dust in the air, may, in the course of years, set up chronic plumbism (Legge & Goadby 1912).

This works out to be somewhat higher but close to current OELs for lead.

Having used air sampling and assessed emissions and exposure, Duckering could see a way forwards to allow control of 'dusty trades' whatever the process causing exposures. There was no need to develop specification standards for each and every process and industry. He put his visionary views thus:

> The most scientific way of regulating a dusty trade would be to impose a limit on the amount of dust which may be allowed to contaminate the air breathed by the workpeople and to leave the manufacturer a completely free choice of methods by which this result may be attained. If such a Regulation were to be adopted, the occupier of a factory would become liable to a penalty in such cases as it was found, experimentally, that the limit was exceeded. There is nothing inherently impossible in such a Regulation (Duckering 1910).

*Photo 3 and 4*
Modern power tools increase the exposure of stone masons. Photograph 3 shows a mason using an electric disc cutter as a saw. Photograph 4 shows a similar handheld powertool being used to polish a gravestone. It is often assumed that conditions in the past were worse than nowadays. In the case of stonemasons this is probably not true.

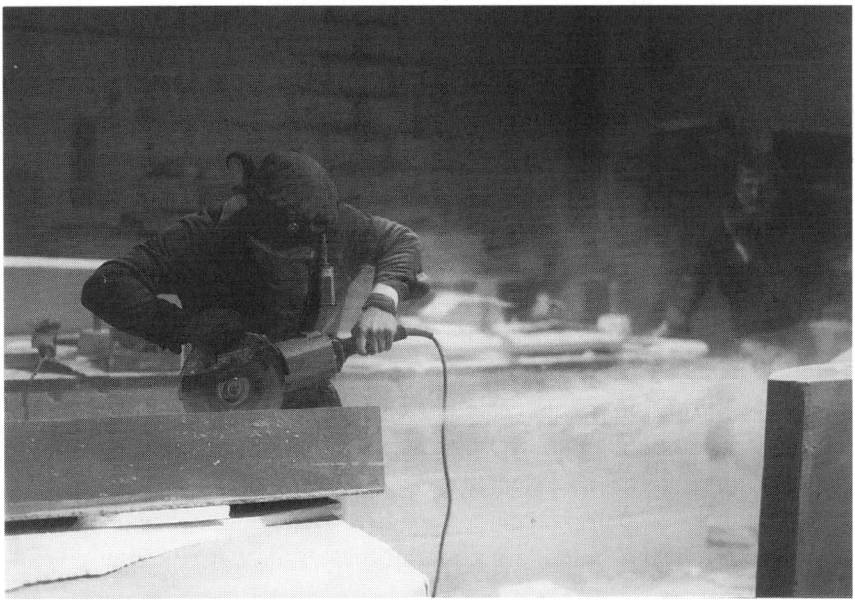

*Photo 4*

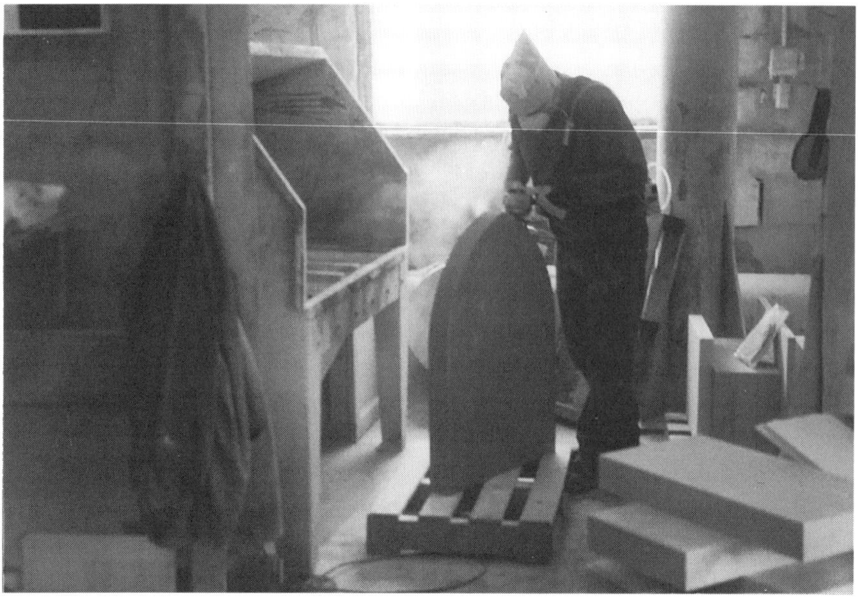

Duckering and Legge's views were ahead of their time and not part of the regulatory ethos in the UK or the rest of Europe which was committed to specification standards (see photograph 3). Although air sampling was used, occasionally, to study some processes in some recognised Dangerous Trades, these findings were invariably translated and transferred into general and sometimes specific Regulations. There are a number of advantages to specification standards especially for small companies and people auditing or inspecting controls. If the controls are clear and known to all, whether a company is complying is fairly straightforward to check both for the company and any external assessor. But the problem is and was: how does one know whether the controls specified are effective enough? (See photograph 4). Without a health-based target to aim for, no answer could be given.

*Industrial hygiene (IH) and OELs evolve in the USA*

Even though attempts were made to control the worst excesses of exposure to toxic substances such as lead and silica, the main threat to public health was still perceived, at the turn of the century, to be infectious diseases. National and local authorities and campaigners were mainly concerned with public health measures to control TB and other infectious diseases. In the USA, sanitary engineering developed as a specialist subject with its own journals. By the turn of the century it was clear that the preventative approach, in combination with better nutrition, was bringing many infectious diseases under control. Some sanitarians, including a few sanitary engineers, wanted to apply this same preventative approach to industrial diseases about which more knowledge was becoming public.

In the USA a few sanitary engineers, chemists and industrial physicians were employed by States such as Massachusetts, and the federal Public Health Service (PHS) set up a Department of Industrial Hygiene and Sanitation in 1913, although initially this was only concerned with infectious diseases. Attempts at preventing the worst excesses of TNT, solvents and other acute poisonings amongst munitions workers and others working in the old Dangerous Trades were made during World War I. But the beginnings of what was to become the new science-based profession of Industrial Hygiene (IH) did not start proper until after the first World War when pioneers such as Winslow, Greenburg, Bloomfield and Sayers, all working for the PHS, began conducting research and field surveys. From the start, these sanitarians were concerned with processes and control and with the developing methods of exposure measurement. Once exposure measurements were made it was completely natural for the sanitarians to ask the question: 'what level of exposure is attainable/safe?' and they wanted and developed practical answers.

> The only standard which can be altogether satisfactory for a sanitarian, is one that deals directly with the actual conditions of the air inhaled by the worker (Winslow 1919).

Winslow echoed Duckering's words some 10 years earlier, but he went further. Rather than making a general recommendation to set limits he set a standard for polishing workshops of 200,000 particles per cubic foot (ppcf) on the basis that this could be attained in the better workshops. Seven years later, in 1926, the final report of the National Safety Council (NSC) committee on benzol (benzene), chaired by Winslow, was published. Winslow's approach to benzene was very similar to his approach to dust in polishing shops. The process was investigated, the controls were examined and ranked in terms of effectiveness and air sampling was performed. By these measures, which were innovatory in 1919 and were by no means in regular use in 1926, Winslow was able to identify the most effective types of control and state, with some certainty, what exposure levels would occur if the controls were applied. But this time the medical evidence showed that over one fifth of people even with the best controls would be affected.

Winslow could not identify a benzene exposure level which was both safe and attainable – an age old dilemma. His committee emphasised that good controls could reduce exposure to 100 ppm and this value became the *de facto* limit. Such limits were very rare at the time, and where published, they contained not one, but multiple standards for the same chemical. One of the first lists of exposure limits was published by the German toxicologist Kobert in 1912. This and other lists published in the 1920s and 1930s always listed multiple limits, which graded the potential health risk from rapidly fatal to levels tolerable for prolonged exposure. Invariably, the concern was with gases and vapours capable of causing acute effects.

One of the last multiple lists in the USA was published in 1935 (Sayers and Dallavalle 1935). Soon after this, multiple limit lists in the USA disappeared and only single number limits were published. This innovation though had to wait upon the creation of the new science-based profession of industrial hygiene, which took concrete professional organisational form in the United States in the late 1930s. The disappearance of multiple limits was a sign of the times.

## INDUSTRIAL HYGIENE, INDUSTRIAL TOXICOLOGY, AND THE OEL PARADIGM

Figure 1 summarises the evolution of the IH profession. It makes clear that this evolution was assisted by the development of another science-based profession, industrial toxicology (IT), and how the evolution of IH relates to the creation of the OEL paradigm.

*Figure 1*
Industrial hygiene, industrial toxicology and the OEL paradigm

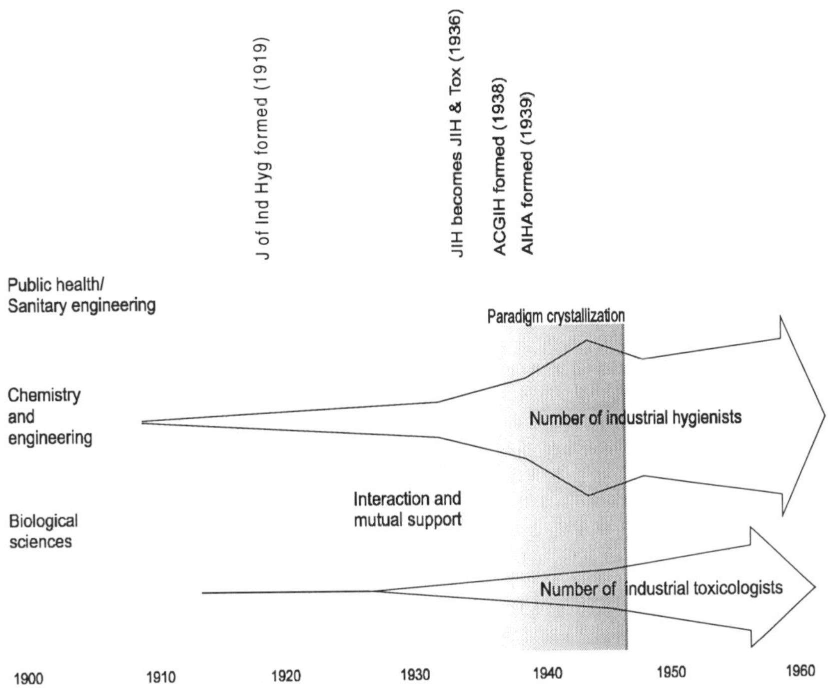


From being a medical sub-speciality in the 1920s, IH had become transformed into a more complex and different science-based discipline concerned with the anticipation, evaluation (including air measurement) and control of exposure to chemical and physical hazards. The ITs, some of whom were also IHs, or worked closely with them, offered the possibility, based on their experiments and theory, of setting risk free threshold exposure levels for chemical substances including new ones and physical agents. The concept of thresholds of toxic effect, developed by toxicologists, had a great effect on the IHs who were particularly receptive. The concept raised the possibility and gave credence to the idea that it should be possible to set a level of exposure, based on animal and human data, below which no danger to health would exist. In the USA there was a synergy between the two newly developing science-based professions of IH and IT (Piney 1989: 452-59). The newly formed partners outflanked the occupational physicians who, in the main, were concerned with the provision of general medical services, the treatment of acute trauma and, sometimes, chemical poisoning. In the USA there was a need for this new science-based profession. IHs changed from being groups of isolated individuals practising a somewhat esoteric and new approach to controlling chemical risk, to making an independent claim as a new science-based profession in the late 1930s when both of the ACGIH (initially called the National Conference of Governmental Industrial Hygienists) and the AIHA (American Industrial Hygiene Association) were formed.

## THE OEL PARADIGM

From the late 1930s onwards, multiple limit setting stopped and single number occupational exposure limits (OELs) were developed. Limits were developed by individual State Bureaux, the PHS and the American Standards Association (ASA). The partnership with industrial toxicology and the use of animal toxicology was quite explicit in some cases. Waiting for health effects to happen and picking up the pieces afterwards as had been the usual practice was not now seen tolerable by IHs. They, and ITs believed it was possible, not just in theory but in practice also, to identify thresholds and prevent harm occurring.

The partnership thus was seen as the way forward to a truly preventative approach, as can be sensed in Frank Patty's preface to the first edition of the by now standard reference work *Industrial Hygiene and Toxicology*:

> ... industrial hygiene has laid aside its swaddling clothes and entered a vigorous stage of advancement... the safeguarding of industrial health is on a business basis of evaluation and control and is recognised as such by both labour and management. The purpose of the industrial hygienist is no longer merely to 'lock the door after the horse has been stolen' but to anticipate and prevent harmful situations, or to control them before serious injury results (Patty 1948).

The 'harmful situations' were of course to be avoided by combining the skills of industrial toxicologists and hygienists to produce OELs.

Before IH took organisational form in the late 1930s, IHs used concepts and developed technical practices and did original research which were to become exemplary for the profession. When it came to limits they were tentative and they hedged any numbers quoted with, sometimes, long lists of caveats. From the early 1940s onwards all this changed. With the creation of the profession of IH a paradigm crystallised in the minds of IHs and ITs. Before this time IHs practised in what could be described as a pre-paradigmatic period. After the paradigm crystallised, only single figure limits were produced, and they were produced as definitive lists. They were given names including words such as 'maximum' or 'threshold' and IHs confidently broadcast them to their employers, other organisations and, within a short time, to many other countries. All this activity and confidence can be seen as the productivity one might expect from a scientific community which had recently come to accept a particular paradigm, organised itself like a profession and whose members were being employed.

Understanding the nuances of how a scientific community sees and uses a particular paradigm is not simple. Strictly speaking a completely self-contained Occupational Exposure Limit paradigm does not exist: there were, and still are, important criticisms of the OEL paradigm, not the least in the IH community. However, as an analytical device a *working definition* of the OEL paradigm is useful. Based on the work of sanitarians and proto-toxicologists as they developed into IHs, and at the same time developed IH as a subject area, it is possible to identify six fundamental tenets of the working definition of the OEL paradigm. These can be summarised as follows:

1. Toxic substances can be used safely;
2. IH control measures are adequate for all toxic substances;
3. threshold doses exist for all toxic substances;
4. standard setters can identify threshold exposures (doses);
5. the major consideration in the setting of OELs is the health effects of toxic substances; and
6. OELs are set at or around the threshold exposure or dose.

## THRESHOLD LIMIT VALUES (TLVS) – THE EXEMPLARY OELS

> What is Industrial Hygiene? Industrial Hygiene is a non-exact science which attempts unsuccessfully to show an exact relationship between the Utopian

> cohabitation of Capital and Labor from which springeth Brotherly love (Extract from a joke *Handbook of Industrial Hygiene – Seminar Extraordinary*, Washington DC, 1936).

TLVs have been, and still are, the most influential OELs in the world. They were taken up unofficially and then officially by many authorities in South America and Europe and their use also quickly spread to Canada, Australia and Japan (see Table 1; further information can be found in Piney 1989: 557-73). Apart from the countries listed, many of the developing countries have adopted TLVs via the International Labour Organisation (ILO) Model Code of Safety Regulations which was published in 1949. The OEL paradigm developed in the USA by the IH profession, interpreted by the ACGIH TLV Committee, rode on the back of the widespread use and acceptance of the TLV List. But what did each country or profession buy when it imported TLVs?

*Table 1* – First use of TLVs in countries other than the USA

| *country* | *first use (unofficial)* | *official use* |
|---|---|---|
| Australia | 1948 | 1956 |
| Canada | 1946 (?) | 1971/72 |
| Denmark | early 1960s | 1968 |
| Netherlands | mid 1950s | 1978 |
| Finland | late 1950s | 1962 |
| France | 1960s (?) | 1980s |
| Italty | 1969 | 1975 (?) |
| Japan | 1952 | 1952 |
| Norway | 1950 | 1950 |
| South America | late 1940s | 1950s (?) |
| Spain | 1962 | 1962 |
| Sweden | 1950s | 1969 |
| Switzerland | 1946 | 1946 |
| UK | early-/mid 1950s | 1960 |
| West Germany | 1958 | 1958 |

*Figure 2*
Sampling results for 3 types of process emitting the same contaminant, based on real data

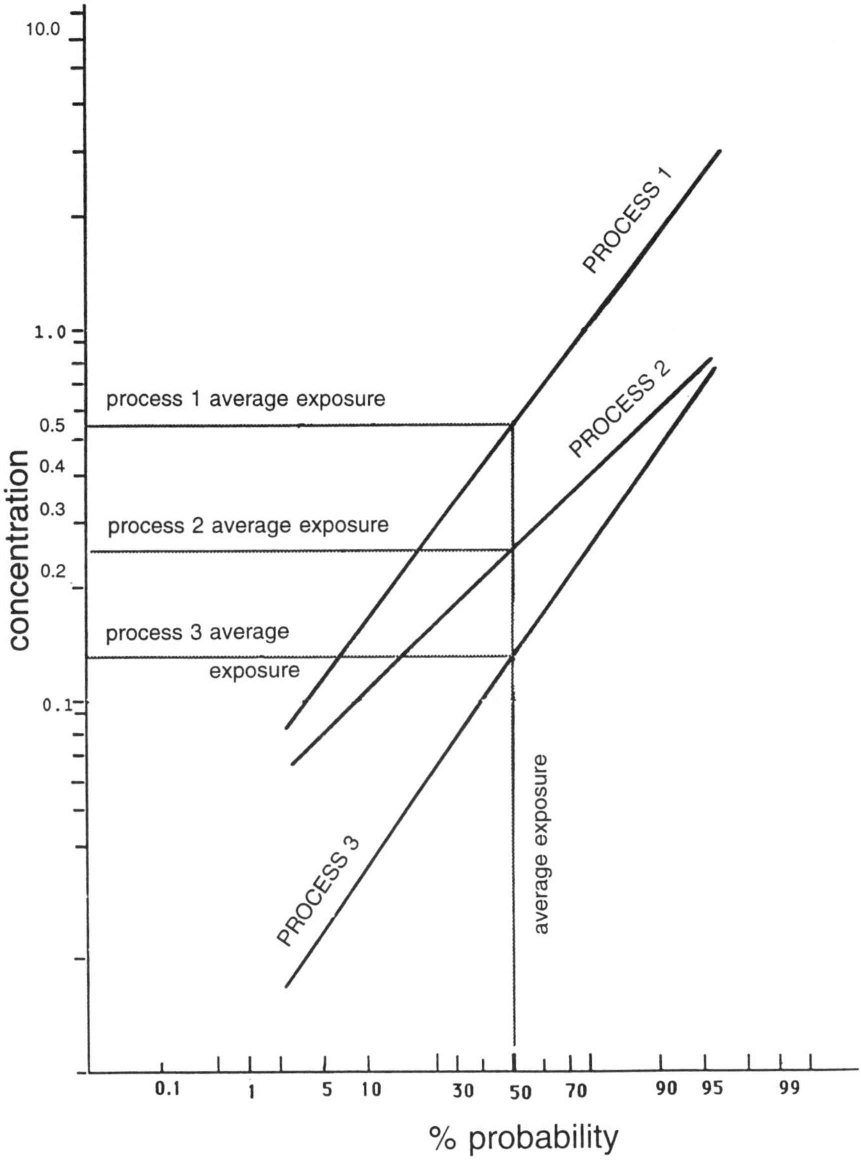

*The definition and meaning of the ACGIH TLV*

Fairhall, the second chairman of the Committee on Threshold Limits (1947-1951) addressed the problem of defining the limits, the year after the first list was published in 1946, as follows:

> As I view the matter I would define the maximum allowable concentration value as 'that amount of gas, vapour, fume or dust which can be tolerated by man with no bodily discomfort nor impairment of bodily function, either immediately or after years of exposure' (ACGIH 1947).

Fairhall's definition is absolute; TLVs (or MACs as they were then called) were health-based OELs which not only protect exposed individuals' health now, but also offer protection over many years of exposure. But these standards were to be applied, and Fairhall had to deal with the question of practicability which he did later in his 1947 report to the Conference as follows:

> There is also one further point I should mention, although it is rather obvious. That is the necessity for preserving a balance between a suitable maximum allowable concentration value and the effect of attaining this value upon the manufacturing operation or process itself (ACGIH 1947).

Fairhall's dilemma echoes that of Winslow, Hatch, Drinker and other IHs. But difficult as the dilemma might be in the practice of setting standards, according to him "there is no industrial poison so potent, so virulent that it cannot be manufactured safely under carefully controlled conditions" (ACHIH 1948). He is in effect touching base with the bedrock of the paradigm by which his profession works and quoting the first two tenets of the *working definition.*

From 1946 to 1952 the TLV list was published with no comment as a simple table of figures. Calling them threshold limit values and publishing them as a bald table of figures conveyed a strong symbolic message. The title and the single numbers invited the reader to believe that the values were thresholds and that exposures below these values were safe. Almost immediately, the ACGIH was criticised for conveying this impression (Yant 1948) and again a year later for using such words as 'maximum' and 'allowable' (Smyth 1950). Smyth made the same points again in mid-1950s in a long paper with some very cogent criticisms of ACGIH TLVs. He objected to tables of figures with no information on how the Committee arrived at the numbers listed, saying that: "no oracular or *ex cathedra* statement on health deserves serious attention" (Smyth 1956). Seven years after the first table of limits was published, a Preface was added but this only served to reinforce the message of the table. TLVs are described as levels to which workers could be exposed "without injury to health" (ACGIH 1953). As if the absolute definition were not enough, other parts of the Preface served to re-assure the reader. The exposure limits were described as "based on the best available information" which at the time was, and still is, highly variable in quantity, quality and relevance. Furthermore, TLVs were described as "reviewed annually by the Committee." This suggests a certain fine tuning and that each value was considered afresh each year. The reality was, and still is, that the process of change was slow and no reconsideration of a TLV value would occur unless strong new evidence was presented or discovered by a committee.

The wording of the Preface and the effect of single numbers meant that the user was almost bound to ascribe a magical quality to the numbers and to do just what the Committee warns against, and what Smyth feared was happening: most if not all people using TLVs believed that exposures below the TLV were safe and above them were dangerous.

Five years after the first Preface was published it was rewritten to cope with complaints and misunderstanding and, "... apparent confusion which has developed in respect of the interpretation of TLVs" (ACGIH 1958). One of these 'confusions' was the belief that exposure below the TLV was safe. The new Preface tries to clear up this confusion by taking a sentence from the earlier Preface and making it the first sentence of the new Preface: "threshold limits should be used a guides in the control of health hazards and should not be regarded as fine lines between safe and dangerous concentrations" (ACGIH 1958). And the next sentence, which has had very similar wordings since 1958 to the present day and which words are often used by other OEL setting committees, defined the protection offered by TLVs:

> They represent conditions under which it is believed that nearly all workers may be repeatedly exposed, day after day, without adverse effect (ACGIH 1958).

Protection is not promised to all workers, as in the first Preface in 1953 but to 'nearly' all workers. The one word represents an important shift in the TLV definition and marks a break with the past. The inclusion of the word 'nearly' could be seen as a faltering in the confidence of the Committee in the claims they previously made for their TLVs. This all depends, however, upon how they, and others, define the word 'nearly'. It can be interpreted in many ways and its inclusion in the second Preface, which was similar in content to the first Preface, together with a tabular TLV list probably did little to change the message conveyed to most TLV users. After all, 'nearly' can mean 'most' and 'most' can soon come to mean 'all'. For the Committee itself, the phrase probably did not have any exact meaning at first except to say that 'some people' would be affected in some way when exposed at the TLV, to some substances. As long as 'nearly all' was not defined, the Committee could rely upon most users interpreting the phrase as meaning small to vanishingly small.

Apart from the 'nearly all' phrase and the almost obligatory 'fine lines' disclaimer, there was another significant addition to the second Preface and that was a sentence emphasising it was, "enlightened industrial hygiene practice" to work to below the TLV value (ACGIH 1958). The OEL paradigm allowed early IHs to reconcile the ideas that thresholds of effect must exist and the need to set attainable standards. By 1958 the exhortation to reduce exposures below TLVs is an indication that it perhaps was not always possible to reconcile these two ideas.

### *TLVs are 'reasonably practible' OELs*

In reality many, if not most, TLVs have been set to take into account the practicability of the controls and there is a great variety of evidence to support this claim. Through an analyses of the minutes of the TLV-committee, it can be established that of the 354 TLVs set between 1962 and 1984, in about 40% of the cases industrial data was sought or supplied, and in 13% of cases the TLV was based mainly on data supplied by industry (Piney 1989: 151-2; 520-56). On the basis that no industry sets limits it cannot comply with, practicability will have been a major factor in the setting of between 13 and 40% of TLVs. This is a similar finding to that of Castleman & Ziem (1988).

Another way of getting some measure of how far TLVs are from being health-based is to compare the ACGIH list with NIOSH Recommended Exposure Limits (RELs), which themselves are supposed to be solely based on health risk assessment (but see below). A comparison of 86 pairs found the following:

REL > TLV – 3
REL = TLV – 33
REL < TLV – 50

Not all NIOSH RELs are lower than ACGIH TLVs but the majority are. On average, RELs were 40% lower than TLVs (Piney 1989: 192-200).

A third way of assessing the status of TLVs is to compare them with standards which are highly likely to be 'reasonably practicable'. A reasonably practicable OEL is a limit which has ostensibly been set by balancing risks to health against the perceived costs of control. Almost by definition, reasonably practicable OELs are standards which can be met by large swathes of industry. With many such limits there may be significant residual risk at exposures below the limit. By 1956 the ACGIH had set 216 TLVs. Imperial Chemical Industry (ICI) had set 55 internal OELs from which 48 paired comparisons are possible. They break down as follows:

ICI OEL = TLV – 15
ICI OEL > TLV – 16
ICI OEL < TLV – 17

There is considerable overlap between the two lists; roughly one-third of the TLVs are the same as ICI's internal OELs, one-third were lower and one-third were higher. Overall, TLVs were somewhat more stringent than the in-house ICI company's OELs but the considerable overlap would indicate that, in 1956, TLVs were reasonably practicable OELs pitched towards the lower end of the spectrum of reasonable practicability.

A yet further way of answering the question is to systematically examine the evidence on which the Committee made its judgements. Smyth did this in 1956 and Henschler and co-workers did so as an internal exercise for the West German DFG Committee in 1984 (Henschler et al. 1984). Roach (1980; also Roach & Rappaport 1990) examined the Documentation of 612 substances with TLVs. One of his conclusions is "that TLVs are generally higher than the no-effect threshold of many people and TLVs for irritant substances are particularly high."

The conclusion is compelling: the majority of TLVs are 'reasonably practicable'. The potential risks to health have been balanced against the practicabilities of control. While this chapter so far has focussed on TLVs the same logic and lessons apply to almost all if not all OEL setting committees. The proof of the pudding is in the OEL numbers. Generally OEL values are the same or similar whatever the make-up of a committee and however it defines its OELs.

## Reasonably practicable OELs in practice

The slow rate of change coupled with the relatively small reductions in numerical value of TLVs have all been presented by the Committee as evidence that the TLVs are close to the 'threshold of effect'. This has reinforced the image that TLVs are more or less health-based OELs. Viewed from the standpoint of reasonable practicability there is, however, an additional and dominant reason for the low rate of change: the difficulties of controlling exposure down to a particular level for certain key processes.

Most substances are used in a variety of processes and operations. If exposures are examined by process/operation a pattern is often evident. Figure 2 represents the reality of the work environment facing any OEL Committee wishing to set reasonably practicable limits. The reason why certain processes or operations become the focus of attention is clear. Process 1 in the Figure causes the highest exposures. Exactly where the OEL is set will depend upon how the Committee balances its perception of the seriousness of health effects, the likelihood that the effect will occur at a certain level of exposure, and its perception of how difficult it will be to control exposures at the top end of Process 1's distribution. A reasonably practicable OEL is not necessarily the same value in every country. There is a narrow spectrum of options implying relatively stringent or lax controls on process 1 activities. Whichever level is chosen, they are all reasonably practicable with greater or lesser effort and cost. If a figure lower than can be achieved by the best control methods or techniques is set, then automatically a proportion of processes using the substance will not be in compliance with the standard, and no standard setting committee sets OELs which are impossible to comply with. Unless the industry fundamentally changes the process or develops more effective controls it will always be out of compliance. This also explains why, when OELs are reduced, the reductions are rarely large (Mendeloff 1988) and when exposures are measured they rarely exceed OELs (Senn 1995).

The tension between wanting to set a standard which protects health, which exercises some control over the highest exposures, and which at the same time can be complied with was evident in the early work of sanitary engineers in the United States. The same unresolved dilemma exists today. It is a contradiction at the heart of the OEL paradigm. At this point it is worth returning to the *Working Definition* and modifying it. It is now much less absolute and more prosaic but it is important to be clear about the basic tenets which standard setters have either explicitly or implicitly been working to, before considering how the paradigm could be changed. A modified *definition* would run something like:

1a Some, perhaps many, toxic substances can be used safely;
2a IH control methods are adequate for many but not all toxic substances;
3a threshold doses exist for some, perhaps many, toxic substances;
4a standard setters can sometimes identify some threshold exposures or doses;
5a a range of considerations, apart from health-based, are taken into account when setting OELs;
6a some OELs may be set at or around a threshold or low risk level of exposure but usually this is not known.

## Single number OELs and their effect

It is important to understand the standard setting process before trying to change it. Therefore, before considering how the OEL paradigm could be re-shaped and re-cast, the effects of reasonably practicable single number OELs are worth examining, as are the range of factors which can come to bear on the standard setting process.

*The effects of OELs*

The single number OEL has existed and been applied since the late 1930s, early 1940s: well over 50 years. The existence and use of the single number reasonably practicable OELs has had a number of effects, many of which were not foreseen by early IHs and ITs. These effects are:

1. Reasonably practicable OELs enable processes and industries to proceed or continue within certain constraints. They thus may facilitate the use of certain substances or processes.

2. Routine use of reasonably practicable OELs reinforces and maintains the OEL paradigm. They are part of the system which apparently controls risk adequately by means of single number limits.

3. Reasonably practicable OELs limit debate to the discussion of single numbers. The complex range of effects a substance might have all got to be compressed and mapped on to one number. This encourages an over-simple view of a complex world.

4. Given their reasonably practicable nature, they: (a) inhibit the production of health-based OELs, and (b) conversely and perversely they inhibit the identification and promulgation of practically attainable exposure levels at processes and for uses which currently operate below the OEL (see Figure 2). The question of how one might set health-based OELs is discussed below. The intention is not to imply that all current reasonably practicable OELs are above what one might describe as health-based or safe levels, but for a significant proportion there will be significant residual risk at exposure levels below current limits. If this is the case, and the evidence is strong that this is so, it means that exposures in many instances should be reduced below, in some cases well below, current OELs. For the lowest exposure processes which do not determine where the reasonably practicable OEL lies, simple controls will be quite capable of reducing exposures well below current OELs. See, for instance Process 3 in Figure 2 and a practical example of such a Process would be companies making small articles out of GRP (Glass Reinforced Plastic) using styrenated resins. The UK OEL of 100ppm for styrene was based on exposure levels and controls in boat buidling (process 1 in figure 2) but

companies making smaller GRP objects could control to much lower levels. Such companies may well apply no active exhaust ventilation control to moulding operations because exposures never approach or exceed the reasonably practical OEL. Exposures in the 20-50 ppm range commonly occur and with relative inexpensive and simple exhaust ventilation could be reduced in most instances below 10 ppm. The single number over-arching reasonably practicable OEL (Process 1, Figure 2) stops this from happening.

*Photo 5*

The highest styrene exposures occur to people making GRP (Glass Reinforced Plastic) boats (GRP boat manufacture is Process 1 in Figure 2). Working inside boat hulls laying-up glass fibre and styrenated resin causes the highest exposures.

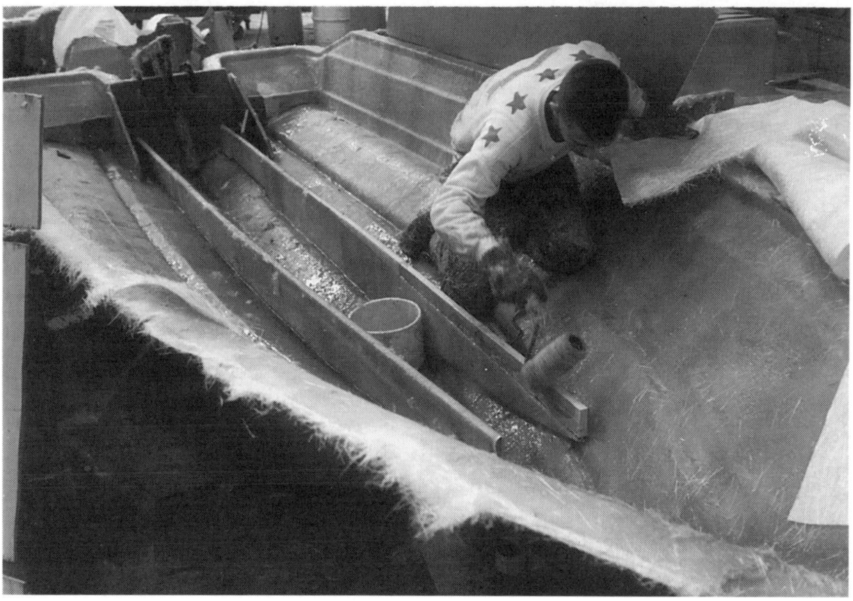

5 They exert restrictions on the uncontrolled use of substances for some processes, but not for others. The people who set the early OELs knew

that they would, if used, restrict the uncontrolled use of a substance or process. They could be achieved, but controls, sometimes involving significant cost, would need to be applied. This has always been a powerful justification for single number reasonably practicable OELs and given the levels of silicosis, lead poisoning etc. in the 1920s and 1930s, IHs promulgating and applying the new limits could see that conditions in the worst industries did improve. Something was better than nothing and nothing was often all that existed.

6 They also probably induce a certain level of informal control, in that, simply by virtue of a substance having an OEL, especially if it is 'low', it tends to become regarded as 'toxic'. Historically, in the UK various industries using and handling lead were regulated, and yet lead poisoning also fell in those industries which were not formally regulated.

7 OELs concentrate attention on substances on OEL lists. The EINECS (European Inventory of Existing Commercial Chemical Substances) data base, set up in the early 1980s lists all chemical substances used in industry in Europe. Over one hundred thousand substances are listed and yet most OEL lists cover seven or eight hundred substances. In reality, the majority will be used in specialist applications, causing potential exposures to small groups of people. One could probably whittle the list down to, say, 10,000 chemicals which are routinely used in industry, causing potential exposures to significant numbers of people. But the point remains that there is a strong tendency for people to only concentrate upon those substances on OEL lists.

8 Conversely, OEL lists deflect attention away from substances which are not listed. There is a tendency for people either to believe that a substance not on the list is not of concern or to be confused about its properties and potential health effects. Either way, there is a tendency not to take substances without OELs as seriously as those with OELs.

## Factors which can influence the setting of OELs

Once one understands how OELs are derived, and one has developed an understanding of their real status and meaning, it is possible to identify a whole range of factors which can influence the standard setting process. The original Working Definition of the OEL paradigm states that the major consideration in the setting of OELs is the health effects of toxic substances. As the history and background of OELs has been explored, this position has become less and less tenable. A range of factors can affect the selection of a particular OEL number and nine broad categories of factor are listed. The impact of health effects on standard setting are considered first.

### *Health effects*

A critical factor which affects any standard setting committee is the health effects reported at current exposure levels and the strength of evidence for health effects below these levels. A large proportion of OELs have been set for substances which have short-term irritant effects or smell strongly. It is not too fanciful to believe that many OELs have been set *because* these substances have irritant effects or smell strongly. Unfortunately, many substances which have long-term effects do not cause significant short-term effects. For such substances there will be little or no warning of potential risk.

Another crucial factor is the type of evidence of health effect, for instance whether it involves a large-scale epidemiological survey or short-term animal test data. The type of evidence of health effect does have an effect on the judgement of people setting OELs. If there is robust epidemiology on a large population of exposed people with long-term follow-up and a strong dose-response relationship this can push decisions on numbers to the stringent end of the reasonably practicable spectrum. But such evidence is rare and if the dose-response suggests clear and significant risk at and below current OELs, the standard setters face a dilemma, and the strong tendency is to fudge the health effects issue and go for a reasonably practicable OEL, perhaps with an exhortation to reduce exposures below the limit by 'enlighted industrial hygiene practice', if possible.

There is also a ranking of value of evidence. In the early days of the OEL paradigm IHs looked to industrial toxicologists (ITs) to guide them, using animal experiments and toxicology. The ASA emergency standard on styrene was quite explicit on this point.

> This standard ... has been established on animal experimentation. It is hoped that by doing so it will be possible to prevent ... the unfortunate and unnecessary exposure to humans which is usually considered necessary ... (ASA 1944).

Unfortunately, this early optimistic view has not been born out in practice and human evidence of harm is still treated far more seriously than animal or toxicological evidence of harm. By demanding unequivocal human evidence one introduces long delays into the standard setting process and drives standard setters into what has been described as the 'generation game': one generation is exposed and not observed, the second generation is observed and harm is demonstrated, until by the third generation some regulatory control is finally exerted. It is true that toxicology does not have clear models of all biological mechanisms which cause human harm. But where reasonable models exist, the results should be used. Interestingly, the ACGIH does appear to use toxicological evidence and to take it far more seriously than OSHA in reviewing and changing its OELs (Mendeloff 1988). Perhaps a sign of the organisation remaining faithful to its historical roots.

### *Other factors*

Factors other than health effect influencing standard setting include:

1 The capabilities of current control technologies and methods. The type and sophistication of control technology and methods varies from industrial sector to industrial sector. Some sectors, for instance pharmaceuticals, can be quite sophisticated and others, for instance woodworking, have adopted relatively crude and erratic exhaust ventilation systems until fairly recently.

2 The costs of control methods. Although this may be seen as a self-evident factor, control costs do not fall evenly on all users of a substance. It is the costs of controls used in the sector causing the highest exposures which matter most and will cause the most argument when a reasonably practicable OEL is set. The costs of applying controls for processes using the same substance but which cause inherently lower exposures are not relevant in current OEL setting practice.

3 The current exposure levels for certain industries and/or processes or operations. This factor has been explored in some detail and it is crucial to any understanding of why an OEL is set and pinned to a limited range of numbers.

4 The perceptions, by the standard setters, of the seriousness of the health effects. Certain diseases are taken more seriously and carry greater weight than others. If the evidence is based on human epidemiology and the effect is cancer this carries more weight than if the health effect is irritation or dermatitis.

5 The importance of the material or process being considered for the industry or the national or local economy. Standard setters are more relaxed about setting stringent OELs if the substance or process is not central to an important industry or to the local or national economy.

6 The development, technical sophistication and financial position of the industries affected. Generally, high tech, modern, profitable industries can develop sophisticated solutions to minimise exposure and can live with stringent OELs. The problems come with sectors which are not technically sophisticated or particularly profitable. These tend to be, but are not always, the older more established industries. In the case of established industries there is the added problem of technical and cultural inertia. Processes and even buildings are organised for production to happen in a certain way. To improve exposure control may require a fairly fundamental reorganisation of both. At an industrial cultural level there is a strong and understandable tendency not to believe that improved controls are needed and that to a greater or lesser extent the regulator is making a 'fuss about nothing'. Achieving a fundamental

change and a stepwise fall in exposure in such industries is difficult, over and above the problem of setting a reasonably practicable OEL which the more progressive members of industry might be able to reach.

7 The relative balance of effects of the proposed OEL between different industrial sectors. A good example of this effect is the setting of the silica MEL in the UK. The eventual outcome of the negotiations over the Limit will be described at the end of this chapter and all that needs to be noted at this point is that the standard setting process and negotiations involved are a good example of how particular sectors running particular processes are differentially affected by the current system which insists upon setting one single number OEL.

8 The relative organisational ability and political power of the various groups involved in the OEL setting process. Certain industrial sectors employ large numbers of graduates and specialists in occupational hygiene, toxicology and medicine. In negotiations over standard settings such sectors can field whole teams of experts, and in some cases a number of regulatory toxicologists and other specialists will have worked for the sector before moving into government. Such sectors can mount technically sophisticated and well argued cases during standard setting which affects their products and processes. If their sector is also an important foreign exchange earner or contributes significantly to a country's GDP the state will be more concerned with decisions which affect such a sector than if it were a small sector making a small contribution.

9 OELs set by other standard setting bodies. The US ACGIH and the German DFG have liaised and tracked each others judgements and other committees have done something similar either formally or informally for decades (Krstic 1994). This judgmental anchoring is important but the anchoring effect of practicability related to specific processes is far more important. One example of this is the case of styrene (Piney 1989: 284-88).

10 Occasionally, the symbolic nature of a substance can become important. For instance, the long-running arguments over the benzene OEL in the USA and the EU took on a far wider, symbolic nature than the properties

of the substance and the degree of exposure would suggest necessary. Such substances become almost talismen, and symbolic battles are fought over them between employer and employee organisations and regulatory authorities. They are in many ways a red herring, a diversion from the real problem of limiting risk from chemical exposures.

### *Are OELs actually used by anyone?*

There has been a lot of debate over the status and meaning of OELs and how they have been and should be set and this Chapter is a contribution to that debate. But the logic behind OELs is that they are supposed to be used to minimise chemical exposure risks. Very few commentators actually consider whether OELs are used. Recent evidence in the UK suggests that most companies do not (HSE 1997). This especially applies to small companies but the approach is similar in all sizes of companies. The researchers found that:

> ... in making decisions about risk prevention most user establishments said they did make use of supplier information along with common sense and experience (of what the rest of the sector did). ... Some regarded monitoring as unnecessary due to the prescence of adequate control measures (HSE, 1997).

It would seem that industry prefers and works to specification type standards, the type of standards which existed before OELs were invented. There is a message and lessons in these research findings.

## MODIFYING THE PARADIGM – UNDERSTANDING THE PAST AND LOOKING TO THE FUTURE

> Mandatory requirements are usually minimum requirements, or representative of the worst permissible conditions. From one point of view, such requirements are a necessary aid to code administration for dealing with recalcitrants; from another viewpoint, they tend to stifle progress and freeze endeavour at the established minimum (Yant 1948).

A different approach is needed to prevent the "freezing" Yant referred to. The earlier parts of this chapter have tried to tease out the contents, beliefs and assumptions of OEL setting committees to get a clear understanding of just what OELs are, what factors may have been taken into account in their production and how well their use might protect peoples' health. We are now in a position to consider how the original paradigm could be modified and how a more effective scheme of minimising risk from exposures to chemicals at work could be developed.

*Turning performance standards into specification standards*

Before OELs existed, standards for a process would, where they existed, be defined in terms of what controls or practices need to be applied. Such specification standards are easier to apply and audit or inspect than performance standards such as OELs. The problem is: how do you know whether the control arrangement specified is good enough? There is also the problem of specifying the controls for each and every process or operation involving hazardous substances. This was the attraction of a performance standard such as an OEL for Duckering in the UK and the early IHs in the USA. If the OEL was well founded, all that the regulator had to do was specify the standard (the OEL) and leave it to the employer to reach it. The problem is that employers don't use OELs and they don't often measure people's exposure and, as we have seen, many OELs will not normally be exceeded even if employee exposure was measured. There is little pressure for improvement in the current system and little practical help for employers, especially small companies, trying to control employee exposure down to 'safe' levels.

What employers need is practical guidance on how to achieve specific OELs and what employees (and employers) need is confidence that the limits applied really do protect health. The proposals laid out below are an attempt to do just that. But at the practical level, although the scheme still relies on exposure zones or limits, the aim is to translate these into control measures. Exposure measurement would be a back-up to ensure that the controls specified actually do work.

*Making a precautionary policy real*

The underlying assumptions which drive the new, modified paradigm include the following:

1. Understanding of the potential health effects of chemicals used at work is limited.
2. A significant number of the thousands of chemicals in regular use are causing health effects, some of them serious.[1]
3. Techniques for identifying such substances are relatively insensitive and have not been routinely applied.
4. The level of proof for identifying the connection between exposure to chemical substances and potential health effects should be based on the balance of probability and not beyond all reasonable doubt.
5. Improved controls, as far as is reasonably practicable, should be applied whenever there is significant evidence of harm and should not wait upon the setting of an exposure limit.
6. Generic standard setting and do-it-yourself sector-based standard setting should be encouraged.

Unlike the current system for setting OELs, which usually involves one committee, the new system will require two separate groups. One to develop *health-based low risk zones* and the other to develop families of *reasonably practicable exposure limits* and associated specification standards.

*Health-based low risk zones*

A health-based low risk zone is an exposure range at which current evidence and understanding suggest there is no significant risk. This may be because dose-response information suggests a no observed effect level (NOEL) and

1 It is incorrect to view all chemicals as toxic and capable of causing significant harm and it is important to relate risk to the degree of exposure which actually occurs. Likewise, the universe of chemicals is unlikely to be divided neatly into mainly innocuous with a few 'bad apples'. That view is too neat, too unlikely and too convenient.

the 'zone' is well below that. Or, if there is evidence that there is a probability of effects occuring down to low exposure levels, for instance a genotoxic human carcinogen, the 'zone' would be set such that the probability of the effect occuring is not significant.

It would be better to signify by name, and in practice, that the process of determining low risk levels of exposure is uncertain by moving away from using the word 'limit' or 'value'. This would move the first committee and its projected message away from the idea of dividing lines and identifiable 'safe levels' once and for all.

A significant number of health-based low risk zones will not be achievable for all the processes using a substance at least in the medium term. The zones represent the pull in the system of reasonably practicable standards and the eventual target to attain. Having said this, the zones must be robust and meaningful and they must in some fashion relate to risk, meaningful risk. Not all exposures to chemical substances are dangerous. Low exposures to many chemicals are probably 'safe' within any meaningful definition of the word. There are few certainties in life but our own inevitable death is surely one. This will happen whether we are exposed to 'chemicals' or not. The additional risk exposure to a particular chemical may cause, has to be put in the context of other risks, otherwise it would be meaningless, both for the people trying to promulgate the standard, and those exposed.

It is difficult to do, but risks from chemical exposure must also be put in the context of other risks at work. Resources available to apply to production and control of risk are finite. It would be distortion, if not a disservice, to pour resources into controlling chemical exposure down to very low levels at the expense of controlling other larger but different risks. The real world of work and risk is messy and practical decisions have to be made. In the past, this messy reality plus reasonably practicable OELs and limited resources have been used as an excuse to do little if nothing. But just because this has been so does not mean that the obverse should apply. The first committee has to set meaningful health-based low risk zones and does not have the option of applying arbitrary safety factors of 10 or 100 or 1,000 'just in case'. If health-based low risk zones are really to be accepted and the ultimate driving force in the system to reduce exposures, the methods by which they are set and their meaning will have to be accepted. The committee setting health-based low risk zones has a difficult job.

*Reasonably practicable exposure limits*

A reasonably practicable exposure limit (RPEL) is a limit tied to a set of control measures (the specification part of the standard). It represents the most cost effective controls which can currently be achieved for a particular set of similar processes. How many RPELs are required will depend on how many sets of similar processes cause exposures to a particular substance above the health-based low risk zone.

*Alternative tenets of a modified paradigm*

Based on what might be called a more precautionary approach the Working Definition of a modified OEL paradigm might read as follows:

1 Threshold or low risk exposure zones probably exist for most, and maybe all toxic substances.
2 Identifying the low risk zones for toxic substances is difficult and has been done for a few substances.
3 Many low risk exposure zones are below current exposure levels and OELs.
4 There should be a continuing effort to reduce exposures below many current OELs.
5 The groups identifying low risk exposure zones should be a different group of people from those identifying reasonably practicable exposure levels.
6 The major consideration when identifying a low risk exposure zone should be potential health effects.
7 The major considerations of the group identifying reasonably practicable exposure levels should be: (a) how far current exposures are above the low risk zone range, and (b) how 'technology forcing' reasonably practicable exposure levels can be for each process.

### *Advantages and objections*

There are advantages and possible objections to the approach proposed. What are the advantages? The main advantage is that it faces the realities of work place exposure and the impossibility of always setting a single number OEL which protects health and is at the same time practicable. Furthermore, it addresses the reality of OEL standard setting; the unequal struggle between the soft facts on health effects and the hard facts of practicability and cost. It also faces four square the uncertainty of decision making on toxic substances. It makes no pretence that the field is understood with any exactitude. In this sense it is more honest than most of the current OEL standard setting regimes.

The health-based low risk zone, moreover, introduces a continual pressure into the system to improve control where it is needed. Without health-based low risk zones, the motivation to improve a practicable limit disappears. Conversely, without the RPELs the phrase 'as far as is reasonably practicable' is vague, debatable and almost unenforceable.

The proposal is dynamic and not static as is the current system. The health-based low risk zone will be refined with time and may fall or rise as knowledge and understanding of the action of different substances increases. Similarly, the RPELs will change as process and control technology changes. The system of health-based low risk zones and RPELs would introduce innovative pressure to develop more cost effective methods of attaining the RPEL, and eventually with many processes, attain the health-based low risk zone. Health-based low risk zones are, furthermore, more easily altered in the light of new evidence in that they have no immediate effect on the RPELs actually enforced.

Sets of RPELs are an improvement on the present system because they represent realistic and agreed targets to aim for in the short to medium term. Coupled to the health-based low risk zone they will encourage innovation in control. They are practical and could draw upon and extend the usefulness of information much of which is already available.

Finally, the proposals combine the advantages of performance and specification standards. The health-based low risk zones are the performance part of the proposal and their status is clear and unambiguous unlike current OELs. And the set of RPELs will be closely tied to types of processes, products and control methods. As such, employers will know what is required of them and enforcing or auditing agencies will have a far easier task assessing compliance with the stricture to reduce exposure 'as far as is reasonably practicable'.

What are the objections to the proposed method? The first objection might be that, with the method proposed, industry does not know where it is. But fixed and certain targets of the type proposed and promulgated by certain standard setting committees are not possible or realistic in occupational health as in many other areas of life for the simple reason that our knowledge and understanding is neither complete or static. Also, it is not as if industry is not used to trying to hit moving targets as markets evolve and production techniques develop. All that the proposal implies is that health-based low risk zones and RPELs become built into the planning process along with other changing factors in production. In these new proposals, industry is not being asked to jump into a bottomless pit and has targets and phased, practical deadlines to work to.

A second objection could be that the proposal is too complicated. Yes it is and no it is not. There are more numbers involved but there are practical achievable targets to attain and once the modified paradigm or approach is accepted it becomes intuitively obvious quite quickly. Setting up formal and agreed procedures for determining HBLs and RPELs will take time. However, once the systems are set up they should be able to function much more rapidly and openly than the current system. On the question of RPELs, the trade unions will not feel so twitchy about one OEL covering all processes. There should be far less trench war-fare between employers' and employees' representatives and less disagreement about where a particular RPEL lies for a specific process. Once care is taken to link exposure data to process and control information, the process of identifying at least the region of an RPEL could almost be automatic using a decision making flowchart. Even if agreement on an exact health-based low risk zone is difficult, identifying RPELs can still proceed on the assumption that the health-based low risk zone is lower than exposures currently being achieved. Once the RPEL setting process is finalised and explicit, there will be large scope for industry to 'do it itself'. The idea of self-regulation so central to the UK Health and Safety at Work Act and the Control of Substances Hazardous to Health Regulations (COSHH) would become more of a reality.

But what will happen to the current OELs? They will assume the same status as the top RPEL. By doing this the reasonably practicable nature of such single number OELs is made clear and the process of identifying health-based low risk zones and RPELs can start. It may be a painful process, but it is necessary.

A further possible objection is that the proposal is unfair, because some people will be put at greater risk than others. This, however, is unavoidable. Take, for example, the conclusion of the Council of Wages and Price Stability in their review of OSHA'a rule making on the on the acrylonitrile OEL. The CWPS was concerned with cost effective regulation and was composed mainly of economists. On the direct question of equal risk they made a clear statement that "... as long as the feasibility of risk reduction methods vary, workers will be exposed to differing amounts of excess risk" (CWPS 1978). The proposal is thus not unfair. Rather, it is this admission of the inevitable differential risk that workers are subjected to that proponents of uniform standards do not wish to acknowledge and, possibly, feel uncomfortable with.

A still further objection to the proposal is that it is so new that it will never gain acceptance. If the contradictions and confusions identified in this Chapter are real and correct, then the OEL paradigm is heading for a crisis if it has not already arrived. If this is the case, then it may not be a question of newness being a factor against the proposal, it could count as a point in its favour – a way out of the current indefensible impasse. Moreover, several aspects of the new paradigm are not new at all: multiple lists, the separation of health based from feasibility OELs, and the idea of a phasing of standards have all been suggested in the past.

The final and probably most important objection to the proposal is that health-based low risk zones will make employers liable, because a proportion will always be out of compliance. The idea of health-based low risk zones will therefor probably meet far more resistance than RPELs. Insurance companies and governments in particular will not like health-based low risk zones as they imply that RPELs are not safe, except where they are within or below the health-based low risk zone. What counter arguments are there and what adjustments in vision will be necessary?

The most cogent argument is that the alternative paradigm and the proposals deal with the actual reality of the workplace. The OEL paradigm hid and confused this reality. The alternative will require people to confront some unpalatable truths and develop a more mature understanding of chemical exposure, OELs and risk. The easy option of claiming and believing that OELs were safe, or nearly safe, is not now available. Conversely, the equally easy claim that all chemicals should be treated as (equally) dangerous is also not available. All parties involved have got to face a more complicated but perhaps more believable view of the work environment. There are no easy black and white, safe – unsafe options.

On the question of liability, this can be split into two questions – one concerns liability for causing illness or disease, the other concerns infringement of legal limits. On claims: exposure above the health-based low risk zone does not automatically make an employer liable. An individual or group still has to demonstrate a logical connection between the illness or disease they have, and exposure in the workplace. If there is a plausible connection then exposure above the health-based low risk zone will make the claim easier, and this is correct. At present, claims that exposures were below reasonably practicable OELs may deflect legitimate claims and prevent connections being made.

On non-compliance: the potential problem is more imaginary than real. It all depends on the legal status of health-based low risk zone. They would be published, in all probability, as advisory levels which manufacturers, employers, designers and suppliers should be aware of and at which they should be aiming. They need not be and probably will not be enforceable limits to have a downward pull on the RPELs. They would, as they are intended to, prevent the claim that the appropriate RPEL had been reached and that no more control effort was needed.

The proposals above would go a long way to making the precautionary policies espoused by HSE (1977), other enforcing authorities and various professional groups real, practical and attainable goals. It is time the single number OEL was given a decent burial and the OEL paradigm which underpins it needs to undergo a shift.

## STONEWORKERS RE-VISITED

What are the implications of the proposal for the exposure to silica, described at the start of this chapter?

### *The silica OEL*

In the UK in the 1970s and early 1980s the quarry industry had done little systematic work to control dust exposures. In sites extracting and processing high silica stone, fine respirable silica dust exposures were high. When the idea of a legally enforceable obligatory OEL was first put forward it was the quarry industry which would be most affected and which probably had most to do to reach the suggested draft standard. Other industries, such as potteries, had developed effective control measures over decades and were not that concerned. The quarry industry was Process 1 in Figure 2 and as such it was the exposure level judged to be reasonably practicable for this industry which determined where the silica Maximum Exposure Limit (MEL) was set. In 1992 a MEL of 0.4 mg/m$^3$ became enforcible. The original OEL published in the UK was 0.1 mg/m$^3$, based on the ACGIH TLV, and the evidence is that exposure at this level for a working lifetime still carries some risk of some people contracting silicosis. The implication is that there is significant residual risk at exposures well below the MEL. It is definitely a limit to work down from and not up to.

The three workgroups described at the start of this chapter were exposed to:

| | |
|---|---|
| Primary crusher workers | 0.8mg/m$^3$ |
| Stonemasons | 2.0mg/m3 |
| Pottery worker | 0.2mg/m$^3$ |

All but the pottery workers exposure exceed the MEL of 0.4 mg/m$^3$ and taking the MEL at face value the pottery employer could be forgiven for thinking that 50% of the limit is reasonable and there is no need for further controls. Unfortunately this would be a mistake. There is significant risk down to 0.1 mg/m$^3$ and probably below this value. NIOSH has published a

Recommended Exposure Level (REL) of 0.05 mg/m$^3$ and this, or below, would probably be a reasonable band for a health-based low risk zone for respirable silica to prevent silicosis. Applying this band puts the estimated (but reasonable) exposure estimates in perspective.

The primary crusher operators clearly exceed the MEL but to attain the low risk zone their exposure would need to be reduced by eight times. While improved controls were designed and applied, the operators would need to wear effective and comfortable respirators but this would probably only need to be a temporary measure.

The particular group of stonemasons are hugely exposed (and at risk of an acute accelerated form of silicosis) and to get to 0.4 mg/m$^3$ could be seen as something of an achievement. The initial control would have to be respirators while controls were devised. It would be tempting to stop at 0.4 mg/m$^3$ having reduced exposure five fold but the low risk zone indicates that it would not be good enough and that there was more to do. It may be that stonemasons doing the sort of work which has the potential to cause huge silica dust exposures (powered tools and high silica stone) should always use a combination of controls applied to the process and respirators. This would become the specification standard for this type of work.

The pottery industry in the UK has done a lot of work on standards of control (i.e. specification standards). If the 0.2 mg/m$^3$ exposures figures were real, this would indicate that the company was not applying methods of control well known to the industry. It should be possible for potteries to attain the low risk zone without resorting to personal protective equipment such as respirators. The specification standards are known.

The UK silica MEL is typical of many reasonably practicable OELs. If used it does stop uncontrolled and gross over-exposure but it can also inhibit necessary and achievable reductions in exposure below the limit. In the case of stoneworkers it is likely that the exposure of all the workgroups mentioned could be brought within the health-based low risk zone. For other substances and processes this will almost certainly not be the case.

## Final comments and conclusions

This chapter has examined how work processes determine the range of exposures people experience and therefore the degree of risk they are subjected to. Before OELs, in the earlier part of this century, regulations to reduce exposures, where they existed, applied to certain industries and processes within those industries. There was a tendency to apply controls to obvious and easy to control sources and not necessarily those causing the most exposure. The problem was that no one could be sure that the controls specified were enough. OELs were seen to be an advance on specification standards as they could be applied wherever a substance was emitted and causing exposure. They constrained the uncontrolled use of substances and they were described and believed to be 'safe' or at least 'nearly' safe. The OEL paradigm forged by the industrial hygienists and toxicologists in the late 1930s more or less guaranteed this was the case. The message of a single number with a name often including the word 'threshold' or 'maximum' gave and still gives OELs a strong symbolic quality from which it has been and still is difficult to escape.

The majority of single number OELs are not solely based on considerations of health risk. They are compromises in which the practicability of achieving the standard and other factors have had a strong influence on the final numerical value selected. Standard setters have to struggle with sets of processes causing different ranges of exposures and yet insist upon setting a single number limit. Inevitably, the range of achievable levels for the process causing the highest exposures defines the terms of the debate. It was ever thus. The soft, uncertain, debatable evidence on health effects stands little chance against this hard, practical reality.

But the fiction that OELs are more or less health-based limits has been maintained by most OEL setting bodies. While it may be not entirely correct to think in terms of a global industrial hygiene community following a coherent paradigm there is a strong continuity of behaviour between standard setting committees in different countries. They certainly behave as if they are following a paradigm. The paradigm has enabled such groups to believe in their project and the correctness of their product (OELs) not only when "the theory wasn't there" (Masterman 1970) but in many instances, when the evidence wasn't there. And yet, standing back from the whole process, there is something unlikely, almost fanciful, about the belief that it is possible to arrive at a set of exposure limits which are achievable now but also protect the health of everyone exposed. In a significant number of cases it is not and will not be possible to identify a health-based low risk zone which is achievable. Trying to consider questions of practicability and health at the same time drive standard setting committees on to the rocks of practicability. There is a need not only to stop setting single number OELs but to change the arrangements by which limits, whether health-based or practical are set. There is a need for a paradigm shift.

Paradigms survive until anomalies central to their workings cannot be resolved and a crisis occurs. At the point at which the crisis is resolved the community undergoes a shift and its 'way of seeing' the subject and how it carries out 'normal science' changes. If the OEL paradigm was purely the construct of a scientific community or research groups the anomalies at its heart would have brought to crisis long ago. But this has not happened because the OEL paradigm is not a scientific paradigm, it is a professional paradigm. While all scientists must have employers who have their own interests there is a sense in which this relationship does not affect the science undertaken, the paradigm to which the group adheres and within which it works. Industial hygienists and industrial toxicologists were different right from the start. Their product, the OEL paradigm, had a direct impact on their employers' activities businesses. The customer, the constituency which used the OELs had a strong interest in maintaining the paradigm. And now it has been taken up by so many countries it has become almost a bureaucratic paradigm. There is a huge amount of inertia and vested interest in the system which has almost frozen, virtually fossilised the paradigm forged over 50 years ago. But even a professional paradigm cannot live with chronic anomalies forever. And some authorities such as the Dutch have made an important shift to a two committee, two limit system (Bal, this volume; Feron, this volume). Even this does not produce the most cost-effective reductions in exposure that a set of RPELs would. And the tension created by not wanting to set a health-based limit too far from the practicable limit may tend to make the health-based committee too conservative. The Dutch system represents a break with the hegemony of the old OEL paradigm and by example may encourage others.

At the start of this century Duckering and Legge in the UK and the early sanitarians/IHs in the USA wanted to prevent chronic ill health. Many of the pioneering IHs had seen too much and knew what over-exposure to dust and 'fumes' could do to people. They did not want to "lock the door after the horse had been stolen" (Patty, 1948) but wanted to "anticipate and prevent harmful situations, or to control them before serious injury results" (idem.). They could see the power of OELs and what an innovative force they could become. They wanted them to be health-based or at least health-linked targets to achieve but this was not possible and limits became reasonably practicable compromises, sometimes very practicable compromises. But the idea, the project of the early IHs and ITs, in my opinion, was correct. What is missing in most instances is truly health-based low risk zones and the link between reasonably practicable exposure limits and the controls (specification standards) they imply.

Companies, especially small companies, have not heard of and do not use OELs and if regulation were organised correctly would not need to. What they do need is clear practical guidance on the controls required now with some idea of where the eventual target is likely to be (i.e. health-based low risk zone). And perhaps this is the clue to developing generic controls for those thousands of chemicals with no OELs. It should be possible to match the degree of controls needed and specified by reference to the potential degree of exposure and broad toxicological categories. Standard setting committees do work exceeding slow and we cannot wait for them to process all the thousands of chemicals in regular use. Otherwise, there is a danger of the whole standard setting process moving into the realms of geological time. Some generic system is required.

Whatever happens and however the debate about how to control chemical risk at work pans out, with the current reasonably practicable OELs, we need to move beyond asking the stultifying question; "Is exposure below the limit?"

*Disclaimer*: the views expressed in this chapter are those of the author as a Visiting Fellow at Aston University and should not be taken to reflect the views of his employer.

## References

American Conference of Governmental Industrial Hygienists (1947) *Proceedings of the 9th Annual Meeting of the ACGIH (26-27 April)*, Buffalo, NY: ACGIH.

American Conference of Governmental Industrial Hygienists (1948) *Proceedings of the 10th Annual Meeting of the ACGIH (27-30 March)*, Boston, MA: ACGIH.

American Conference of Governmental Industrial Hygienists (1958) *Proceedings of the 19th Annual Meeting of the ACGIH*, Cincinnati, Ohio: ACHIH.

American Standards Association (1944) *Allowable concentration of styrene monomer American War Standard Z37.15*, American Industrial Hygiene Standards, New York: ASA.

Castleman, B.I. & G.E.Ziem (1988) 'Corporate influence on Threshold Limit Values', *American Journal of Industrial Medicine* 13: 531-559.

Cook, W.A. (1945) 'Maximum allowable concentrations of industrial atmospheric contaminants', *Industrial Medicine* 14: 936-946.

Council of Wages & Price Stability (1978) *Comments on OSHA's Proposal on a Permanent Acrylonitrile standard on behalf of the Regulatory Analysis Review Group*, Washington DC: CWPS.

Djang, T.K. (1942) *Factory inspection in Great Britain*, London: George Allen and Unwin Ltd.

Duckering, E. (1910) 'Report on an Investigation of the air of work-places in potteries' In: *Report of the Departmental Committee appointed to enquire into the dangers attendant on the use of lead and the danger of injury to health arising from dust and other causes in the manufacture of earthenware and china and in the processes incidental thereto, including the making of lithographic transfers*, Volume 2, Cd – 5219, London: HMSO.

Elkins, H.B. (1948) 'The case for Maximum Allowable Concentrations', *American Industrial Hygiene Association Quarterly* 9: 22-25.

Hale, A.R., M. Piney & R.J. Aylesbury (1986) 'The development of occupational hygiene and the training of health and safety professionals', *Annals of occupational hygiene* 30: 1-18.

Health and Safety Executive (1977) *Toxic substances: A Precautionary Policy,* Guidance Note EH18, London: HMSO.

Health and Safety Executive (1997) *Industry's perception and use of occupational exposure limits*, London: Research International UK Ltd., HSE Books.

Henchler, D. (1984) 'Exposure limits: History, philosophy, and future developments' *Annals of occupational hygiene* 28: 79-92.

Krstic, G. (1994) 'Benzene: Chains of influence in deciding exposure limits', *Indoor Environment* 3: 22-34.

Kuhn, T.S. (1970) *The Structure of Scientific Revolutions*, Chicago: University of Chicago Press.

Legge, T.M. & K.W. Goadby (1912) *Lead Poisoning and Lead Absorption – The Symptoms, Pathology and Prevention with Special Reference to Their Industrial Origin and an Account of the Principal Processes Involving Risk*, London: Edward Arnold.

Lemasters, G.K. et al. (1985) 'Occupational styrene exposure for 12 product categories in the Reinforced Plastics Industry', *American Industrial Hygiene Association Journal* 46: 434-441.

Masterman, M. (1970) 'The nature of a paradigm', in: I. Lakatos & A. Musgrave (eds.) *Criticism and the Growth of Knowledge*, Cambridge: Cambridge University Press; 59-90.

Mendeloff, J.M. (1988) *The Dilemma of Toxic Substance Regulation*, Cambridge, MA: MIT Press.

National Safety Council, Committee on Benzol of the NCS Chemical Rubber Sections (1926) *Final Report*, Washington DC: NSC.

Patty, F., editor (1948) *Industrial Hygiene and Toxicology, Volume 1*, New York: Interscience Publishers Inc.

Piney, M. (1989) *The Development of Chemical Exposure Limits for the Workplace*, thesis, University of Aston.

Roach, S.A. (1980) 'Control limits – Workplace environment' in: *National Conference on Health and Safety Seminar*; 11-20.

Roach, S.A. & S.M. Rappaport (1990) 'But they are not thresholds: a critical analysis of the documentation of TLV's', *American Journal of Industrial Medicine* 17: 727-53.

Russell, J.R. (1983) 'Asbestos: a failure?', in: HSE: *Her Majesty's Inspectors of Factories 1883-1983*, London: HMSO.

Sayers, R.R. & J.N. Dallavalle (1935) 'Prevention of occupational diseases other than those caused by toxic dusts', *Mechanical Engineering* 57: 230-234.

Senn, E.P. (1995) 'Ending OSHAs dependance on exposure limits', *Applied Occupational and Environmental Hygiene* 10: 520-522.

Smyth, H.F. (1984) 'Current confidence in occupational health', *Annals of the American Conference of Industrial Hygiene* 9: 323-329.

Viscusi, W.K. (1982) 'Setting efficient standards for occupational hazards', *Journal of Occupational Medicine* 24: 969-976.

Yant, W.P. (1948) 'Industrial hygiene codes and regulations', *Transactions of the 13th Annual Meeting of the Industrial Hygiene Forum of America*; 48-61.

Winslow, C.E.A. et al. (1919) 'Standards for measuring the efficiency of exhaust systems in polishing shops', *Public Health Reports* 34: 427-449.

# 3

*Roland Bal*

# BOUNDARY DYNAMICS IN DUTCH STANDARD SETTING FOR OCCUPATIONAL CHEMICALS

## INTRODUCTION

Once started as the activity of some individual scientists, and later taken up by professional organisations, standard setting for occupational chemicals has since the 1970s increasingly become a task of government agencies. This shift in the location of standard setting has been accompanied by a growing 'rationalisation' of the process, mainly by structuring the information input, separating the decision making process into two or more pieces, and making legal frameworks for the implementation of standards in workplaces. This has led in turn to the design of assessment protocols, the standardisation of toxicity tests, and has involved the definition of domains of discretion for the actors involved.

In this contribution, I shall concentrate on the organisational setting in which the development of standards for occupational chemicals takes place. I will limit myself to the way in which standard setting organisations have differentiated between, on the one hand 'scientific' and, on the other, 'non-scientific' aspects of the decision-making process, while at the same time permitting the integration of these domains of discretion in one standard. Furthermore, I will concentrate on one standard setting organisation, namely the Dutch

In: R. Bal & W. Halffman (eds.), *The Politics of Chemical Risk*, Kluwer Academic Publishers, Dordrecht 1998: p. 75-103.

procedure for developing occupational exposure limits.[1] By doing this, it will be possible to follow the development of this procedure through time, and thus to venture into the dynamics of boundary creation and maintenance within standard setting organisations. In the next section, I shall first introduce a conceptual framework that enables me to analyse occupational standard setting.

## MANDATE, BOUNDARIES AND REPERTOIRES

Although the organisation of standard setting can differ between countries and regulatory contexts, a common characteristic is that at least some external actors are involved in the decision-making process. These external actors always involve professionals, and, depending on the regulatory tradition, also representatives drawn from interest groups.[2] In practice, standard setting is thus never an activity of government alone, but always involves other actors as well. This phenomenon can be explained by the need for government to secure the compliance capability and readiness of all actors involved (Zald 1978; De Vroom 1990), viz., both interest groups and professionals. Through their participation, a basis for legitimacy is created in all relevant social groups. From the perspective of government, standard setting is itself a risk-prone process, exposing governments to the risks of either under- or overregulation, and the risks involved can be mitigated by transferring responsibility through the inclusion of external actors in the decision-making process (cf. Krücken 1994).

Analysts have usually focused on one of two different aspects of standard setting. First, students of policy-making and administration have focused

---

1 Dutch standard setting for occupational chemicals has mainly been selected for analysis because it has been shown to be one of the more productive organisations of standard setting, both in terms of the number of standards developed, and in terms of the protection these standards offer to workers (Bal & De Vroom 1993).

2 Within countries with a corporatist tradition tripartite commissions are usually installed in which interest groups participate alongside government representatives. Within countries lacking such a tradition, like the US, interest groups usually participate in decision making through some sort of judicial process, like formal hearings (Brickman et al. 1985).

their attention mainly on the organisational context in which standard setting takes place. Some of these have looked at the best way to match different types of policy problems with the 'best' advisory structures (f.e. Barker & Peters 1993). Others have criticised standard setting, or other policy making processes in which experts are involved, as forms of technocratic control (e.g. Fischer 1990). Although this literature has been able to analyse some salient aspects of the organisational structure as well as the ideologies of standard setting, it has left out some other crucial aspects. The main problem in this context is the fact that this literature has tended not to problematise boundaries between scientific and non-scientific elements of standard setting. Rather, it has taken both science and the boundaries between science and non-science for granted.[3] The second type of literature, mainly stemming from the field of science and technology studies, has taken the construction of boundaries within standard setting as its main focus. This literature has tended to take an actor-oriented approach to the issues, following actors in the way they construct scientific facts and boundaries between science and non-science (e.g. Cambrosio et al. 1992). By doing this, however, it has tended to ignore the organisational settings in which standard setting takes place and to incorporate the pressures arising from that setting. Furthermore, while students of policy have had hard times in analysing controversies, students of science and technology have had difficulty in explaining the lack of controversy (cf. Martin & Richards 1995: 518).

In the following, I combine, but shall not try to integrate, these two kinds of literature. On the one hand, I focus on the development of an organisation for standard setting, following this procedure through time and especially following the way in which distinct 'domains of discretion' are created. On the other hand, I go into the way in which these domains are reproduced in the actual practice of standard setting, thus giving them their seemingly unproblematic nature. I shall, furthermore, analyse some of the tools that have been developed to make possible this translation from a contingent practice to a more or less rationalised procedure.

---

3 This does not mean that no problems are considered regarding the use of expertise in policy making, but these problems are seen to arise because of uncertainties within science, and not from structural problems concerning the way in which boundaries are created.

The transfer of responsibilities from government to external actors in standard setting can be done in different ways, but usually takes the form of some kind of mandate. Within this mandate, domains of discretion are differentiated and the discretionary space thus defined is transferred to the mandated actors, usually experts and in some cases also interest groups. Also, the means of integration of the differentiated domains are defined in the mandate. The mandate thus defines what information input is required for the standard setting process, who has the responsibility over this information, and how the different kinds of information are coupled to enable standards to be produced. The main object of this differentiation of domains of discretion is to canalise the information input, and thereby possible conflicts (Schmidt & Werle 1992). The main source of conflict is seen to be the intermingling of the domains, and therefore the rules in the mandate aim at preventing any kind of 'heterogeneity overload'. The mandate does not prevent conflict, nor does it provide for automatic conflict resolution. Rather, through its canalising function, it prevents conflicts from spilling over the boundaries of the differentiated domains. Following Gieryn, I will call this process of differentiation 'boundary work', that is "the attribution of selected characteristics to the institution of science (i.e. to its practitioners, methods, stock of knowledge, values and work organisation) for purposes of constructing a social boundary that distinguishes some intellectual activity as non-science" (Gieryn 1983: 782).[4] However, where Gieryn localises boundary work explicitly in language, I extend this notion to include organisation as well.

Apart from institutionalising a boundary between the scientific and non-scientific, and specifying how the differentiated domains of discretion are to be integrated, the mandate provides a repertoire in which the activities in the practice of standard setting can be presented in a rationalised way. The main function of the rationalistic repertoire is to legitimise standard setting practice. That is, when confronted with questions concerning the way

---

4 In Steve Shapin's definition the concept of boundary work is strechted to include other than science – non-science distinctions: "bounding a practice is a way of defining what it is, of protecting it from unwanted interference and excluding unwanted participants, of telling practitioners how it is proper to behave within it and how that behaviour differs from ordinary conduct, and of distributing value across its borders" (Shapin 1992: 335).

in which specific standards have been set, actors from standard setting practice will refer to the rationalistic repertoire, to legitimise their activities.

Within standard setting practice, however, lots of information circulates which cannot be articulated within the rationalistic repertoire, because of its contingent nature. For example, the quality of different laboratories or researchers, the feeling an expert may have regarding a specific toxicological profile, or the knowledge interest groups may have of the practice of exposure testing at particular company-sites, may not be easily expressed within the rationalistic repertoire. This contingent information, moreover, does not easily fit into either of the domains which have been created in the mandate. At the same time, however, it may be crucial for the 'quality' of the standard. I will argue that within the mandate specific tools have been developed that make it possible to 'translate' information from the contingent repertoire to the rationalistic repertoire. Examples of such tools are the so-called safety factor and the selection of committee members. These tools not only make it possible to translate information from the contingent to the rationalistic repertoire, they also function in the creation of a package – a greyboxed version of a domain – which can be handed down to the other domains.[5] The differentiation and integration of domains of discretion within the mandate can therefore be seen to be dependent on the translation work made possible by these tools.

In the following, I analyse the organisation and practice of Dutch standard setting for occupational chemicals. I first explore the initial build up of the organisational setting and the way in which this has developed through time. It will become clear from this that, both within the organisational setting and within the rationalistic repertoire, boundaries between the different domains of discretion become stricter over the course of time as a result of both internal discussions and more general reorganisations of the advisory structure in Dutch politics. Second, I analyse the mandate for standard setting; in particular, I focus on the tools that have been developed in order to translate the contingent into the rationalistic repertoire.

---

5 See Fujimura (1992) for the notion of 'packages'.

## THE ORGANISATIONAL SETTING

At the beginning of the 1970s, after a period of relative quietness, occupational exposure to chemicals again became part of the political agenda in the Netherlands. In part this was the result of a growing awareness of the 'chemisation' of the environment, but more directly it was caused by new social activity around the discovery that exposure to vinylchloride may cause cancer. Under pressure from, among others, the Industrial Labour Union,[6] the Minister of Social Affairs decided to consider the installation of a procedure for the establishment of Occupational Exposure Limits.

Activities related to such a procedure had already been commencend in the Ministry. In 1973, the Medical Department of the Labour Inspectorate had installed a working group that had advised the installation of a 'national TLV committee' (De Valk & Wink 1974). Part of this advice was a call to include representatives from employers' and workers' organisations in the setting of occupational exposure standards.[7] Before that time, the Labour Inpectorate had already been active in standard setting and had organised contacts with the association of industrial hygienists to work on this (Brokamp 1987; Bal 1996). The establishment of a standing committee on occupational exposure limits would not only formalise and institutionalise these activities, but would also give them a more legitimate structure of corporatist control.

According to the original plan, the 'national TLV committee' would be one committee, of which interest groups, policy-makers and experts would be members, thereby creating no organisational boundary between the health and policy aspects of standard setting. Such a committee, however, never surfaced. Instead, in June 1976 a 'working group of experts', later called the Dutch Expert Committee on Occupational Standards (DECOS) was installed (Ministry of Social Affairs 1976), followed in December of the same

---

6 Interview with Van Hattum, former labour representative in the MAC commission. Also: Geers (1988).

7 Accompanying the publication of the proposal, industrial hygienist Zielhuis published an editorial entitled 'About them, without them', in which he pleaded for the inclusion of representatives of interest groups in governmental standard setting as well (Zielhuis 1974).

year by the installation of a National Committee on MAC values, in which representatives from interest groups and policy-makers would participate (Ministry of Social Affairs 1977). At that time it was thought that DECOS' main role was to summarise and evaluate the scientific information on specific chemicals, in order to facilitate the discussions within the MAC committee. Experts, it was thought furthermore, should not only be selected because of their knowledge and experience, but should also reflect the positions of the interest groups involved: labour and industry.[8]

Although two committees were set up, the organisational boundary between the assessment and the management of chemicals was initially very permeable. The whole organisation of standard setting was embedded within the Ministry. Furthermore, there were many other links between the two groups. For example, the secretariate of both DECOS and the commission were in the hands of one person. It seems that, from the point of view of the Ministry of Social Affairs, the boundary between the scientific and non-scientific stages in the procedure was not at first seen as much of a problem needing to be addressed in its own right, and more attention was paid to the corporatist structure of interest group involvement in the decision making.

With the procedure in place matters changed rapidly. Both DECOS and the National MAC committee felt the need for a more clear-cut task differentiation. Their work on this resulted in the publication of their 'starting points' (National MAC committee & DECOS 1978), in which the boundaries between risk assessment and risk management became more visible, although nothing changed organisationally. What did change, however, was that a repertoire became available in which the procedure could be put forward in a rational manner. With this repertoire, furthermore, a more normative stress was put on the boundary, which had previously only been talked about in organisational terms. Central to the repertoire is the notion that standard setting for occupational chemicals should be seen as a three-step process, and that the three organisations that make up the procedure are all responsible for one of these steps. In the first step, a scientific assessment is made of the health effects of occupational exposure to chemicals, leading to the formulation

---

8 This is apparent from the letter that was send to invite experts to become a member of the Working Group of Experts (Director General of Labour 1976).

of a health-based standard. This health-based standard should, in the second step, be evaluated in terms of its economic and technical feasibility, leading to a so-called feasibility standard. This feasibility standard then forms the input to the third step, in which the government, in particular the Directorate General of Labour of the Ministry of Social Affairs and Employment, adopts it and transforms it into a regulatory standard. A central feature of the repertoire is that the differentiated domains of discretion are hierarchically integrated, in the sense that the outcomes of each step form the input to each next step and cannot again be discussed.[9]

Although the hierarchical integration of decision making has been preserved, several changes have been made to the organisation of the standard setting process since 1978. In the first place, in 1986, the evaluation of the feasibility of health-based standards has been taken over from the National MAC committee by a committee of the Labour Council. Although presented as part of a general restructuring of advisory boards (Labour Council 1985), the externalisation of interest representation is also part of an attempt to decrease the amount of discussion between the risk assessors and the risk managers within the MAC procedure (Brokamp, personal information). Increasingly, discussions about the risk assessment within the 'second step' came to be discouraged. One of the former members of the Labour Council committee expressed this as follows:

> At first I had trouble with that. What did I know... They send me a report with 'draft' on it in big letters. So I read it well and didn't agree with some of it, and I expressed those comments in the meeting. But everyone fell down on me, because a lay person should not mingle with the risk assessment. Only DECOS was allowed to do that.

As a consequence of the new organisation, DECOS formally no longer advises the MAC committee directly. Instead, the risk assessment is sent to the

---

9 In a strict sense, we should speak of a four-step procedure, in which the first step consists of the production of priority lists for the rest of the steps. However, I will use the term 'three-step', first because this more closely follows the rationalistic repertoire of Dutch occupational standard setting, but second, and more importantly, because this more clearly reflects the organisational differentiation between domains of discretion as implemented by the procedure.

Director General of Labour, which then formally requests advice from the Labour Council (Directorate General of Labour 1986). Furthermore, in order to acquire a richer information base for the evaluation of feasibility of the health-based standard, a rudimentary cost-benefit analysis complements the request for feasibility advice. The new procedure, however, slowed down the standard setting process considerably, mainly as a result of a lack of manpower at the Directorate General. In order to overcome this an informal procedure developed, in which the old procedure is mimicked: reports from DECOS again form the direct input to the deliberations in the second step of the procedure (Brokamp 1991).

The externalisation of the MAC committee was also accompanied by a new phenomenon in the procedure: the publication of a draft report by DECOS which is publicly available for critique. Through this, the possibility of interest group reactions to the risk assessment is maintained, but is now organised as a consultation process. Another difference from the old procedure concerns the membership of the Labour Council's committee. Formerly, the MAC committee only consisted of representatives drawn from organised interests, but in the new procedure policy-makers also have a place in the committee.

The next major restructuring of the organisation of the MAC procedure found place in 1994, when DECOS became part of the Health Council. Also, the activities of the Labour Council were discontinued and its advisory work was taken over by the Social Economic Council. Again, these changes were part of a general restructuring of advisory councils, but there were some substantive arguments as well. For example, it was felt that the advisory process on labour conditions should be more integrated with the totality of social-economic policy (Social Economic Council 1993). Concerning DECOS, it was also felt that expert advice on occupational chemicals should be brought more in line with that on environmental chemicals. An earlier attempt in this direction had been made with the publication of the Health Councils' advice on standard setting in 1985,[10] which had presented a com-

10 In his request for the advice, the then Minister of State for Health wrote: "in the establishment of regulatory standards, different methods are often used and different criteria are employed to evaluate the toxicological information. This lack of agreement in the risk assessment has consequences first and foremost for the

prehensive set of starting points for occupational as well as environmental standard setting. But despite this, expert advices from the Health Council and DECOS continued to differ. This was seen as problematic. As a policy maker from the Environmental Ministry expressed it: "how can I sell to the public that two groups of experts each hold a different opinion?"

A further influence on the organisational restructuring came from overseas, with the strong criticism that was levelled against the Threshold Limit Values (TLV) Committee of the American Conference of Industrial Hygienists (ACGIH). This organisation, and its anual list of TLVs, was (and still is) very influential. At the start of the MAC-procedure, as has been the case in almost any standard setting organisation, especially in the field of occupational standards (Salter 1988; Piney, this volume), MAC values had been taken over from the TLV list. These standards had gradually been replaced by MAC values, but at the beginning of the 1990s, most MAC values were still taken from subsequent TLV lists.

To many it came as a shock that several articles were published at the end of the 1980s in the *American Journal of Industrial Medicine* that greatly criticised the standard setting procedure within the ACGIH.[11] The ACGIH, according to the critics, had been captured by industrial interests (Castleman & Ziem 1988), and its standards could no longer be seen as health-based but were to be seen as feasibility-based (Roach & Rappaport 1990; also Piney 1989, and this volume). This was denied by the ACGIH and by its (former) members (Breysse 1991; Stokinger 1988), pointing to methodological errors in the critique and to their experience in serving on ACGIH committees. Throughout the discussion, however, the theme ran, that, within the standard setting process, a strict separation can and should be made between con-

---

health-based standards. The standards for one and the same substance are often difficult to compare and the totality of exposure from different sources is hardly ever taken into account" (Health Council of the Netherlands 1985: 15-16).

11 The main articles are Castleman & Ziem (1988), Robinson (1989), Zielhuis & Wibowo (1989), Roach & Rappaport (1990), and Robinson et al. (1991). That the criticisms really were felt as a shock can be seen from the huge number of 'letters to the editor' that were published, especially in response to the Castleman & Ziem and the Roach & Rappaport articles. In 1986, the DECOS still had expressed its trust in the ACGIH TLV committee (DECOS 1986).

siderations of health and of policy or economics.[12] The only difference of opinion was whether the TLV committee did or did not differentiate sufficiently between the two domains of discretion.[13]

This call was repeated in the Netherlands when the American critique of TLVs was translated into the Dutch situation in 1991. An important moment here was the publication of a thesis by Ulenbelt (1991) and a conference that was held for the occasion. Although it was generally felt that the American situation was not directly applicable to the Dutch, some fierce criticisms were levelled at the MAC procedure. One of the criticisms was that the scientific expert group did not live up to its own standards, for example by having an inconsistent policy on the assessment of reproductive risks (Stijkel 1992; also Stijkel et al. 1996). The critique especially gained momentum with the discussion over the standard for Man-made Mineral Fibres, for which DECOS had just published its first draft report. Pointing to some large inconsistencies in the report and to the fact that the then chair of DECOS had links with the fibre industry, the MAC procedure stood accused of being captured by industrial interests.[14] In the subsequent discussions, the separation between the assessment and management of chemicals was

---

12 Both sides to the discussion, however, had differing views on what was to be seen as 'scientific' information. For example Castleman and Ziem (1988; also Ziem & Castleman 1989) argued that what can be regarded as truly scientific has to stem from academic or industry-independent scientists, and has to be publicly available. In contrast, both Stokinger (1988) and Cox (1988) argue that information that has been collected from the workplace by occupational hygienists is essential to the standard setting process. The fact that this knowledge is often not publicly available should not prohibit its use by standard setting organisations. Note that the critics of the TLV have a very strict view of the kind of knowledge that can be used for standard setting, stressing global criteria of assessment, whereas proponents of the TLV system argue instead for localised knowledge.

13 Those that answered the question in the affirmative (e.g. Breysse 1991) did not plead for any changes in the process, while those that argued otherwise did. Woitowitz (1988), for example, argued for the establishment of ethical codes for TLV committee members. Although, according to the ACGIH nothing was wrong with the existing procedures, they were changed after the publication of the criticisms. The effects of these changes are controversial, but Rappaport (1993) claims that they have improved ACGIH standard setting.

14 Ulenbelt's critique was expressed, among others, in an interview with one of the largest Dutch newspapers (Didde 1991). See Bal & Spit (1994) for an extensive analysis of the Man-made Mineral Fibre controversy.

stressed once again. The critique had a great impact within the MAC organisations, where it was felt that the criticism was unduly directed at a procedure that was one of the best of its kind.[15]

In sum, since its establishment, the organisational distance has increased between the three domains of discretion that are distinguished in the mandate for the setting of MAC values. Moreover, within the rationalistic repertoire more emphasis has been laid on the desirability of a separation between considerations of health, economics, and policy. These changes in the procedure can be linked to developments in the general policy on advisory boards and on labour conditions, but are at the same time reactions to tensions within the standard setting procedure.

## BOUNDARY ORDERING DEVICES

Setting occupational health standards in the Netherlands has increasingly come to depend on the organisational separation of science, interests and policy. This boundary has become one of the main sources of legitimacy for the procedure. However, as we know from the extensive literature on the subject (among others Jasanoff 1990; Wynne 1992; Cambrosio et al. 1992), the practice of standard setting usually does not entail clear-cut boundaries between these domains. Furthermore, in interviews, (former) members of the committees of the MAC procedure often point to aspects that cannot easily be phrased in the rationalistic repertoire, such as the feeling they have concerning certain toxicity profiles, or the trust they put in the measurements originating from certain companies. These aspects, though sometimes crucial to the standard setting process, cannot easily be ascribed to one of the officially differentiated domains. This leads to a discrepancy between the mandate for and the practice of standard setting. How, then, is this discrepancy compensated for?

---

15 Only two years earlier, this statement was made by Noordam and Maas (1990), and it was repeated by Zielhuis, the founding father of the procedure, at the conference mentioned earlier (Zielhuis 1992).

My suggestion is that, within the mandate, certain tools are developed that enable participants in the procedure to translate the heterogeneous information found in practice to the more-or-less homogeneous information required. These tools function as 'boundary ordering devices' (Shackley & Wynne 1996), by fascilitating translations between the contingent and the rationalistic repertoire, and thus co-constructing domains of discretion. In the following I analyse three such boundary ordering devices in the mandate for the production of MAC values; the so-called safety or uncertainty factor, the person of the expert, and the so-called company visit.[16]

*Safety factors*

DECOS' task as laid down in the establishments decree, is to: "prepare and report on the scientific data with regard to hazardous substances, on the basis of which insight can be given into the toxicological aspects of the substances" (Ministry of Social Affairs 1976). While it is established that the working group should report on the "toxicological" or the "health" aspects of occupational chemicals, these notions are not specified. Nor is the way in which the advice should be drafted, or whether or not a health-based standard should be proposed or not. At first glance, then, the formulation of the official mandate leaves DECOS wide discretion. This has been narrowed down by the working group itself, however, and by other organisations such as the Health Council, in further (semi-)official publications.[17]

---

16 These three are by no means the only boundary ordering devices to be found in standard setting mandates. In my thesis, which I hope to complete later this year, I shall provide a more systematic overview.

17 The main reports in this case are the 'starting point' documents concerning both MAC values (Working group of experts & MAC committee 1978) and standard setting in general (Health Council of the Netherlands 1985). Both documents have been accepted by the Directorate General of Labour. In the 1978 report this is stated explicitly: "The Directorate General of Labour fully agrees with the vision of the National MAC committee and the working group of experts concerning the principles for establishing MAC values as laid down in this document" (National MAC committee & DECOS 1978: 1). Although this official recognition has not been published in the case of the Health Council report, in interviews with officials from the Ministry of Social Affairs this document is identified as having been very influential in establishing guidelines for setting MAC values.

As becomes clear from these publications, the expert group's task is first to evaluate all the scientific literature concerning a specific chemical. This evaluation should lead to the establishment of a 'critical effect', being the first adversarial effect to arise with higher concentrations of the chemical, and to the establishment of a 'no-adverse-effect-level', or a 'minimal-adverse-effect-level'. Because of the many uncertainties that have been introduced into the process of establishing such a level, however, it is claimed that it cannot be directly put forward as a health-based standard. Instead, the level is divided by a so-called safety factor that should compensate for these uncertainties.

The idea of a safety factor was coined in 1954 by Lehman, a German toxicologist, then working at the United States Food and Drug Administation (Lehman & Fitzhugh 1954). The factor he introduced was meant to reduce the uncertainty that information obtained from experiments with small groups of genetically relatively homogeneous animals, who are exposed to high concentrations of chemicals, had to be used in creating standards for a large and hetergeneous human population. Certainty that the standard could actually protect humans was to be obtained by dividing the concentration at which no effects were seen in the laboratory by a factor of 100. Since then, the application of a safety factor, or uncertainty factor, as it is nowadays called, has become common pratice within standard setting, but the rational of applying a factor of 100 has changed.

The most important change has been that the factor 100 itself was devided into different factors. So, for example, at the beginning of the 1970s it was argued that the factor 100 was actually made up of two factors 10, one to compensate for uncertainty arising because of the translation from animal data to humans, and the other to compensate for uncertainty arising out of the extrapolation from homogeneous to heterogeneous populations (Bigwood 1973). This division implied that it had become possible to differentiate safety factors into other factors, thereby bringing in more contingent knowledge. So, for example, at the start of the MAC procedure, it was argued that the factor 10 which was used for compensating heterogeneous populations could be lower for occupational populations than for the general population, because the former was more homogeneous in nature.

Furthermore, because of the fact that no definitive rationale could be given for the make-up of the safety factor, it was argued that its magnitude was to be determined by experts on a case-by-case basis and based on their knowledge of the effects of a certain chemical and their experience with standard setting in general. Though it was argued by the working group that the factor would therefor always have some degree of arbitrariness, they were sure that the experts would be able to provide a rationale for every factor they came up with (MAC committee & DECOS 1978).

In later years, the rationale for setting a safety factor was worked out further. So, in 1985, a committee of the Health Council – made up in part of experts who were also members of DECOS – provided a further articulation of the rationale for setting a safety factor. They argued that not two but three factors could be distinguished. Not only were there the two already existing factors, but a factor concerning the "variation that arises because of the whole complex of environmental influence and observational errors" was added (Health Council 1985). The committee kept insisting on the need for a case-by-case assessment of the safety factor, to be employed by competent experts.

In the course of 1992 there was a discussion within DECOS, in which two committee members proposed to create a more or less standardised rationale for the application of safety factors. Such a system would lead to a more controllable expert assessment of chemicals, making the assessment more transparent. The proposal met with considerable criticism from the other committee members, however, and was not adopted. In an article the reason for this rejection was stated as: "the weakness of such a system is that it may be used not as a supplement to, but at the expense of, the input of expertise and experience. Hundreds of evaluations conducted over the years have shown that expertise and experience are indispensable" (Feron et al. 1994: 262; Feron, this volume).

Paralleling the changes in the organisational setting in time, we can thus see a further articulation of the safety factor. However, this has not lead to a shift, in Ted Porter's (1995) terms, from 'expert knowledge' to 'mechanical objectivity'. Although the need for a further protocolisation and standardisation of the expert assessment is stated, this has not lead to the abolition of expert knowledge.

The main point here is that the safety factor allows experts to pragmatically integrate information that is contingent on the use of a certain chemical into standard setting, while at the same time enabling them to present this as a *scientific* result. So, in setting an environmental standard for formaldehyde at the beginning of the 1980s, Zielhuis noted:

> ...120 microgram was very important in the case of those houses. This standard was already in use. (...) You cannot say that a standard should be exactly 120, it might just as well be 90 or 150. The number 120 is only reached by a certain method of multiplying and dividing. The argument is given in the report to reach 120; it is also correct with regard to the experimental outcomes of the carcinogenicity experiments.[18]

Using safety factors, experts are thus able to integrate information that is contingent on the chemical they are assessing, on its use and on their feelings about this in the scientific assessment. It enables them to translate these contingencies in the rationalistic repertoire, thereby at the same time producing a standard and constructing the scientific domain.

### *Boundary ordering people*

How does one become a member of DECOS? According to the mandate, experts are installed *à titre personel*. Members of DECOS are expected not to represent the organisations for which they do their daily work,[19] but to be representatives of knowledge. That is, they should be experts. But what, then, is an expert? If an expert is to represent knowledge from a scientific speciality within the policy community, this entails the translation of that knowledge into usable terms. And it entails that the expert has to legitimise his actions within both the scientific and the policy communities.

This problematic position as a science-policy hybrid sets specific criteria for the person of the expert. Members of DECOS therefore speak in much

---

18 Cited in Van Eijndhoven & Groenewegen (1991: 277), and commenting on the work of the Special Advisory Committee on Formaldehyde, which was installed after the 1980 CIIT studies reporting the carcinogenicity of formaldehyde. See Jasanoff (1986) for an extensive account of this study, and its subsequent route through several national bureaucracies.

19 Although, as noted before, at the start of the procedure mention was made of some kind of representation of interests within the committee.

broader terms than knowledge *perse* when they refer to experts. According to Kolk, at that time chair of DECOS:

> (...) the expert possesses more than enough relevant and up-to-date factual knowledge; has enough experience in positions in which he or she has been confronted with the societal consequences of the advice he or she gives for individuals, groups or institutions; and can and will on this basis take the moral and intellectual responsibility for those advices (Kolk 1993: 114).

On this basis, he states that young, recently graduated scientists cannot be seen as experts. Although their factual knowledge is very up to date, they have insufficient experience "to advice on standards with often far-reaching societal consequences" (idem.). Older scientists are also excluded from the definition of expert, since they have "mostly insufficiently been able to keep their factual knowledge up to date, and because the societal context has changed considerably since they entered the field a quarter of a century ago" (idem.).

Being an expert thus not only entails the possession of specialised knowledge. Although this is a prerequisite, it is not sufficient for expertness.[20] Members of DECOS should, in their own view, have knowledge of the societal context in which they operate. Furthermore, they should keep both their factual and societal knowledge constantly up to date. Moreover, they believe it important to addopt an attitude in which they are able to weigh the consequences of their advice for society. The ultimate consequence of that is that they should be prepared to expose themselves, or even their children, to the concentration advised, as is regularly expressed in interviews.[21] They should furthermore be prepared to translate their considerations into an advice, and to defend it against critics.

---

20 According to Notten, former scientific secretary of DECOS, specialist knowledge is even a disadvantage for members of DECOS. What is needed is an overview over different specialty fields. Interview, March 10 1994.

21 For example, Joosting states that: "one who is not willing to expose himself, is not entitled to have employees who must be exposed, nor to judge upon that." Interview, March 30 1994. Zielhuis tells a story of an experiment at the beginning of the 1970s, in which the research group (containing a number of later DECOS members) exposed themselves to chloride ion. Interview, June 15 1993. See Verberk et al. (1975) for an article on the experiment.

The expert is thus revealed to be a typical hybrid, moving between the domains of science and policy. An expert is not just an intermediary between these domains, but forms an interface as well as a boundary between them. In other words, (s)he can be seen as a 'boundary ordering person'.

But even this combination of skills, knowledge and sense of responsibility are not enough. Members of DECOS are supposed to work in a *group*, and so the mandate presupposes that they can function in and as a group, even more so since DECOS always strives for consensual advice. From interviews, therefore, a picture arises of a process of socialisation in the group, comprising both social and cognitive aspects. Joosting, for example, states that: "people from companies might have a very one-sided attitude at the start, but once they are members of DECOS this changes. They learn how to see things from an hygienic perspective" (interview, March 30 1994). Kummer, himself an epidemiologist, states that: "you also change yourself through the contribution of the laboratory workers. We will say that 'your rat is not a human being' (...). But you see it going in both directions. Everyone is going to understand what the other does and from that understanding one tries to reach a consensus" (interview, April 15 1994). Reflecting on the introduction of a new member into the committee he states: "in the beginning he thought he had to defend himself (...). He was responsible for the writing of documents and stood very far from reality. In the course of a couple of months he transformed into a completely different person. He began to make jokes, an important thing, and took a vulnerable attitude, also an important thing" (idem).

The importance of this socialisation process, which makes members of DECOS take a vulnerable attitude, make jokes, share a common culture, and state themselves in a common, hygienistic repertoire, puts great pressure on the size of the committee and on the length of membership. At the start, in 1976, only eight members were selected, and though the committee grew in later years, its membership never exceeded twelve. Members of DECOS are furthermore to be found in many other expert bodies, like committees of the Health Council. Members moreover usually hold their seats for a long time: four of the members selected in 1976 were still serving in 1990, and the last of these only retired in 1994. This does not necessarily mean that members are selected from an *old-boys' network*, as Salter has noted with reference to membership of the TLV committee (1988: 44-45), although personal contacts are mentioned in interviews as a relevant and often-used selection criterion. Rather, the analysis above leads to an explanation in terms of the enabling function – concerning both the daily activities of DECOS and the productivity of the mandate in general – of the use of a shared repertoire. This, of course, still leads to the creation of a 'boundary elite' (Hoch 1989), since experts who do not share this repertoire are being excluded from the committee.

*The company visit*

As we have seen, although the mandate for the health assessment of chemicals has been increasingly articulated over time, it still leaves ample room for expert discretion. This is even more so for the second step of the MAC procedure: the assessment of the feasibility of the health-based standard. The MAC committee is mandated to advise the Directorate General of Labour, taking account of the health assessment, and "all further relevant aspects" (Ministry of Social Affairs 1977). In his speech at the installation of the committee, former Minister of Social Affairs Boersma mentioned that these 'further relevant aspects' were to be understood as all possible consequences of a proposed standard "for employment and the economy" (Boersma 1977). In the *starting-points* document furthermore, the MAC committee's task is seen as assessing the "socio-economic consequences, technical feasibility, international agreements, etc." of the proposed standards (National MAC committee & DECOS 1978: 4). The ways in which the MAC committee should proceed in the gathering of information or in deliberating upon it are not specified.

Although the mandate is not very specific as to the task of the MAC committee, in practice a procedure has developed that is aimed at consultation with the groups that are represented within the committee, that is, industry and labour. At the start of the procedure, consultation with industry was co-ordinated by the Dutch Chemical Industry Association, which published the proposed MAC values in a couple of newsletters and then awaited reactions. This so-called 'peep-system' became formalised from 1991 onwards. From then on, all relevant industry associations are informed of the possible implementation of a new MAC value and it is left to their discretion to inform their members. Although this has led to a growth of reactions, suggesting a greater awareness in industry of the new MAC values, the method still has some problems. In most part this is caused by the fact that industry associations or companies often do not know exactly which chemicals are used in the production process, let alone the concentrations to which workers are exposed (Brokamp 1996; Halffman & Van Raalte 1996). Furthermore, starting in 1986, a second method of collecting feasibility-information has been developed. These so-called 'workplace analyses' are performed by order of the DG of Labour, and contain a more detailed and systematic analysis of the technical and economic feasibility of the proposed standard. This method has also run into some problems. First, they are perceived as being too expensive and to take too much time. Second, there has been some conflict over who is the responsible actor for performing feasiblity analyses, since the MAC committee found that the 'workplace analyses' duplicate the work that should be done by the committee itself (Brokamp 1991). Because of these problems, the workplace analyses are only performed in some 15 percent of cases, leaving the (formalised) peep-system the most commonly used method of feasibility assessment.

The deliberations in the committee are anything but adversarial. In the twenty years since its establishment the committee only failed to reach a consensus on three occasions. Several tools have been developed to enable the committee to reach consensus. One of these is the 'company visit', which is performed by the representatives of industry in the committee. Whenever a complaint is filed against a proposed MAC value, the industry representatives will visit the company in which the problems will arise, to assess the validity of the complaint. This often leads to the withdrawal of the complaint. Nijland – a former member of the committee – for example, tells the story of a visit to a large firm processing formalin:

> This big firm (...) handles thousands of tons of the substance per year. Every day a couple of big trucks arrive. The critical point is during the connection of the tube to the truck. Lots of data were collected on this during the years. This was all nicely demonstrated at the company visit, and it seemed alright. Only, Zuber – then head of the industry representatives – didn't trust the measurements and so we went back a week later to check on them. And indeed, they had done it all wrong and all the data they collected were useless. And so we couldn't bring the complaint to the committee either (interview, 9 March 1994).

On other occasions, the working conditions are so poor in a company that complaints are withdrawn all the same, because the firm would be in trouble if this were to be brought to light.

Through the company visit complaints are filtered before they are brought into the deliberations of the committee. The visit is therefore an element in the construction of interest by the committee: interests are not given from the start, but have to be made in the process of assessing feasibility. Moreover, and more importantly in this context, the contingencies of the company visit are not easily mapped onto the differentiated domains of discretion. Constructing interests through the company visit requires a lot of technical skill and knowledge. It is only through the deliberations in the committee and through the wording of the advice that these technical skills and knowledge are transformed into a package containing the interests concerning a particular chemical.

## CONCLUSIONS AND DISCUSSION

In order to be productive it seems that standard setting organisations cannot function without the dual movement of differentiation and integration of domains of discretion. While the rationalistic repertoire makes sure that, from the outside, the boundary between risk assessment and management seems strict, internally a more flexible, contingent repertoire can be used in order to negotiate about inconsistencies and to establish consensus. This is not to say that there are no boundaries in standard setting. The different committees in the case of Dutch standard setting for occupational chemicals really do different things, and use different methods to arrive at their conclusions. But the separation of domains of discretion cannot be as strict as is suggested in the rationalistic repertoire. Rather, they are reproduced in practice through the use of tools that have been designed for the task of translating the heterogeneity of practice into the orderly world of the mandate.

The fact that both the experts and the MAC committee consistently strive for consensus reinforces the image of *a priori* existing domains of discretion. For both committees this entails playing upon the expectations and wishes of government, for it is mostly government that wants both the domains of health and interests to speak with one voice.[22]

Concerning the MAC committee, it is interesting to note that whereas the committee's make-up is to represent dominant interests in the field of labour conditions, the workings of the committee are not coined in terms of interests. Apparently, it is not done in the Dutch context to express one's interests in a direct way. Instead, discussions on interests are rephrased in terms of the technical or economic feasibility of proposed standards. Paraphrasing Wynne's (1982) study on the role of science in the Windscale Inquiry, one could argue that interests are ritualised in the Dutch context of setting exposure limits for occupational standards. Through this ritualisation, interests are objectified, while at the same time it enables actors to make compromises.

Within the MAC procedure we have seen that in the course of time, as a result of both reorganisations within Dutch advisory councils and internal struggles, the boundaries between the domains of discretion have become stricter. In the organisational setting, the domains have been separated from each other, while within the rationalistic repertoire, more emphasis has been put upon their distinctions. At the same time, the boundary ordering devices have themselves in part become more rationalised and articulated. This has not lead to a complete protocolisation of practice. Instead, the actors are left with ample discretion, enabling them to translate the heterogeneity of practice into the homogeneity of the mandate.

The above analysis suggests that the dualistic organisation of standard setting for occupational chemicals is productive both in terms of the number of standards set and the protection they offer to workers. Standardisation thus seems to be something to be avoided, while at the same time the public should have the impression that the organisation guarantees strict boundaries. There are, however, two dangers in this. First, the discrepancies between the mandate and the practice of standard setting can at times become points of criticism by outside watchers. This might lead to a further articulation

22 This becomes even more apparent when a consensus cannot be reached. For example, in the few cases that the MAC committee has not been able to reach a consensus, the Ministry of Social Affairs and Employment has refrained from implementing a MAC value (Bal & De Vroom 1993).

of the mandate, thus endangering the productivity of the procedure. Second, in times of controversy, the actors within the procedure tend to fall back on the rationalistic repertoire with its strict boundaries, since this repertoire is used as the legitimation of practice. This is, for example, precisely what happened in the controversy on MMMF. Instead of becoming a resource for the closure of the controversy, however, this falling back on the rationalistic repertoire tends to hamper the discussion, leading to a further polarisation of the respective positions.

The analysis presented above should not be read as saying that what happens in Dutch occupational standard setting cannot stand the light of day, as would be suggested by an analysis using the mandate as the normative yard-stick for standard setting (e.g. Abraham 1993). Nor can it be said that what happens in practice is the 'real thing' and that the rationalistic repertoire is just a rationalisation of practice, as is often suggested by actor-oriented students of science and technology. As Shapin has noted about science:

> 'Stories about science' might, in principle, be separable from the realities of 'science itself', but officially sanctioned stories function to pour value over science, to specify its boundaries, to mark it off from other forms of culture. In just that sense, myth is *realized* through its uses and 'stories about science' belong – contingently, problematically, but consequentially – to some versions of what might be meant by 'science itself' (1997: 340).

Likewise, both the mandate and the practice of standard setting, and both the rationalistic and the contingent repertoires used in either of these, cannot be easily or unproblematically be separated from one another. Analyses of standard setting should take them both into account.

## REFERENCES


Abraham, J. (1993) 'Scientific Standards and Institutional Interests: Carcinogenic Risk Assessment of Benoxaprofen in the UK and US', *Social Stusdies of Science* 23; 387-444.

Bal, R. (1996) 'De grenzen van het mandaat: over de problematische omgang met carcinogene stofffen en de contextualiteit van politiek', *Kennis & Methode* 20: 235-64.

Bal, R. & B. de Vroom (1993) *De Vaststelling van MAC-waarden*, Leiden: Leyden Institute for Law & Public Policy.

Bal, R. & A. Spit (1994) 'De Risicopolitiek van Man-made Mineral Fibres', *Tijdschrift voor Toegepaste Arbowetenschap* 7: 63-72.

Barker, A. (1993) 'Patterns of Decision Advice Proccesses: A Review of Types and a Commentary on some Recent British Experiences', in: Peters & Barker (eds.) *Advising West European Governments: Inquiries, Expertise and Public Policy*, Edinburgh: Edinburgh University Press; 20-36.

Bigwood, J. (1973) 'The acceptable daily intake of food additives', *CRC Critical Review of Toxicology*, June: 41-93.

Boersma (1977) Toespraak ter gelegenheid van de installatie van de Nationale MAC-Commissie, Ministery of Social Affairs: Voorburg, pressrelease nr. 77/19.

Breysse, P.A. (1991) 'ACGIH TLVs: A critical analysis of the documentation', *American Journal of Industrial Medicine* 20: 423-8.

Brickman, R., S. Jasanoff & T. Ilgen (1985) *Controling Chemicals: The Politics of Regulation in Europe and the US*, Ithaca: Cornell University Press.

Brokamp, J.J.A.M (1987) *MAC-waarden: zin of onzin?*, Masters Thesis, Erasmus University Rotterdam.

Brokamp, J.J.A.M. (1991) 'De haalbaarheid van MAC-waarden', *Maandblad voor Arbeidsomstandigheden* 67: 735-37.

Brokamp, J.J.A.M. (1996) 'Bedrijven meten te weinig', *Arbeidsomstandigheden* 72: 532-35.

Bus, J. & J. Posthuma (1992), editors, *MAC-waarden op de arbeidsplaats*, Alphen aan den Rijn: Samsom H.D. Tjeenk Willink.

Cambrosio, A., C. Limoges & E. Hoffman (1992) 'Expertise as a Network', in: N. Stehr & R.V. Ericson (eds.) *The Culture and Power of Knowledge*, Berlin: Walter de Gruyter; 341-61.

Castleman, B.I. & G.E. Ziem (1988) 'Corporate influence on Threshold Limit Values', *American Journal of Industrial Medicine* 13: 531-59.

Castleman, B.I. & G.E. Ziem (1994) 'American Conference of Governmental Industrial Hygienists: Low Threshold of Credibility', *American Journal of Industrial Medicine* 26: 133-43.

Committee on Hazardous Substances (1989) Letter to Directorate General of Labour concerning working program of 1989, 31 May 1989, reference R-1853/JB/smp.

Cox, G.V. (1988) 'Threshold Limit Values: A Balanced Report', *American Journal of Industrial Medicine* 14: 233-4.

Dalderup, L.M. et al. (1976) 'Angiosarcoma of the liver and vinylchloride', *Tijdschrift voor Sociale Geneeskunde* 54: 333-35.

De Valk, J.H.C.M. & A. Wink (1974) 'Naar een Nationale TLV-Commissie', *Tijdschrift voor Sociale Geneeskunde* 52: 186-187.

Didde, R. (1991) 'Gezondheidsnorm op werk is vaak een slag in de lucht', De Volkskrant, 25 May 1991.

Director General of Labour (1976) Letter to candidate members of working group of experts, 2 March 1976, reference 80.882.

Directorate General of Labour (1986) Letter to the Labour Council concerning procedure for establishing MAC values, 30 May 1986, reference DGA/MD/7203.

Dutch Expert Committee on Occupational Standards (1986) 'MAC-waarden nader beschouwd', in: Labour Inspectorate, *Nationale MAC-lijst 1986*, The Hague: labour Inspectorate, supplement.

Eijndhoven, J. van & P. Groenewegen (1991) 'The Construction of Expert Advice on Health Risks', *Social Studies of Science* 21: 257-78.

Feron, V.J., C. Hoeksema, J.H.E. Arts, P.C. Noordam & C.L. Maas (1994) 'A critical appraisal of the Setting and Implementation of Occupational Exposure Limits in The Netherlands', *Indoor Environment* 3: 260-65.

Fujimura, J.H. (1992) 'Crafting Science: Standarized Packages, Boundary Objects, and "Translations"', in: A. Pickering (ed.) *Science as Practice and Culture*, Chicago and London: University of Chicago Press; 168-211.

Gilbert, N.G. & M. Mulkay (1984) *Opening Pandora's Box*, Cambridge: Cambridge University Press.

Halffman, W. & A. van Raalte (1996) *De registratieplicht gevaarlijke stoffen geëvalueerd*, Den Haag: VUGA.

Health Council of the Netherlands (1985) *Advies inzake uitgangspunten voor normstelling*, The Hague: Health Council of the Netherlands, nr. 85/31.

Hoch, P.K. (1989) 'The Crystalization of Stratetig Alliance: The American Physics Elite and the Military in the 1940s', in: Mendelsohn, Rue Smith & Weingart (eds.) *Science, Technology & The Military*, Dordrecht: Kluwer; 87-116.

Jasanoff, S. (1986) *Risk Management and Political Culture*, New York: Russell Sage Foundation.

Jasanoff, S. (1990) *The Fifth Branch: Science Advisers as Policymakers*, Cambridge, MA: Harvard UP.

Jasanoff, S. (1995) *Science at the Bar: Law, Science, and Technology in America*, Cambridge, MA: Harvard UP.

Joosting, P.E. & R.L. Zielhuis (1962) 'Pragmatisme of Dogmatisme', *Tijdschrift voor Sociale Geneeskunde* 40: 479-85.

Joosting, P.E. & R.L. Zielhuis (1963) 'Nogmaals: Pragmatisme en Dogmatisme', *Tijdschrift voor Sociale Geneeskunde* 41: 177-80.

Kolk, J.J. (1993) 'MAC-waarden in Nederland: verleden, heden en toekomst', *Tijdschrift voor Sociale Gezondheidszorg* 71: 112-4.

Krücken, G. (1994) 'Risk Regulation: some remarks on its (socio-)logic with specific reference to drug safety', manuscript, University of Bielefeld.

Labour Council (1985) Besluit tot instellen van een Commissie Grenswaarden Gezondheidsschadelijke Stoffen, Zoetermeer, 17-10-1985.

Lehman, A. & O. Fitzhugh (1954) '100-Fold margin of safety', *Association of Food and Drug Officials; Quarterly Bulletin* 13: 33-35.

Magnuson, H.J., D.W. Fassett, H.W. Gerrarde, V.K. Rowe, H.F. Smyth & H.E. Stokinger (1964) 'Industrial Toxicology in the Sovjet Union – Theoretical and Applied', *American Industrial Hygiene Association Journal* 25: 185-97.

Mik, G. de (1993) 'De advieswaarden: wikken en wegen', *Tijdschrift voor Sociale Gezondheidszorg* 71: 120-1.

Ministry of Social Affairs (1976) 'Instelling werkgroep van deskundigen ten behoeve van de in te stellen Nationale MAC-Commissie', *Staatscourant*, 1976, 115.

Ministry of Social Affairs (1977) 'Instelling Nationale MAC-Commissie', *Staatscourant*, 1977, 10.

National MAC committee & Dutch Expert Committe on Occupational Standards (1978) 'Uitgangspunten bij advisering inzake MAC-waarden', *Tijdschrift voor Sociale Geneeskunde* 56, supplement 1.

Noordam, P.C. (1993) 'Internationale aspecten van grenswaarden', *Tijdschrift voor Sociale Gezondheidzorg* 71: 122-3.

Noordam, P.C & C.l. Maas (1990) 'Nederlandse MAC-waarden: wijze van vaststellen en niveau's zijn toonaangevend!', *Intermediair*, 30 November 1990.

Piney, M. (1989) *The Development of Chemical Exposure Limits for the Workplace*, Thesis, University of Aston, Birmingham.

Porter, T.M. (1995) *Trust in Numbers: The Pursuit of Objectivity in Science and Public Life*, Princeton, NJ: Princeton UP.

Rappaport, S.M. (1993) 'Threshold Limit Values, Permissible Exposure Limits, and Feasibility: The Bases for Exposure Limits in the United States', *American Journal of Industrial Medicine* 23: 683-94.

Rip, A. (1992) 'Expert Advice and Pragmatic Rationality', in: N. Stehr & R.V. Ericson (eds.) *The Culture and Power of Knowledge*, Berlin: Walter de Gruyter; 363-79.

Roach, S.A. & S.M. Rappaport (1990) 'But They are not Thresholds: A Critical Analysis of the Documentation of TLV's', *American Journal of Industrial Medicine* 17: 727-53.

Schmidt, S.K. & R. Werle (1992) 'Technical Discourse in International Standarization', paper presented at 4S/EASST joint conference, 12-15 august 1992, Göteborg.

Shackley, S. & B. Wynne (1996) 'Representing Uncertainty in Global Climate Change Science and Policy: Boundary-Ordering Devices and Authority', *Science, Technology & Human Values* 21: 275-302.

Shapin, S. (1992) 'Discipline and Bounding: The History and Sociology of Science as Seen throuhg the Externalism-Internalism Debate', *History of Science* 30: 335.

Shapin, S. (1997) 'Signs of the Times', *Social Studies of Science* 27: 335-49.

Social Economic Council (1993) *Advies inzake het Voorstel van wet houdende wijziging van de Arbeidsomstandighedenwet en de Kernenergiewet in verband met opheffing van de Arboraad*, The Hague: SEC, nr. 93/32.

Star, S.L. & J.R. Griesemer (1989) 'Institutional Ecology, Translations and Boundary Objects: Amateurs and Professionals in Berkeley's Museum of Vertebrate Zoology', *Social Studies of Science* 19: 387-420.

Stijkel, A. (1992) 'Ook het nageslacht beschermen', in: J. Bus & J. Posthuma (eds.) *MAC-waarden op de arbeidsplaats*, Alphen aan den Rijn: Samsom H.D. Tjeenk Willink; 65-75.

Stijkel, A., J. van Eijndhoven & R. Bal (1996) 'Drafting Guidelines for Occupational Exposure to Chemicals: The Dutch Experience with the Assessment of Reproductive Risks', *American Journal of Industrial Medicine* 30: 705-17.

Stokinger, H.E. (1988) 'Threshold Limit Values: Any Alternative?', *American Journal of Industrial Medicine* 14: 231-2.

Ulenbelt, P. (1991) *Omgaan met blootstelling aan chemische stoffen*, Thesis, University of Amsterdam.

Verberk, M.M., P.E. Joosting & B. Bink (1975) 'Effecten van chloor bij proefpersonen', *Tijdschrift voor Sociale Geneeskunde* 53: 106-12.

Vroom, B. de (1990) *Verenigde Fabrikanten*, Groningen: Wolters-Noordhoff.

Wynne, B. (1982) *Rationality and Ritual: The Windscale Inquiry and Nuclear Decision Making in Britain*, Chalfon St Giles: British Society for the History of Science.

Wynne, B. (1992) 'Carving out science (and politics) in the regulatory jungle', *Social Studies of Science* 22: 745-58.

Zald, M.N. (1978) 'On the Social Control of Industries', *Social Forces* 57: 79-102.

Zielhuis, R.L. (1974) 'Over hen, zonder hen', *Tijdschrift voor Sociale Geneeskunde*, 52: 157.

Zielhuis, R.L. (1992) 'Algemene inleiding', in: J. Bus & J. Posthuma (eds.) *MAC-waarden op de arbeidsplaats*, Alphen aan den Rijn: Samsom H.D. Tjeenk Willink; 28-33.

Zielhuis, R.L., P.C. Noordam, C.L. Maas, J.J. Kolk & H.P.A. Illing (1991) 'Harmonisation of Criteria Documents for Standards Setting in Occupational Health', *Regulatory Toxicology and Pharmacology* 13: 241-262.

Ziem, G.E. & B.I. Castleman (1989) 'Threshold Limit Values: Historical Perspectives and Current Practice', *Journal of Occupational Medicine* 31: 910-8.

## DISCUSSIONS

### *The Risk Assessment – Risk Management Boundary*

Questions and comments following the presentation by *Mayer*

*Somers*. The mechanist separation between risk assessment and risk management is basically incorrect. It places scientists in a quiet, pleasant space and then the rest of us have to do the work of regulation. This was clear with the example of saccharin, where science extrapolates from tumors in rats to carcinogenicity in humans. The separation between 'pure scientific assessment' and 'non-pure regulation' is rather simplistic.

*Mayer* answers that she agrees but that there is still a strong political pressure to maintain the separation.

*Jasanoff*. There is a kind of schizophrenia in the Royal Society report, already mentioned. What is interesting is the interpretation of the Red Book (NAS 1983). A lot of people involved in writing the Red Book have now disavowed the rigid separationist model that the Red Book stands for. In the US, the National Academy has done a lot of back-pedalling from the rigid separation, for instance in the 1994 report on science and judgement (NRC 1994).

Questions and comments following the presentation by *Bal*

*Jasanoff*. Is there a causal relation between repertoire and organizational change? Or is there an intermediate step?

*Bal.* During controversies the normative stress on a separation between risk assessment and management becomes stronger. This implies that within the repertoire the distinction between the two is more heavily stressed. My analysis suggests that there is a tendency to formalize this into a greater organizational distance between the domains of discretion, but it would be wrong to suggest that there is a causal link implied. For standard setting to be productive, the domains of discretion cannot be separated too much, so in the end the continuation of controversy might lead to a reframing of the issues.

*Passchier.* I would like to add a bit to the point of restructuring of the expert advice in the Netherlands. The Health Council has got other tasks, but the real debate is about the role of the scientists. It is possible that the entire Health Council will be abolished. Then the next step will be that scientific input to the policy process will be given on a kind of project basis, in reaction to specific questions from the governement, rather than the possibility that scientists now have, which is to give their own input. The role of scientists in advisory work is still very clearly being questioned.[23]

## General discussion

*Nilsson.* It is important to clarify the distinction between risk assessment and risk management. Some members of the workshop seem to doubt the possibility of making such a separation, or think that such a distinction should not be made. I agree that this separation is fuzzy, not always clear from the actions of regulatory scientists. There is uncertainty and unless it is clearly stated how this uncertainty is dealt with, there is space for interpretation, and influences of interest. However, there are statistical rules for dealing with the uncertainty. The division between risk assessment and risk management can be done, and it should be done, for otherwise the door is open to arbitrary judgements.

23 Editors' note: in 1996 the Health Counil obtained a new mandate from the government to continue its advisory work.

*Calow*. The first question is what we want to protect by risk assessment and the other is how to do it. It is a question of relevance, where scientific considerations and other issues – social, political – are involved. Once you have decided what the targets are, the science of achieving them can be fairly clearly defined. It can be rather precise. Now there is fuzziness between 'what' and 'how' questions. I agree to some extent with Sue Mayer that there is not enough open involvement by society at large in the question of what to protect. Scientists see that as their problem, but in my view that is not entirely their problem.

*Smit* (in respons to Nilsson). One should distinguish two types of uncertainty. Often it is stated that uncertainty creates room for conflict, controversy. But uncertainty can be both the cause *or* the result of controversy. In the first case the uncertainty is shared by all participants. The second type of uncertainty is the uncertainty to the outsiders, such as politicians. They are confronted with two positions, with different certainties, opposed to each other. Here the controversy results in uncertainty. It is important to establish these different types of uncertainty for the policy process, because they involve different types of social processes, and require different measures to deal with them.

*Millstone*. I am struck by the remark of Nilsson about statistical ways of dealing with uncertainty, because there are also conflicts between the different methods one can use. There is a multitude of methods. Simply turning to statistics is not going to deal with the problem of uncertainty.

There is a fear for the risk of arbitrary decisions, once the separation between risk assessment and risk management is questioned. I want to avoid that risk, but still question the simple separation between risk assessment and risk management. We find social assumptions imbedded in scientific activities. That opens the opportunity to lay them out, disentangle them, and then the possibility rises that one can reassemble them. Make decisions, interests etc. explicit. That reconstruction is not arbitrary in the sense that the evidence is explicit.

*Mayer*. In risk assessment, science is making the assumption that it is dealing with closed environments. It is not fully acknowledged that in fact there are a lot of interactions in the environment. When you open this up, showing a variety of different ways that risk-assessors are not really dealing with the things they thought they were dealing with, that seems to be too challenging for those in the risk assessment. Then they don't take a step forward to a more rigid science, but, in my experience, fall back on the industry and its interests. This is almost the opposite of Nillson's comment.

*Younes.* I see the danger of arbitrary decisions, but there is even more danger when you are mingling the risk assessment and the risk management phase. Then you would overburden the natural scientists with societal judgements. I am really for a clear disctinction. For example, what to do with carcinogens? Would you give scientists the responsibility of making a judgement on what dose is acceptable? We have seen this in the UK: in the assessment of particles. With the scientific knowledge we have, you cannot set a threshold. So it is a societal judgement which choice you make.

I see three steps in the process of regulating chemical risk, which all should be looked at from a scientific point of view: biological issues, social issues and economic issues. I have been involved in a number of committees, and I haven't experienced that scientists were put under pressure to take cost-benefit analysis into account.

In addition, the terminology raises problems. To speak of safety, and safety factors, is a different approach than talking about risk, and risk assessment. Safety assessment can be done when you are dealing with occupational exposures, food additives, and the like. But with chemicals in the environment, you must assess the risk with the aim of risk reduction. These are two approaches, which we should keep seperate.

*Feron.* Risk assessment should be as far from risk management as possible. Risk assessment involves a lot of uncertainties. That implies a debate and therefore you need a group of people to look at the entire body of data. This should be an open process, showing the decisions made and with an invitation to others to come up with better ideas.

The second step, after the health based recommendations, should also be as scientific as possible, but with different scientists, considering social and economic factors.

*Krücken.* There is also a legal dimension to the sharp distinction between scientific risk assessment and political risk management. For example, in

German law there is a clause referring to the 'state of the art' in science and technology. I would warn against the idea that the boundary is pure rhetoric, just a myth: it also has legal consequences.

*McCutcheon* (adding to remarks of Nilsson and Feron). The separation between risk assessment and risk management makes for regulatory efficiency, and is also efficient for the regulator. I think that (eco)toxicologists would not be very comfortable if they have to do cost-benefit analysis as well as effects- and exposure assessments.

*Somers*. Those who wrote the Red Book did not quite mean what they said, or at least not in that way. But it led to a great belief in quantification and so we spent a lot of time pushing science in that direction, towards in my opinion trans-science (Weinberg, 1972). But prognostications are not measurable: is it really true that this limit will lead to five Canadian deaths in a million? That is not measurable.

Another issue concerns the uncertainties in science. Take the example of dioxins: on the basis of the same data the acceptable daily intake is 1600 times lower in the USA than in Canada. You have to accept this range. That is the gap with the Red Book policy where a medical expert would say: 'this is safe, this is unsafe'. But that is difficult to explain to the public.

*Stijkel*. It is a good idea to distinguish both stages and to be as scientific as possible. But I also propose building in more involvement possibilities in both stages, through more transparency and systematic decisions, open discussion on uncertainties, which in my view is absent at the moment. The case-by-case approach, central to standard setting, needs to be discussed. We need a more systematic approach to gather data, analyze data, and to discuss what we have and what we miss.

*Heyvaert* (concurring with the remark made by Krücken). I was struck by Piney's suggestion that we should have two standards: one practically manageable level and one more linked to the health-based level. As a lawyer, I would say that this creates a lot of nervousness in industry, because they have to indicate to the employees one the one hand that there is a known health risk, and on the other that they are managing it to another level.

Another consideration: it is important to create more awareness about the distinction between risk assessment and risk management. The scientist is also a social person and this should be laid bare. Particularly on the European level, when you acknowledge this, you are no longer just a scientist but you are a policy maker and then you have a legitimacy problem. This is especially a problem in Europe. Therefore you often see the tendency to stress that 'this is science, not policy'.

*Bijker* (summing up the discussion so far). One question is whether a distinction between risk assessment and risk management is possible at all. That is an essentialist issue, which we cannot settle here. A second issue is that when we, as most of us do, accept that this distinction is made, we acknowledge that this distinction is not always that clear and simple, but that it generally makes sense to divide the process in this way. The question is then how it is done, how fixed or how dynamic the distinction is.

*Nilsson* (refering to the remarks by Calow). Because there are a lot of uncertainties, it seems as if toxicologists don't know what to do at all. But in the case of pesticides regulation we confronted agencies in a lot of countries with questions about how and why they adopted certain regulations, and there was a lot of agreement among them (Nilsson, Tasheva & Jaeger 1993). So we do not alway disagree, but some areas are more problematic than others, such as cancer. We should not pretend to be scientific when we try to quantify certain endpoints, because with different models you will end up with different numbers. What is possible, however, is to make procedures more open and transparent.

*Sedee*. In my experience, the distinction between risk assessment and risk management can be made. In our Ministry two different departments are involved with these two processes. The assessment has to be transparent. The same procedures in the same expert group should be followed, so that a comparison is possible. In that way you get a risk assessment and at least a reliable qualitative ordering of substances.

In the Dutch environmental policy context we work with health zones, produced by the RIVM. We have two limits: a maximal permitted limit and a target limit. After setting these two limits, we can think of setting a standard. So with the information from the scientific institute and the Dutch

Health Council on the upper and lower limit, we can discuss the standard, considering costs and feasaibility.

*Millstone.* My view is not that the distinction between risk assessment and risk management is too complex to be made. They can be distinguished, but often they are not. For example, when McCutcheon says that 'we want decisions, we want to set standards', that is already a political decision. Studying expert groups, what we find in practice is that all kinds of social-political considerations are involved in assessment.

What I expect of more transparency is that it will provide a means to lay out how in practice empirical evidence and political considerations have been involved in the decision making. Then experts say something like: 'Given the evidence, different recommendations are possible, depending on different assumptions.' That range would then go into the risk management phase.

*Van Damme.* How can one guarantee objectivity in expert groups? First, they have to be competent. Second, experts should be desinterested, independent. No social partners should be in the expert group. Third, they should not be neutral, their mandate should stress that they have an approach of likelihood of safety, not likelihood of effect. This is a basic option.

Transparency is not guaranteed with robot-like systems. I believe more in persons trying to be objective, not neutral. Data that come out of this process can be used in more political considerations, for instance on how many workers will be protected by a limit value.

*Jasanoff.* I want to underscore contradictions in discussions on the boundaries. One the one hand we are discussing it in essentialist terms – is it in some epistemiological way possible to seperate science and politics? But alternatively, that we all know that things are not so pure – as Bijker stated – seems to me not totally correct. I think the contrast is between, on the one hand, thinking that it is possible and, on the other hand, the belief that what you are saying about science and politics is something like the product of a language game, embedded in society.[24] Then it is not possible to distinguish between risk assessment and risk management in a general way.

Referring to Lewis Carolls' Humpty Dumpty, I would say that it is of course possible to distinguish between risk assessment and risk management, depending on consensus on the definitions. These may be shared by all of us in this room, but may have little resonance elsewhere in the world. We can either do that, defining risk assessment and risk management for the purpose of further talk, or we are more concerned with what happens with our ideas in the world of institutions. In that case, we would be more concerned with issues of transparency.

In the further discussion it is important for everyone who says that the distinction can or cannot be made, to ask the next question: what is the meaning of 'can', whose language game is it, who is using these words?

---

24 The concept of 'language game' is taken from Wittgenstein (1958) and refers to the idea that language is embedded in the way we live the world, that is in our practices and institutions, and does not refer to an objective world 'out there'.

## REFERENCES

National Academy of Sciences (1983) *Risk Assessment in the Federal Government: Managing the Process*, Washington, DC: National Academy Press.

National Research Council (1994) *Science and Judgment*, Washington, DC: National Academy Press.

Nilsson, R., M. Tasheva & B. Jaeger (1993) 'Why different regulatory decisions when the scientific information base is similar? – Human risk assessment', *Regulatory Toxicology & Pharmacology* 17: 292-332.

Weinberg, A. (1972) 'Science and trans-science', *Minerva* 10: 209-22.

Wittgenstein, L. (1958) *Philosophical Investigations*, Oxford: Oxford University Press.

# PART II

## THE INTERNATIONAL ARENA

# INTRODUCTION

The European Union has been a particularly important source of new, supranational regulations concerning chemical risks. Numerous EU Commission Directives and Regulations concerning environmental and occupational exposure have re-shaped national regulatory systems. Given that these developments have involved decisions of high political importance, these shifts from national governments to the European Union have been extensively discussed and contested. Attention from policy analysts has thusfar concentrated on the political aspects of harmonisation. However, from the perspective of risk regulation, the internationalisation of regulatory science is equally important.

Firstly, expert advice can be structured along different lines. At the level of the European Commission, standing advisory committees exist, such as the Scientific Committee for Occupational Exposure Limits to Chemical Agents (SCOEL), specifically to serve the Commission. In addition, the Commission can rely for advice on ad hoc committees, or national sources of expertise. For instance, the 'old chemicals' program relies on national expert groups that re-assess industrial chemicals that are already on the market, so-called 'rapporteur countries'.

Secondly, these developments may have important implications for the risk assessment – risk management distinction. The European Commission seems to favor 'technocratic' forms of expert advice. While this is partly due to its size, it can also be attributed to the absence of a well-developed arena of skilled policy contestants, at least as compared to national policy arenas, occupied by environmental movements, media attention and the like. In sharp contrast to national contexts, the European Union has hardly any institutionalised form of public or policy debate, and less resourceful policy actors have difficulty participating in the highly lobby-oriented policy making system of the European Union.

Thirdly, the European Union has created opportunities for new international networks of expertise and research. New EU research programs support important innovations in the regulatory arena, such as the development of new ways of assessing environmental impacts. Expert communities have supported the development of such programs and have shown a willingness to accommodate new international policy developments. Not only is the European arena a relevant domain for professional organisations (e.g. the Society for Ecotoxicology), but the latter also support initiatives to develop expertise suited for the purposes of regulatory policy.

These new networks of research and expertise are only partly an integration of existing national resources. More often than not, they are concerned with new policy domains and questions at the European level, and run parallel to national expertise. Drawing on expertise across Europe, these networks may provide a transnational knowledge base for EU regulatory policy, one that in time could alter existing patterns of regulatory organisation in different countries.

The above considerations raise a number of questions: what different models of organising expertise are being used within the EU, and what are their advantages and disadvantages? Will it be possible to harmonise assessments without losing contact with the national policy implementation process? What are the consequences for future participation of interest groups in decision making? What are the obstacles to developing a common research background, given different national regulatory contexts?

In his chapter, Vic Feron reflects on his experiences in risk assessment at a national (Dutch) as well as a European level. He suggests that differences between experts in the international arena that may arise because of nationally specific practices, such as the assessment of carcinogens or the use of extrapolation factors, do not necessarily lead to insurmountable problems. Crucial in this regard is the extent to which certain organisational as well as personal demands are met. Overcoming national differences, for example, is, according to Feron, dependent on experts getting to know each others' peculiarities. This is best achieved in standing committees. Furthermore, experts should be open to being convinced by the arguments of their colleagues, and should be willing to strive for consensus. Feron also argues against speeding up the process of setting exposure limits by using uniform systems for the assessment of substances. In his view, a careful analysis, made by a group of experts in a transparent process, remains the best guarantee of the credibility and validity of exposure limits, both at a national as well as an international level.

Karel van Damme shares this last conclusion. In his contribution, he compares two standard setting procedures of the EU: the setting of occupational exposure limits by the SCOEL, and the classification of substances by the working group on Carcinogens, Mutagens and substances toxic to Reproduction (CMR). Van Damme evaluates the workings of these procedures by comparing them to what he calls the 'Saracci paradigm'. According to the latter, expert assessments of chemicals should be objective and impartial, but should not be neutral; that is, they should be geared towards workers' protection. Whilst the SCOEL procedure compares positively with the Saracci paradigm, the CMR procedure does not. Van Damme illustrates this by means of a detailed case study of the classification of Man-made Mineral Fibers, and argues that this is due primarily to a lack of clarity about the boundary between the scientific evaluation of data on the one hand, and national or industrial interests in the CMR procedure on the other. Moreover, this procedure lacks transparency, and is so dependent on lobbying that industrial interests easily prevail. Van Damme concludes by highlighting some of the pitfalls of international standard setting, and suggesting alternatives.

Nilsson discusses the consequences of the new EU membership of Sweden for chemical risk assessment. According to him, Sweden has a long-standing tradition of a political, rather than scientific, evaluation of chemicals, which is based on the assessment of hazard rather than risk. Moreover, Swedish political culture is more inclined towards protecting the environment than protecting the interests of industry and employment. This is illustrated by the great influence of the environmental movement on policy making. Given this, harmonisation with the EU has to take place on at least three levels, namely: the scientific basis for the assessment of chemicals, the procedures according to which chemicals are assessed and managed, and political culture. Although Nillson believes that Swedish regulation of chemicals can benifit from the integration in the EU, based upon his conviction that the scientific assessment of chemicals should prevail over politics, he is rather pessimistic as to whether this will succeed.

Sheila Jasanoff differs radically from Nilsson on the prevalence of science over politics, but like him stresses the multi-layered nature of harmonisation. Jasanoff starts by discussing the role of Science and Technology Studies in showing that standards are not just technical measures, but represent negotiated forms of social understanding, arguing that what is to be called scientific in the assessment of chemicals is not just a technical, but a deeply political question. She then goes on to show that the methodology of quantitative risk assessment was developed in response to the specific, controversial context in which the regulation of chemicals in the USA is embedded. She argues that the EU's adoption of this approach may be an inadequate reaction to the challenge of harmonisation. Moreover, she suggests ways in which a process of 'reciprocal commentary' between experts and non-experts, between different member states, and between science and policy can be encouraged.

# 4

*Vic Feron*

# RECOMMENDING HEALTH-BASED EXPOSURE LIMITS IN THE NATIONAL AND INTERNATIONAL ARENA: A PERSONAL VIEW

## INTRODUCTION

Risk is the measured or estimated probability of injury, disease, or death inherent in our daily activities (Johanssen 1990). Thus, the health risk of chemicals is the measured or estimated probability of injury, health or death inherent in the use of chemicals. Estimation of the health risk associated with the use of chemicals requires an identification of the potential health effects (toxicity or hazard identification) as well as a determination of the amount of a chemical to which humans are exposed (exposure assessment). Careful assessment of these ingredients of health risk allows scientists to define the conditions under which the risk is sufficiently high to cause concern, as well as the conditions where the risk would be sufficiently low as to be of no health concern (Johanssen 1990).

Hazard identification, including dose-effect/response evaluation and extrapolation of experimental data obtained in either animals or man to projected human exposure scenarios, constitutes the basis for recommending health-based exposure limits (HBELs). This first step in risk assessment or standard setting should involve toxicological data and considerations only; it should not be contaminated with data and considerations on actual exposure levels or on technical and/or socio-economic feasibility (Feron et al. 1994).

The present paper describes the author's experiences with recommending HBELs at the national and international level. As an example, the three-step procedure for recommending occupational HBELs in The Netherlands will

In: R. Bal & W. Halffman (eds.), *The Politics of Chemical Risk*, Kluwer Academic Publishers, Dordrecht 1998: p. 121-129.

be discussed. Other major topics that will be addressed are the characteristics of national versus international committees, and the criteria for selecting the members of such committees. The importance of discussions among experts, the advantage of time-out periods, the way to deal with poor databases, the problem of time-consuming procedures, and the reason for seemingly inconsistent recommendations within and between committees are also briefly discussed.

## SETTING OCCUPATIONAL EXPOSURE LIMITS IN THE NETHERLANDS: AN EXAMPLE

Since 1978 occupational exposure limits, designated as maximum accepted concentrations (MACs), have been established by a three-step procedure in The Netherlands. In the first step, the Dutch Expert Committee on Occupational Standards (DECOS) establishes a health-based recommended occupational exposure limit (HBROEL). Until recently, the DECOS was an advisory group of the Ministry of Social Affairs and Employment (MSAE), but since January 1994 it has become a committee of the Health Council of the Netherlands. The members of DECOS are experts drawn from research institutes, universities, ministries and industry, who participate in the committee on a personal basis. Under the responsibility of DECOS, a Criteria Document is produced, containing all relevant toxicological data, together with a critical evaluation of these data and, finally, the HBROEL. A draft of the Criteria Document, called the Public Draft Document, is submitted for comment to experts from industry and the trade unions, and is available to experts worldwide. The DECOS studies all comments made and, if these are justifiable and desirable, amends the draft document including the HBROEL. If the fundamental basis and the value of the HBROEL are significantly altered, the draft document goes public again. The final Criteria Document is then published by the Health Council. To date about 100 Criteria Documents have been published, in English, with an executive summary in Dutch. In our view, two aspects of this first step are of crucial importance: (a) the HBROEL is based on toxicological data and considerations only, and (b) the HBROEL is not ratified until the Draft Criteria Document has been made public to experts (in principle from all over the world) who may send in their comments.

In the second step of the procedure, the DECOS document is made available to the Subcommittee on MAC values of the Social Economic Council. This Subcommittee consists of representatives of employers' organizations, trade unions and government departments. It discusses and evaluates the technical and/or socio-economic feasibility of the HBROEL after consultation with the supporting organizations. In some cases, a 'workplace document' containing information on exposure concentrations in the workplace is made available by the MSAE. Finally, the Subcommittee recommends an operational MAC to the MSAE. This recommendation, complete with arguments, is available to the public. Crucial to this step is that it shows whether the recommended MAC is identical to the HBROEL and, if not, the reason for the difference.

In the third, administrative step, the MSAE sets the MAC. This value may be different from the HBROEL. So far, this has happened only for cadmium, lead, nitrogen dioxide, sulphur dioxide, carbon disulphide and wood dust. Clearly, the aim is to have all MAC levels identical to the HBROEL, preferably immediately, but if this is not feasible, then in the near future.

Essential to this three-step procedure is the strict separation of the three steps. The first step is purely health-based, the second step is a feasibility step, and the third administrative step leads to the MAC, a legally binding value. The transparency of the entire process is also crucial to this three-step procedure, including openness and the availability of documents to all of the individuals involved, a procedure which best serves the health and well-being of workers.

At the European level HBROELs are established in a way which is very similar to the first step of the Dutch procedure. The two other steps are much more complicated in the international arena, because of larger technical and socio-economic differences between countries and the protection of national interests. Maybe they are too complicated, and, thus, will never be taken!

## GROUPS OF EXPERTS

HBELs are established by permanent or occasional committees of experts, who participate on a personal basis. Different disciplines and subdisciplines are represented in the committee; from chemistry to pathology, epidemiology and biostatistics; from inhalation toxicology to neurotoxicology, reproductive toxicology, genetic toxicology, etc. Recommending HBELs cannot be done by two or three individuals; a group of, for example, 10 to 15 experts is needed; discussion among experts is essential. If very specific expertise required for a proper evaluation of certain crucial data is lacking, specialists in that particular area should be called in, and indeed are.

The tools of the committee members are toxicological data, expertise and experience. All relevant toxicity data, including data on biotransformation, epidemiology, studies on volunteers and casuistic information, should be available in a readable document that also contains a critical evaluation of the data. Experience of the experts in many aspects of hazard identification and extrapolation of available data to projected human exposure scenarios is essential to a successful discussion resulting in a balanced view and consensus within a reasonable period of time.

Does the situation outlined above exist in the everyday practice of recommending HBELs? Is this a true picture of reality? According to my experience, both questions can be answered in the affirmative. In the national as well as in the international arena, the key elements are groups of experienced individuals with expertise in different areas discussing the available data on a personal basis with the intention of reaching a consensus. The discussion may be trenchant and feelings may run high, but consensus is nearly always reached on the basis of convincing argumentation. To reach consensus may take a couple of meetings, the time-out periods being used to collect additional data or to consult other experts. The time-out period is a practical way to avoid minority views, and to offer the opportunity to re-examine reports and papers. In my experience an HBEL is hardly ever recommended after a single committee meeting. All of a sudden a member may raise a question or touch upon an aspect that has so far not been considered but which turns out to be highly relevant. So, a time-out period - which is the rule rather than the exception - is indeed extremely helpful.

## AREAS OF ATTENTION

The areas to be discussed in this section are poor toxicological databases, time-consuming procedures and seemingly inconsistent recommendations.

*Poor toxicological database*

It is not exceptional for the toxicological database for a widely used, high-production-volume chemical to be too poor, for justifying the setting of a HBEL. In these cases, application of large safety factors has been suggested to compensate for the lack of data and to encourage industry to provide more information (Stijkel 1995). However, such a recommended HBEL would not be purely health-based but would be politically motivated. Recommending very low HBELs as a means to put pressure on industry is clearly beyond the responsibility of a committee for setting HBELs. When the database of a chemical is too incomplete to justify the recommendation of a HBEL, the committee should just say so.

*Process too time consuming?*

The complete procedure for setting MAC values in the Netherlands may take several years. Such a long period of time is incompatible with concepts of speed, forcefulness, promptness and responsiveness (Kolk 1993). However, in our view, care and quality should prevail in order to maintain the credibility of the process and of the experts involved, and, most importantly, the credibility of the established MAC value. Since there are always constraints of finance and the availability of experienced and skilled manpower, fewer carefully established MAC values are to be preferred over more MAC values of doubtful repute. Moreover, the relatively long time period between the publication of the (draft) DECOS value and the setting of the MAC value gives industry the opportunity to take measures, if necessary, to meet the new value. When reliable exposure data clearly show that a (much) lower exposure limit than the one being discussed by DECOS would not involve any technical or economic problems, it has been suggested (De Mik 1993) that it would save time if a low (exposure-based) OEL were recommended. In my view this is wrong and DECOS should complete its deliberations and recommend a health-based rather than an exposure-based OEL. Of course, in step 2 or 3 of the procedure, an exposure-based MAC value can be suggested or established without affecting the openness or transparency of the process.

*Inconsistencies*

The setting of HBELs should be as consistent as possible, but there is little consensus about the way to achieve this. There is some support for a uniform system for the evaluation of substances: a classification by types of effects and types of studies, and using more or less fixed correction, extrapolation and safety factors (De Mik 1993; Stijkel 1995). The weakness of such a system is that it may be used not as a supplement to, but at the expense of the input of expertise and experience. Hundreds of evaluations conducted over the years have shown that expertise and experience are indispensable. Databases differ both qualitatively and quantitatively, are often far from complete, and contain studies that vary widely in their relevance and adequacy. The consultative process nearly always involves intense discussion on matters such as the toxicological relevance of certain effects, the overall 'no-observed-adverse-effect-level' and the size of the safety factor. In my view, this latter should be decided from the total weight of the evidence. It is my conviction that fixed factors for all kinds of (theoretical) situations are not very helpful, will reduce flexibility and cannot guarantee objectivity. I believe in consistency based on good data evaluated by competent, experienced individuals with expertise in different disciplines (see also Van Damme, this volume).

## NATIONAL VERSUS INTERNATIONAL COMMITTEES

Are there remarkable differences between national and international committees with respect to the way a committee works? Is it easier to reach consensus in a national than in an international setting? In a global sense, in my experience, both questions can be answered in the negative. Of course, there may be country-specific approaches to matters such as the use and size of safety factors, adjustment for differences in body size, the policy in dealing with carcinogens or with subpopulations at excess risk. Such differences may broaden and intensify the discussion but do not prevent experts from expressing their personal views and drawing their own conclusions on the basis of avalaible data and considerations on the spot.

Of course, it happens that consensus cannot be reached, but the minority will nearly always accept the viewpoint of the majority, and, thus, there will not be a recorded minority statement. If the minority strongly disagrees with the majority view, the minority view should be recorded and documented. Transparency and openness of the process dictate this. On the other hand, it is not easy, if not impossible, to stick to a (prejudiced) opinion if scientific arguments suggest its incorrectness. The laws of science and logic cannot be ignored, and scientists do not want to lose their scientific credibility. I once experienced that, after consensus had been reached about the precise phrasing of a statement during a two-day meeting of an international *ad hoc* committee, two members changed (or were forced to change?) their mind sometime after the meeting, and a minority view was included in the report, specifying that in the first instance full consensus had been attained during the meeting. This is bad practice but, fortunately, the exception which proves the rule.

Overall, *in my experience*, there are no consistent differences in recommending HBELs between national and international committees. Differences that might occur are incidental and 'statistically insignificant', generally being within the 'standard deviation' of the results (recommendations) of expert committees.

## PERMANENT VERSUS OCCASIONAL COMMITTEES

In my perception there is quite a difference between permanent and occasional committees. Members of standing committees gradually get to know each other, learn each others' expertise and are willing to accept each others' peculiarities, all of which promotes mutual confidence and a relaxed atmosphere. Such settings warrant openness and a vulnerable attitude during the debate, leading to optimum results. In my experience, *ad hoc* committees, be it on a national or an international level, hardly ever reach such a relaxed atmosphere characterized by openness and vulnerability. There is more reluctance to speak up, and there is less willingness to listen to scientific arguments.

## SELECTION OF MEMBERS FOR COMMITTEES

What type of individuals do we need in a committee for setting HBELs? The best one in each discipline or subdiscipline, but with:

a) at least a feeling for and some experience in risk assessment and standard setting;
b) the willingness to listen to their fellow members' scientific arguments, and to look for consensus; and
c) the time and opportunity to study documents and to attend meetings.

Thus, expertise, experience and opportunity (rather than social background and position) should be and in my experience are the criteria for selecting the members of expert committees. When a member does not take the job seriously, this is extremely disturbing and insulting to the other members, and also irresponsible towards society. Thus, the selection of committee members is a rather important issue.

## CONCLUSION

In conclusion, recommending HBELs, the first step of health risk assessment and standard setting, can best be performed by permanent committees consisting of experienced, international experts representing a variety of relevant disciplines and subdisciplines.

## References

De Mik, G. (1993) 'De advieswaarde: wikken en wegen', *Tijdschrift voor Sociale Gezondheidszorg* 71: 120-21.

Feron, V.J., C. Hoeksema, J.H.E. Arts, P.C. Noordam & C.L. Maas (1994) 'A critical appraisal of the setting and implementation of occupational exposure limits in the Netherlands', *Indoor Environment* 3: 260-65.

Johanssen, F.R. (1993) 'Risk assessment of carcinogenic and noncarcinogenic chemicals', *Critical Reviews in Toxicology* 20: 341-67.

Kolk, J.J. (1993) 'MAC-waarden in Nederland: verleden, heden en toekomst', *Tijdschrift voor Sociale Gezondheidszorg* 71: 112-14.

Stijkel, A. (1995) *On Managing Reproductive Risks of Occupational Exposure to Chemicals*, Thesis University of Amsterdam, Amsterdam.

# 5

*Karel Van Damme*

## SOME CONSIDERATIONS ON THE EUROPEAN UNION AND THE POLITICS OF CHEMICAL RISK FOR WORKERS' HEALTH

### INTRODUCTION

The European Union has established major tools for the protection of workers, consumers and the environment in relation to the use of chemicals. Some of these will be discussed in this paper, in particular with respect to the setting of limit values for chemicals in the workplace and with respect to the classification and labelling of existing chemicals, using the example of Man-Made Mineral Fibres. We will start with the identification of different kinds of uncertainties that can be encountered in the data used in the regulation of chemicals. Moreover, a general code will be introduced for regulators who have to face scientific data and their uncertainties, labelled the 'Saracci paradigm', and compliance of different Commission procedures with the paradigm will be assessed further in the paper. In the third part, some procedures related to chemicals and health protection under the mandates of the articles 100A and 118A of the Treaty of Rome will be introduced, and a comparison between these procedures will be made. The paper will then continue with an empirical analysis of the way chemicals are assessed under these two articles, which will take us into the workings of the Scientific Expert Group (now called Scientific Committee for Occupational Exposure Limits to Chemical Aspects (SCOEL) for the setting of limit values for chemicals in the workplace, and into the classification of Man-Made Mineral Fibres, respectively. In this analysis, our attention will be directed at the way uncertainties are handled within the two frameworks, and at the transparency of the procedures. We will end with some focused

---

In: R. Bal & W. Halffman (eds.), *The Politics of Chemical Risk*, Kluwer Academic Publishers, Dordrecht 1998: p. 131-157.

conclusions concerning the politics of chemicals within the European Union and some suggestions of how the regulation of chemicals should proceed. The paper is also based on personal past experience as a regulatory scientist, operating in different European Union regulatory frameworks.

## UNCERTAINTIES IN SCIENTIFIC DATA: THE EXAMPLE OF LIMIT VALUE SETTING

We will start with a short description of the nature of the scientific uncertainties of two different types of data used in limit value setting, trying to illustrate the challenges to be faced in order to strive for objectivity and to demonstrate the irrelevance of neutrality when using these data for regulatory purposes. First, data obtained from animal studies will be discussed, and second, we will investigate problems with the interpretation of human data.

### *Limit values based on animal experiments*

Animal experiments can offer interesting information that can be used in limit value setting. We should, however, be very aware of the possible traps in extrapolating the results of such experiments to humans. In particular if no reliable human data are available and the aim is nevertheless to provide limit values, then 'being aware' stands for using effective safety factors when extrapolating from animals to humans. Some important traps to be avoided by applying safety factors are the following:

- related to the pharmacokinetic aspects of toxicity: the same exposure level may lead to a different dose in humans compared to the test in animals, and to a different dose in different animal species and in different strains within one species;
- related to the pharmacodynamic aspects of toxicity: human beings may have different metabolic pathways compared to the animal species under study. They may show a different sensitivity to the toxic effect than animals;
- related to other interfering variables: the animal group used for a toxicity study is usually genetically well known, without sick individuals, housed

in optimum conditions and treated to a balanced diet, while for the human population such variables may differ considerably.

Moreover, to study certain less frequent effects and effects of low doses, animal experiments are often not appropriate. Sometimes they are even totally inappropriate, because it is difficult to arrive at significant statistical differences between the exposed and the non-exposed animals, given the limited number of animals used. If one extra rat out of a hundred contracts cancer in the population of exposed rats compared to the non-exposed animals, this is not a statistically significant figure and this variation may be due to chance. If this difference is in fact not due to chance (and if we assume that the risk can be directly extrapolated from this species to man), this could mean that one per cent of the workers exposed could suffer from cancer as a result of equivalent exposure.

Extrapolating dose-response relationships from high doses to low doses is also an unreliable practice. At exposure levels where a clear dose-response relationship can be shown, one is operating in the more linear part of the curve. Setting a NOAEL by extrapolating from the linear part does not deal with the fact that biological effects appear to be non-linear at the onset of the curve. In principle, extrapolating in this way may especially be a problem for the substances which need metabolic activation.

### *Limit values based on epidemiological studies*

In the best of all cases, limit values are based on properly conducted epidemiological research. It is selfevident that limit values determined in this way are never more precise than the epidemiological studies from which they are deduced. Other uncertainties simply result from extrapolating human data to persons other than the group under study. Uncertainties should be addressed by using safety factors. The reliability of dose response relationships and NOAELs or LOAELs based upon human data can be limited for several reasons.

The first are shortcomings in the determination of airborne exposure levels. Epidemiological studies rarely give precise data on exposure. Several problems or questions crop up regularly in this respect:

- how representative are the ambient measures compared to the real exposure?;
- what is the accuracy of the measurement method itself?;
- in the case of particles, what was the configuration of the particles of a given substance and what fraction of them was inhalable?

The replies to these questions and to others force us to moderate the dose-effect ratio one way or another.

Further ways in which epidemiological studies can be flawed have to do with insufficient control of variables interfering with the correlation between airborne exposure level and dose:

- is it possible that, apart from exposure through the respiratory tract, absorption also occurred through the skin or through oral ingestion?
- what was the workload of the population studied? In other words, at what frequency and to what extent was a substance breathed in from the ambient air? It could be dangerous to extrapolate a NOAEL from a population with a moderate workload to a population with a heavy one.
- did the persons in the study group use respiratory protective equipment or not?

Furthermore, different diagnostic approaches used to discover early effects may have a different sensitivity and will thus lead to a different NOAEL or LOAEL for the effect under study. This should also be taken into consideration when a health-based limit value is deduced from epidemiological data. A few examples of this are:

- when studying early effects of asbestos induced pulmonary fibrosis, the use of radiological changes as a diagnostic criterion will lead to a higher NOAEL or LOAEL than if alveolar gas exchange had been studied.
- when studying the NOAEL or LOAEL of a non-genotoxic carcinogen for mainly curable cancers, the study of cancer mortality as an outcome could lead to the value being set at a higher level than if the incidence of cancer had been used as the outcome.

Moreover, for some adverse health effects such as cancer, epidemiological research only allows us to detect pronounced risks in human populations available for research. One of the reasons for this is that to detect excess risk, reference always has to be made to a reference population, such as the population of a country or a region. Quite often, this reference group is (more) exposed to other factors which may have the same effect. In this case, a false impression may be given that the exposure studied does not have a harmful effect on the health of workers or that respecting a certain exposure limit offers adequate protection.

It is true that there are epidemiological techniques to take account of the differences which distinguish the observed group from the reference group, but it is then necessary to have prior knowledge of these other risk factors. Epidemiological studies cannot provide an entirely satisfactory solution to this problem. In addition, the conditions under which the study is performed are not determined by the researcher. The epidemiological study method is based on complex reality and tries to answer questions by seeking associations in the jungle of data for a given exposure and a given risk.

These are difficulties in defining a NOAEL or a LOAEL for a given exposure and a given effect. But even then, some remaining questions have to be addressed:

1 To what extent is it precluded that other harmful effects which have not been studied will appear at concentrations lower than the limit value indicated? The history of certain exposure limits, such as those for vinyl chloride and benzene, has shown a free fall over time. This is mainly due to the fact that other possible effects have been studied or considered which were not incorporated in earlier standards. When analysing criteria documents on existing exposure limits it is striking to find that the majority of them are still based on the protection against acute effects, e.g. instantaneous irritation of the mucous membranes. For a large number of substances, other effects are rarely studied.

2 Do the interactive factors of the working environment, the ambient surroundings or life-style have an influence on the effect? It is sometimes extremely difficult to answer this question. It is nevertheless necessary to take it into account if one wishes to set reliable, which in most cases means lower, limit values.

All the above mentioned considerations must be a major incentive to define carefully the safety margins to be taken into consideration when establishing health-based limit values, even if they are based on epidemiological research with exposed humans. A safety factor should take into account the varying degrees of extrapolation uncertainties on the one hand, and the severity of the adverse health effect on the other. As extrapolation is a risky activity, with lots of elements to be balanced, safety margins should therefore or be set on an *ad hoc* basis, or be extremely large.

## FROM SCIENTIFIC DATA TO REGULATIONS: THE 'SARACCI PARADIGM'

Within the setting of limit values or the classification of chemicals, diverging viewpoints may arise between the actors. It is remarkable that differences in viewpoints sometimes concern the same data. This is not so much due to the uncertainties in scientific data, but to a different attitude towards risk between actors, in dealing with uncertainties. While the former may explain the basis for diverging viewpoints, the latter explains the reason why diverging viewpoints may arise using the same data.

Subjectivity in science and in the interpretation of scientific data is often put forward as a basic problem in regulatory work with respect to chemical risk. This subjectivity has been described as an often unconscious process. The fact that the same scientific data are used to draw different conclusions is thereby often the prevailing argument (Nilsson et al. 1993). We have to disagree with the statement that scientists involved in regulatory activities are usually not conscious of the subjectivity in their arguments.

In our opinion, rather the opposite is true: it is precisely the fact that scientists are able to identify the uncertainties in the data they are using that makes it possible for them to develop the arguments intentionally in view of their moral objectives which will definitely not be neutral. Either they aim to protect workers and will take into account the uncertainties 'on the safe side', or they are ready to serve a different interest and will consider the absence of a clear proof of an effect at a given level of exposure as the absence of an effect at that level of exposure.

In our experience, when a discussion of scientific data reveals at the outset very different interpretations for the same data, two things can happen. Either the discussion leads to a common conclusion based on a scientifically sound agreement on the interpretation of the data, despite differences in moral objectives between the scientists, or the discussion of the data does not lead to agreement and thus makes the differences in moral objectives explicit.

Paraphrasing R. Saracci's presentation at a workshop on ethics in occupational health in Como in 1994 (satellite workshop of the ICOH Conference on Occupational Epidemiology) one can say that for a regulatory scientist:

- objectivity is something always to strive for, knowing one can never be totally objective;
- impartiality is a must and should always be met;
- neutrality is something to avoid: if the aim is health protection, for instance, the regulatory activity should unequivocally serve this aim, and no other aims.

This paradigm should guide regulatory scientists, and is a workable tool in assessing compliance of regulatory practices with the official objectives. In order to illustrate this, we will use the example of the 118A activities with respect to limit value setting, and the I00A debate with respect to the classification of Man Made Mineral Fibres (MMMF, also called Manufactured Mineral Fibres, Synthetic Mineral Fibers, and Man-made Vitreous fibers, which is preferred by industry). Before we come to this, the procedures for the regulation of chemicals under these two different mandates will be explained very briefly, and only in so far as is necessary for our purpose.

## Different legislative frameworks: I00A and 118A of the Treaty of Rome

Some of the regulations with respect to chemicals are based on article I00A of the Treaty of Rome, and they aim to harmonise protection for citizens (in their capacity of workers or consumers) against health and safety risks due to chemicals, and also to protect the environment. These regulations are decided in view of the free circulation of goods – in this case existing and new chemical substances and preparations – in a single European market. Decisions taken in this legislative framework have to be applied by all Member States. With respect to health and environmental protection, no marketing restrictions other than the ones forming part of these European regulations can be imposed by any of the Member States, once a decision has been taken. So the classification of chemical substances and preparations and how they should be labelled is nowadays decided at a European Union level. Recently developed regulations and those still being drawn up with respect to risk assessment for 'existing' chemicals (100,102 substances which were already on the market and listed in the so-called EINECS Inventory, as distinguished from 'new' substances) will result in decisions to be applied strictly in the single European market.

Other regulations with respect to chemicals concern the protection of workers as part of the social activities of the European Union. These regulations are based on article 118A of the Treaty of Rome. These are minimal social requirements with which all Member States have to comply in their national regulations. This means that Member States are allowed to have stricter regulations, but not less severe ones. In principle, Member States are not allowed to lower their current level of protection for workers when transposing the European Social Regulations into national legislation. Some workplace exposure limit values for chemical substances are part of these regulations, as well as regulations concerning protection against carcinogens, maternity protection, and the so-called Seveso Directive on the prevention of industrial chemical accidents (82/501/EEC; 87/216/EEC; revised in 1996: 96/82/EC).

In contrast to the imperative consequences of decisions taken within the I00A framework, the activities of the European Union within the 118A framework have resulted in both the above mentioned strict, albeit minimal requirements and in what we might call the elaboration of guiding principles.

### *The preparation of decision making in the I00A and the 118A Framework*[1]

In both legislative frameworks, final decisions are taken either by the Council or by the Commission. One of the relevant differences between Council Directives and Commission Directives is that the latter instrument is quicker by far. It should be noted that the use of Commission Directives has been a more common practice within the I00A 'single market' framework than within the 118A 'social affairs' framework.

With respect to the politics of chemical risk, it may be relevant to consider that the early preparation of decisions within the I00A framework is basically

---

1 We will not address the early stage preparatory activities, prior to expert meetings organised by the Commission.

done in well structured but unofficial meetings. The epicentre of it is the CMR Working Group.[2] All Member States have their representatives, often affiliated to the ministries dealing with environmental protection, who together draw up the conclusions. Industry (the producers of chemicals) and also trade unions (in a very modest way) are represented in the informal working groups in an advisory capacity. The decisions finally resulting from this preparatory work are mandatory for all Member States, and are very concise: a label will figure on receptacles, providing some key information to the user.

In contrast, the 118A initiatives are prepared by the Commission, within a strictly formalised negotiating framework. A strictly tripartite Advisory Committee on Health and Safety at Work comprising representatives of Member States (from Labour Ministries, national employers' and trade union organisations), sets up Ad Hoc Groups, also on a tripartite basis. Every initiative with respect to health and safety at work is first discussed in these Ad Hoc Groups. There is also the Scientific Expert Group on Exposure Limit Values, the key body in a transparent procedure of the Commissions activities in the field of limit value setting.[3] The decisions which may finally result from this initiating tripartite process are not necessarily compulsory and are less precise than those resulting from the 100A process. They indicate options with respect to the general approach to be adopted in a national workplace prevention policy rather than indicating (precise) quantifiable measures. This is to some extent the logical consequence of the matter being dealt with, but also the expression of a lack of interest of the different negotiating partners to be more precise. Some of the reasons for this may be the following:

1 Member States are interested in not having to make considerable changes to their current national policy, for instance because their policy or organisational framework with respect to health at work is the expression

---

2 Carcinogens, Mutagens and substances toxic to Reproduction.

3 In the meantime, the SEG became an official body of the Commission, and is now called Scientific Committee for Occupational Exposure Limits to Chemical Agents (SCOEL).

of their socio-political tradition and part of an institutional framework which applies a much larger field than workplace prevention only.

3 In principle, employers' and employees' representatives in the Tripartite Advisory Committee also represent Member States. Their attitude towards the 118A framework is co-ordinated by UNICE (an international union of confederations of European industries and employers) and ETUC (the European Trade Union Confederation) respectively. These European employers and trade union institutions are seeking a compromise between the different interests of the national organisations. This often results in positions which aim to avoid centrifugal forces, overwhelming centripetal forces within the employers' and workers' groups respectively.

3 On the employers' side, this enhances a dynamic in which UNICE will rather be forced to brake, while national employers' representatives may sometimes tend to support the establishment of new regulations, often in order to comply with agreements between social partners decided at a national level. They will, however, rarely insist firmly in this respect.

4 On the trade union side, the dynamic is somewhat different: some of the national trade union representatives tend to seek the best possible compliance with their national policy. They either oppose European initiatives as they are afraid these might somehow constitute a threat for what are considered to be their well established achievements or aims[4] at national level, or – with the same objective – try to enforce a European regulation that fits their national situation. Other national trade union representatives are faced with a lack of national regulations. They therefore seek European tools which allow for national action to provide better protection. The complexity of these dynamics makes it difficult to reach agreements, but this can be overcome through subtle wording in regulatory proposals, a tactic requiring a far-reaching technical competence, in particular from the trade unions' and Member States representatives' side, both official delegates and additional experts (if any). This requirement is not always met.

---

4 The aim can also be to reduce or limit health and safety regulations, pretending or assuming that these can obstruct employment, and hoping that health and safety will not be affected.

Within the 100A framework the dynamics in the preparatory stage process of regulations is different. It is not UNICE but CEFIC (European council of federations of chemical industry) that is the main permanent representative here on the 'employers' side, which stands for producers of chemicals in this case. Trade unions participate in some of the meetings, sometimes represented by one single ETUC expert.

Producers have an ultimate interest in enforcing the single market and even in regulating chemical risk issues. Their concern in decisions will therefore be balanced against their fear that 'severe' regulatory decisions might in some cases have economic consequences which they would prefer to avoid.

ETUC representation in this very technical field is a rather unusual experience for trade unions, and given the nature of the expertise required for these meetings, the trade union impact on the decision process depends above all on the training and experience of the persons acting as the experts. The authority of such a person as a regulatory scientist seemed to be important for the influence that this person may have on the activities of the working groups, also as a representative of workers' interests.

### *Some aspects of the interface between 100A and 118A regulations*

The decisions taken within the I00A framework might affect the protection of workers against adverse health effects, both directly and indirectly. Although huge efforts are being made by the European Union to make information on risks available to users of products and especially workers, in the practice of daily working life, the receptacles' label – resulting from decisions taken within the I00A classification process – is often the only direct information workers and employers of very small enterprises will have access to. Therefore this may be the only source of information with respect to possible adverse health effects and precautions to be taken when using a substance or product, through its Risk and Safety sentences.

Decisions taken on the basis of I00A Directives to some extent also affect 118A Directives. For instance, in the so-called Carcinogens Directive (90/394/EEC, OJEC L196, 1990, page 1; 28/06/90) this Directive is subject to revision probably resulting in a new Directive in 1997) clear reference is made to the classification of substances as carcinogens of category 1 or 2 within the I00A framework. For these substances, the Directive requires substitution by other products whenever possible.

With respect to risk assessment for existing chemicals in particular, it is not surprising that tensions may arise between actors in both frameworks, as they may represent different institutions and interests. One field where these tensions might become more explicit in the future is risk management, as this is not only addressed in the 118A framework, but will also become a future activity within the I00A framework. In particular, the identification of No-Observed-Adverse-Effect-Levels within the framework of risk assessment for existing chemicals (I00A) on the one hand, and the establishment of exposure limit values for chemicals in workplaces (118A) on the other may lead to divergence of decisions. Such outcomes, however, can be avoided. If that is the objective, the different parties will have to face the fact that there is a substantial difference in approach towards risk assessment between I00A and 118A decisions. Since the beginning of the classification activities of the European Commission, industry has successfully asked to have a 'substance-by-substance' approach within the I00A framework. This means that the possible adverse effects on human health and the environment will be considered as if the substance were the only one possibly affecting health or the environment, and exposure limits will be set accordingly. It is obvious, however, that the human body or the environment may be subject to several exposures which may increase the risk of the same adverse health effect. A combination of substances may even enhance an effect which is not seen when substances are tested separately. As risk assessment does not take this possibility into account, either for existing substances or for new substances, the information on which protective measures are based in the I00A framework may often be incomplete.

## COMPARING REGULATORY PRACTICES

In this section we compare the regulatory practices of the 100A and 118A frameworks. As for the 118A framework, attention will be focused on the workings of the Scientific Expert Group (SEG or SCOEL: Scientific Committee for Occupational Exposure Limits to Chemical Agents). We will look mainly at the way the SEG deals with scientific uncertainty in the setting of health based occupational exposure limits. The transparency of the procedure is also discussed. To get some grasp of the way chemicals are regulated within the 100A framework, we will go into some comments on the classification and labelling of so-called Man Made Mineral Fibres.

## Occupational exposure limit value setting for chemicals

### *The transparency of the limit value setting procedure and the SEG*

Although defined as health-based, many of the current limit values are known to be based largely if not exclusively on feasibility considerations. A first requirement to avoid this ambiguity is a two step procedure, as adopted now by Member States and social partners in the European Union within the 118 A framework, with a clear separation between health-based and feasibility considerations. This is a first condition for transparency. In the European procedure, a Scientific Expert Group (SEG) takes care of the first step. An extensive SEG criteria document is published for every substance, together with a health-based limit value. Making this information available to all interested parties and persons is a second element in the transparency of the process. Because there is one unique evaluation by a credible scientific body, the second step will become more transparent as well, because any deviation from the single health-based limit value put forward by the SEG will have to be argued without challenging the validity of the scientific health-based evaluation. As a consequence, a confusing mixture of arguments created by the existence of different health-based limit values can be avoided. The political fact that Member States do not seem to want the establishment of compulsory European limit values, but instead prefer to set their own legally binding values, if any, might make the SEG an even more crucial body in the transparency of the whole process. This will be the case if Member States are forced to use the same European SEG Health-Based Limit Value as a starting point in their national procedures for setting limit values. Any deviation should thus be argued and these arguments should be open to all parties concerned, and notified to the European Commission.

Within the context of a unified European market, it is unclear how it can be argued that a more decentralised limit value setting process, including the evaluation of scientific data, might make the process more transparent

than with the current European procedure. Although such a more 'local' decision process may seem to be more democratic and to offer a better opportunity for the participation of those directly concerned, we believe that it will lead to a situation in which the scientific arguments and even the feasibility arguments will be much more subject to the influence of interested parties, while such influence can be controlled more easily when applying the current European strategy.
The foreseeable diversity in evaluations and health-based limit values that will result from a more decentralised approach might do considerable damage to the credibility of limit values as a tool for improving working conditions.

### *Safety factors and the SEG*

The considerations concerning uncertainty in risk assessment outlined above are illustrative of the fact that negotiating chemical risk is very demanding in terms of the ability to analyse scientific data of a very heterogeneous nature. It also illustrates the need to assess how uncertainties and even gaps in knowledge should be taken into account when assessing risk. There has been a repeated request to the Commission, mainly from the employers' side, to make the way the SEG is dealing with uncertainties in data 'more transparent', by adopting strict rules for the application of safety factors. Such requests can be explained as part of industry's wish to have a system for limit value setting which is highly predictive with respect to its outcomes and therefore in accordance with their need for planning policy. As we may assume that industry is not always aiming to be extremely protective, the question should be raised as to what extent predictiveness may be in compliance with protectiveness.

A strict safety factor approach, however, would be synonymous with denying that uncertainties are due to a huge variety of elements which differ very much from one substance to another. There are no magic formulas for dealing with uncertainties in data when it comes to using these data for regulatory purposes (see also Feron, this volume).

However, there are principles or criteria to be adopted by a body such as the SEG, for instance with respect to the selection of data (e.g. for reasons of validity or credibility), with respect to the strict exclusion of technical feasibility considerations from their criteria (in view of their mission to give guidance to the protection of workers' health), and also with respect to the clarification of what might be considered as adverse health effects.

When these principles and criteria are clear, and the competence and the autonomous judgment of the SEG is guaranteed by its composition, as has been the case, then it would be strange to request that the SEG should adopt strict principles for applying safety factors. Safety factors would be the only major tool left for dealing with the totality of uncertainties in the totality of available data, also in view of the diversity in susceptibility in exposed workers' populations and in view of the protection of more vulnerable individuals. The evaluation of existing data and the setting of limit values cannot become a mathematical activity. Simplifying the approach will not make the data more reliable.

The request for fixed safety factors could therefore only be met through setting extremely severe safety factors, as illustrated by Anne Stijkel (1995), a solution that would definitely not be in accordance with the wishes of some of the partners in the regulatory process who request such safety factors. An analysis of possible consequences of the idea of using an extremely severe safety factor may reveal possible drawbacks of such a solution:

1 low credibility of the resulting health-based limit value, entailing that such a limit value would hardly be taken into consideration in the final regulatory decision making process. As a consequence, one might arrive at a situation one should avoid: feasibility considerations will be the prevailing argument in limit value setting;
2 within the current context of a growing involvement of industry in research fields which were traditionally subject to independent research, as epidemiology (industry has the data and now also has the scientists) and animal experiments (industry has the resources for these), such a solution might result in increasing emphasis on the development of research strategies aimed at 'proving the absence of an effect', leading to a dynamic of the production of more 'precise' data of such kind for regulatory purposes;
3 such a strategy might in addition compromise the correct identification of a series of priority research concerns either on a particular substance or on some more basic or general aspects, and simultaneously the availability of resources for independent research on these topics.

In our understanding, transparency is largely met by the above mentioned principles and criteria of the SEG.

*The SEG and the Saracci paradigm*

The above considerations should allow us to make an evaluation of the compliance of the Scientific Expert Group on Limit Values of the European Commission with Saracci's paradigm. In order to do so, some specific problems have to be identified with respect to the terms of the paradigm. In relation to health-based limit value setting one can argue that objectivity is not fully possible because of the remaining uncertainties in available data which will need interpretation for regulatory purposes. Striving for objectivity is possible when dealing with the uncertainties. This is a basic requirement for the credibility of the setting of health-based limit values. Furthermore, impartiality requires that the researchers report the data taken into account in a way that is correct and verifiable by third parties. Pressure coming from interested parties should have no influence on the decisions. Finally, non-neutrality implies that as the group is dealing with uncertainties in deciding upon the protection of workers' health, its members should take decisions which are on the safe side.

Guarantees with respect to the abovementioned requirements may be that in its composition, the SEG has the highest possible level of competence as a group in the very different scientific fields related to limit value setting. Furthemore, its members are carrying out their activities in full professional independence and have neither a direct economic or social interest, nor direct commitments with the parties involved (member states, employers, employees). SEG members might lose more than they gain if they did not comply with the requirement of impartiality: they would indeed compromise their high credibility in the international scientific community when not respecting their independence towards the interested parties. Finally, its members are generally known to be concerned with the protection of workers' health, and have shown that they play safe where uncertainties are concerned.

It is our belief that the common judgement of such a group, clearly meeting the above mentioned requirements, is the best guarantee of a credible and workable first step within a two-step procedure for limit value setting. Within this context, it is also in the interests of the credibility of the scientific community to have a single European scientific authority, the

SEG, at the end of the first step of the procedure for the evaluation of existing data and the establishment of health-based limit values.

## A I00A CLASSIFICATION STORY: MAN MADE MINERAL FIBRES

To get to grips with the regulatory activities within the 100A framework, we will go into some detail concerning the classification and labelling of one group of substances, the so-called Man-Made Mineral Fibres. MMMF are very important substances from a commercial point of view, and there is a great deal of data available on MMMF, especially concerning their carcinogenic potential. This still ongoing, controversial and seemingly never-ending debate, although it is rather an exception in this respect, may offer a very relevant and illustrative opportunity for making an evaluation of current possibilities and limits – and also politics – of the European Union's classification system.

Several aspects of this debate are relevant in this respect. First, the relevance of different types of animal experiments with respect to the effect on humans was the focus of attention, while little attention was paid to human epidemiology. In fact, epidemiology as a discipline was almost exclusively represented by the trade unions and the manufacturers, and occasionally by some other special experts in a separate working group. Biology and chemistry were the major training fields of Member States' representatives. Epidemiological studies had already revealed the probable carcinogenic potential of insulation wool fibres (Saracci et al. 1984; Marsh et al. 1985; Simonato et al. 1986a; 1986b; 1987; Enterline et al. 1987).

Second, industry had set up their own animal experiments, which were different from other animal experiments (Hesterberg et al. 1993; McConnel et al. 1994; Rossiter et al. 1995). As the former were inhalation experiments, they were presented by industry as far more relevant than any other animal experiment such as intraperitoneal injection (Pott et al. 1989; 1991) or intratracheal instillation. These inhalation experiments were very badly reported, however – although published in scientific journals – and interpreted as negative in a scientifically unacceptable way (Infante et al. 1994; 1996; Van Damme et al. 1995).

Third, manufacturers were highly involved in the debates, and different manufacturers sometimes apparently had different and even opposite positions and interests. An example of this is the fact that the rockwool industry was ready to accept a category 3 classification (lowest positive ranking) for cancer risk of respirable rockwool fibres, but the manufacturers of one Member State disagreed with this because their national legislation might in that case no longer enable them to sell the product to ordinary consumers. Another example is the fact that the insulation wool industry and ceramic fibre industry organisations, respectively, have made very different proposals for the classification of the different types of MMMF in the CMR Working Group.

Fourth, trade unions were usually represented by a single expert delegated by the ETUC. Moreover, there were different viewpoints within the trade union world. Trade unions with affiliates in the asbestos industry were in favour of classifying MMMF as carcinogens, while trade unions with their affiliates in the MMMF industry were very concerned about the effect of a possible classification on employment. Trade unions having the users of the products among their members were in favour of a correct classification and labelling as a first step towards adequate protective measures. The different viewpoints were not expressed through different trade union representatives. Trade union representation was clearly aimed at contributing to a scientifically sound classification. In practice, this depends mainly upon the ETUC expert in person.

Fifth, international meetings, announced as scientific meetings, were organised by industry, who found partnership for this in the scientific world. On one of these occasions, statements by speakers which were not in accordance with industry's presumed commercial interest were challenged in an aggressive way, such as was hardly ever been seen before during scientific meetings: collective and well organised whistling from a considerable group of participants who had nothing to do with science was the welcome given to Professor Pott when he began his presentation at the MMMF Workshop in Paris in February 1994. In other scientific forums statements were made which were clearly incorrect. For instance, the Hesterberg study was reported at the ICOH Conference, held in Nice in 1993, as if no cancers were seen in the inhalation experiments for insulation fibres. This does not correspond with the data published later on. Not only were cancers seen, reinterpretation of the data on these badly reported experiments also revealed that the results were positive (Infante et al. 1994; 1996; Van Damme et al. 1995).

Sixth, a lot of pressure was exerted on some of the Member States' representatives by their own governments to take a position which was not in accordance with their scientific conviction; there was a complete change in position of representatives of one Member State regarding carcinogenicity of ceramic fibres in two consecutive meetings, while there was no change in position on scientific evidence.

Seventh, two very opposite approaches towards the use of data for risk assessment were shown. Industry representatives and some of the Member States' representatives considered each experiment separately, arguing that it was either not a relevant approach, or that the results were statistically not significant. According to them, these experiments were to be considered as proof of the absence of effect. The other approach was adopted by other Member State representatives and strongly argued by the ETUC representation, who compared the consistency of all available data with the hypothesis that respirable fibres of insulation wools may cause cancer and may not cause cancer, respectively. The authors of a document following a scientific and regulatory workshop organised with Trade Union support concluded that all data considered were compatible with the hypothesis that all respirable MMMF, including different types of insulation wool fibres, have a carcinogenic potential in humans.

Eight, at one point during the debate, the labelling debate became mixed up with the issue of setting limit values. The idea was raised to establish a workplace exposure limit value for MMMF which – if respected – was assumed not to constitute a risk of cancer. As a consequence, classification as carcinogens would no longer have to be considered. Such an approach would imply that the classification system no longer refers to the intrinsic carcinogenic properties, but to a risk of lung cancer at an exposure level which is assumed to be respected. The next step of such a concept of classification might then be to set up animal testing for possible effects at that level of exposure only, a practice which would make no sense from a scientific point of view, for many reasons that will not be discussed further here. It should otherwise be stated that this event is illustrative of one of the possible motives behind the idea of having limit values established in the framework of this I00A procedure, rather than leaving this to the SEG in the 118A framework. Such an approach is typical of a particular interpretation of the risk assessment concept which was introduced into the I00A legislative framework. Together with the introduction of risk management in the I00A framework, this will have to be the focus of attention by persons concerned with the politics of chemical risk.

And last, during the debate on MMMF, a request about obtaining an eco label for insulation wools was discussed in the Commission and was almost approved. Those discussing the classification were not aware of the fact that a parallel discussion had taken place in the Commission, with participation of employers' and trade union representatives.

*The MMMF classification procedure and the Saracci paradigm*

The above considerations should allow us to make an evaluation of the compliance of the classification activities of the European Commission with Saracci's paradigm.

- Objectivity: data are to a large extent provided by industries having a direct interest; this constitutes a challenge to objectivity which can broadly be overcome through very critical evaluation of data by the Working Group members. However, the competence of the CMR Working group is not sufficient to cover all relevant disciplines. This is solved either by consultation of national experts by the delegations, or by setting up specialised expert groups who advise the CMR Working Group.
- Impartiality: although its members are willing to perform their activities in full professional independence, pressure is often exerted by their governments, giving priority to assumed economic interest and thus not health protection. This may considerably impair impartiality in some cases.
- Neutrality: the CMR Working Group is definitely contributing to the better protection of human health and the environment, and is willing to do so. However, in the case of a major economic interest, it seems that difficulties may arise.

The MMMF story dramatically reveals a particular aspect of the 'politics of chemical risk', namely that the main problem in the future may be the lack of resources for independent research activities, in contrast to the availability of resources in industry. This has been true for a long time for animal experiments. A more recent phenomenon is that epidemiological research is also increasingly being carried out by industry, which has the data, the money to set up studies, and the money to pay the epidemiologists. Industry should not be discouraged from conducting further research, but a dramatic imbalance may arise between the industry's potential in conducting research and the possibilities to conduct research independent of industrial interest. A dramatic example of this is that the International Agency for Research on Cancer (IARC) had no other possibility for financing the updating of the European study on cancer risk and MMMF than accepting important co-financing from industry (Boffetta et al. 1995). Such imbalance has to be corrected, and with it the probability that this situation might further stimulate the 'production' of negative data (see also Van Damme et al. 1995), as was done for instance in the study of Wong et al. (1991).

## CONCLUSIONS

Both in the field of health protection at work (118A Directives) and the classification and labelling of chemicals (100A Directives), the European Union has developed workable tools to improve the protection of workers and the general public against risks related to the use of chemicals. However, the success of the policies developed in this respect depends on the determination of all parties involved to protect humans and the environment. Parties involved should thus not be neutral in this respect. Each of the parties involved in the decision making process may show a lack of determination for different reasons related to assumed (real or imaginary) interests. It is important to identify both the weaknesses and the strong points in the current framework for regulation in the field of chemicals in the European Union. As the effectiveness of a policy is not stronger than its weakest points, we will identify a (far from complete) number of possible pitfalls or drawbacks of the current policy, and some suggestions for improvement.

First, a transparent procedure for setting limit values for workplace exposure to chemicals has been established. The principle adopted, that of an impartial group of highly competent experts in different, relevant fields providing the decision making process with an extensive document with only health-based limit value proposals, is of utmost importance. The transparency of the process requires not only that these documents are made available to all interested parties or persons, but also that any decision taken on a limit value either at a European or at a national or sector level which is different from the SEG proposal, should be accompanied by an extensive explanatory document discussing in particular all the reasons for the difference as well as the possible consequences of opting for a different limit value, including a detailed description of the health risk management policy. Such a document would complete the transparency of the procedure and, together with the SEG criteria document, constitute a permanent tool and thus indirectly an incentive for rationally striving towards better protection whenever possible.

Second, classification with respect to intrinsic hazardous properties should not be mixed up with limit value issues: the idea of testing and classifying substances for their hazardous properties only if these effects can be demonstrated at expected dose levels – even if based on worst case situations – is to be rejected. The mutual interference of limit value setting procedures and classification of substances is the wrong solution to the problems with relevance to testing procedures for intrinsic hazardous properties to humans. The hazard identification process would thus not be done independently of the risk assessment process, but become part of it. This might imply that, where animal experiments are done, a tendency may arise to give preference to the application of dose levels which are considered relevant to humans. However, at lower dose levels, animal experiments may become largely insensitive both *per se* and as predictors of human risk. Therefore, such mutual interference is making the 'grey zone' of uncertainties with respect to what might happen in humans much larger in both directions -because of added uncertainties – and this is especially problematic because a simple 'yes' or 'no' decision will ultimately result from the procedure: when a 'yes' or 'no' may relate to the outcome 'irritation', the problem is of lesser importance. In contrast, when it relates to mutagenicity, carcinogenicity and toxicity to reproduction, an erroneous 'no' may have dramatic consequences. In addition, the 100A procedures are based on a substance-by-substance approach, which does not take account of the possible effects of likely or incidental co-exposures. This limitation too, may contribute to a lack of reliability with respect to the conclusions of the procedure for the protection of humans.

Third, the debate on MMMF shows the difficulties which may occasionally arise when roles are mixed up between representation of national interests and scientific evaluation of data. Even occasional signs of role confusion may considerably hamper the credibility of a system which has its merits.

The nature of the bodies that elaborate regulatory proposals does not always make it easy to respect all three requirements of the Saracci Paradigm. The fact that the CMR Working Group decided to have specialised expert group meetings in which experts other than those who are members of the CMR Working Group have been invited, may be illustrative of the need to occasionally go into the direction of the 'SEG principle'.

And last, the biggest threat to the regulatory actions of the European Union is related to the input of data into the preparatory work: there seems to be a growing impact of interested industries on the available data. Again, there is no objection to industry contributing to the generation of data, but the resources in terms of both data and allocation available to industry and more independent scientific research institutions respectively seem to become increasingly disproportionate to the disadvantage of independent research. Because the decisions cannot be more precise than the available data, the impact on the decision making process of a party with other interests than purely health protection may thus become too important. Since the protection of workers' health is a societal issue, data which may be relevant in this respect should – as a principle – be object of disclosure to scientific research or evaluation that is not controlled by industry.

In this paper we have tried to illustrate the need to take a clear position in regulatory activities in the field of chemical risk, unequivocally aiming at the protection of health. We illustrated the importance of such a position in regulatory practices when it comes to dealing with uncertainties. With respect to transparency of the procedures – which is another important concern – it should first of all be stressed that this is already a problem for many of the experts themselves: they often have difficulties in keeping an overview of the whole picture related to chemical risk regulations. Not only are various scientific fields involved, but the regulatory framework *per se* is also very complex. Of course, one should avoid simplifying the problems: in a 'chemical society', accurately dealing with chemical risks will inevitably require complex frameworks. The problems and their solutions should not be simplified, but clarified.

It is obvious that if the protection of health is the unequivocal aim of the European Union policy in this respect, as it should, transparency is a key tool for attaining the aim. In practical terms, making the procedures transparent will mean that continuous efforts must be made first of all to clarify the issue to the European and the national parliaments.

*Acknowledgements:* The author wishes to thank Dr Ludwine Casteleyn and the editors for their critical and helpful remarks, and Ms Hazel Cook for her loyal and accurate technical assistance.

## References

Boffetta P., R. Saracci, G. Ferro, A. Andersen, P.A. Bertazzi, J. Chang-Claude, J. Cherrie, R. Frentzel-Beyme, J. Hansen, T. Hemmingson, J. Olsen, N. Plato, L. Teppo, P. Westerhohlm, P. Winter & C. Zocchetti (1995) *IARC Historical cohort study of Man-made vitreous fibre production workers in seven European countries; extension of the mortality and cancer incidence follow-up until 1990*, Lyon: IARC Internal Report 95/003.

Enterline, P.E., G.M. March, V. Henderson & C. Callahan (1987) 'Mortality update of a cohort of U.S. man-made mineral fibre workers', *Annals of Occupational Hygiene* 31: 625-656.

Hesterberg, T.W., W.C. Miller, E.E. McConnell, J. Chevalier, J.G. Hadley, D.M. Bernstein, P. Thevenaz & R. Anderson (1993) 'Chronic inhalation toxicity of size-separated glass fibers in Fischer 344 rats', *Fundamental and Applied Toxicology* 20: 464-476.

Infante, P.F., L.D. Schuman, J. Dement & J.E. Huff (1994) 'Fibrous glass and cancer', *American Journal of Industrial Medicine* 26: 559-584.

Infante, P.F., L.D. Schuman & J.E. Huff (1996) 'Fibrous glass insulation and cancer', *American Journal of Industrial Medicine* 30: 113-120.

Marsh, G.M., P.E. Enterline, R.A. Stone & V.L. Henderson (1991) 'Mortality among a cohort of U.S. man-made mineral fiber workers: 1985 follow-up', *Journal of Occupational Medicine* 32: 594-604.

McConnell, E.E., O. Kamstrup, R. Musselman et al. (1994) 'Chronic inhalation study of size-separated rock and slag wool insulation fibers in Fischer 344/N rats', *Inhalation Toxicology* 6: 571-614.

Nilsson, R., M. Tasheva & B. Jaeger (1993) 'Why different regulatory decisions when the scientific information base is similar? Human risk assessment', *Regulatory Toxicicology & Pharmacology* 17: 292-332.

Pott, F., M. Roller, U. Ziem, F.J. Reiffer, B. Bellman, M. Rosenbruch & F. Huth (1989) 'Carcinogenicity studies on natural and man-made mineral fibers with the intraperitoneal test in rats' in: Bignon, Pet & R. Saracci (eds.) *Non-occupational exposure to mineral fibers*, IARC Scientific Publication No 90, Lyon: International Agency for Researrch on Cancer; 173-179.

Pott, F., M. Roller, R.M. Rippe, P.G. Germann & B. Bellman (1991) 'Tumors by the intraperitoneal and intrapleural routes and their significance for the classification of mineral fibers' in: Brown, Hoskins & Johnson (eds.) *Mechanism of fiber carcinogenesis*, NATO ASI series, Series A, Life Sciences, vol. 223, New York: Plenum Press; 547-565.

Rossiter, C.E. & J.R. Chase (1995) 'Statistical analysis of results of carcinogenicity studies of synthetic vitreous fibres at Research and Consulting Company Geneva', *Annals of Occupational Hygiene* 39: 759-769.

Saracci, R., L. Simonato, E.D. Acheson, A. Andersen, P.A. Bertazzi, J. Claude, N. Charnay, J. Esteve, R.R. Frentzel-Beyme, M.J. Gardner, O.M. Jensen, R. Maasing, J.H. Olsen, L. Teppo, P. Westerholm, P. & C. Zocchetti (1984) 'Mortality and incidence of cancer of workers in the man made vitreous fibres producing industry: an international investigation at 13 European plants', *British Journal of Industrial Medicine* 41: 425-436.

Simonato, L., A.C. Fletcher, J.C. Cherrie, A. Andersen, P.A. Bertazzi, N. Charnay, J. Clause, J. Dodgson, J. Esteve, R. Frentzel-Beyme, M.J. Gardner, O.M. Jensen, J.H. Olsen, R. Saracci, L. Teppo, R. Winkelmann, P. Westerholm, P.D. Winter & C. Zocchetti (1986a) 'The man-made mineral fiber European historical cohort study: an extension of the follow-up', *Scandinavian Journal of Work, Environonment & Health* 12: 34-47.

Simonato, L., A.C. Fletcher, J.C. Cherrie, A. Andersen, P.A. Bertazzi, N. Charnay, J. Clause, J. Dodgson, J. Esteve, R. Frentzel-Beyme, M.J. Gardner, O. Jensen, J. Olsen, R. Saracci, L. Teppo, P. Westerholm, R. Winkelmann, P.D. Winter & C. Zocchetti (1986b) 'Updating lung cancer mortality among a cohort of man-made mineral fibre production workers in seven European countries', *Cancer Letters* 30: 189-200.

Simonato, L., A.C. Fletcher, J.C. Cherrie, A. Andersen, P.A. Bertazzi, N. Charnay, J. Clause, J. Dodgson, J. Esteve, R. Frentzel-Beyme, M.J. Gardner, O. Jensen, J. Olsen, L. Teppo, R. Winkelmann, P. Westerholm, P.D. Winter & R. Saracci (1987) 'The International Agency for Research on Cancer historical cohort study on MMMF production workers in seven European countries: an extension of the follow-up', *Annals of Occupational Hygiene* 31: 603-623.

Stijkel, A. (1995) *On Managing Reproductive Risks of Occupational Exposure to Chemicals*, Amsterdam: Coronel Laboratory.

Van Damme K., L. Casteleyn & E. Heseltine (1995) *The carcinogenicity of Man-Made Mineral Fibres; a workshop report to the attention of the European Commission Working Group on the Classification and Labelling of Dangerous Substances*, Brussels: European Trade Union Technical Bureau for Health and Safety.

Wong, O., D. Foliart & L.S. Trent (1991) 'A case-control study of lung cancer in a cohort of workers potentially exposed to slag wool fibres', *British Journal of Industrial Medicine* 48: 818-824.

# 6

*Robert Nilsson*

# INTEGRATING SWEDEN INTO THE EUROPEAN UNION: PROBLEMS CONCERNING CHEMICALS CONTROL

## CHEMICALS REGULATION IN SWEDEN

### *Early developments*

In Sweden the main stimulus for improved chemicals control originally came from the scientific community. Although media coverage certainly played an important role, during this early phase the debate was to a large extent based on research, and many respected scientists appeared as figureheads of, or collaborated with the environmental movement. During the period 1970-1985, balanced and gradual progress was made in various fields of products control that on the whole was based on scientific principles. A notable exception was the dioxin hysteria which provoked direct intervention at the ministerial level to restrict, and later ban several of the chlorinated phenoxy herbicides, and to prohibit pesticide application from aircrafts, as well as all the use of pesticides in areas open to the general public.

However, as time passed, and in spite of significant progress in toxicology and ecotoxicology, the role of high quality science has gradually become less important in shaping not only Swedish national policy priorities for chemicals control, but also in influencing the environmental movement. Nurtured by a general distrust in 'experts', and coupled with little understanding for the economic realities that provide the basis for modern society, it is perhaps not surprising that lately Greenpeace often seems to have more influence on the Swedish Ministry of the Environment than the Swedish

In: R. Bal & W. Halffman (eds), *The Politics of Chemical Risk*, Kluwer Academic Publishers, Dordrecht 1998: p. 159-171.

National Academy of Sciences. Naturally, such tendencies have affected agency policies to a high degree.

The task of Swedish government agencies is to implement the laws enacted by parliament. By tradition the agencies have enjoyed a rather independent position. However, during recent years ministerial manipulation has increased mainly due to a system of political appointments of compliant managers, which in some cases has reached even as far down as the technical level in some of the agency hierarchies.

However, it would not be fair to put all of the blame on ill-educated laymen, or opportunistic bureaucrats and politicians. The scientific community itself must share part of the responsibility for this unfortunate development. In many cases researchers with little knowledge of toxicology have acted far outside their field of competence and have provided fallacious interpretations of their results while exploiting the news media to promote their own interests. Even when such excesses are discounted, professionals in (e.g.) medicine and epidemiology often tend to overextend interpretations of their own data in order to secure continued funding for certain 'grant-dense' areas, such as health risks from chemicals. *Science* recently quoted a scientist affiliated with the US National Institute of Environmental Health Sciences who bluntly asserted that:

> Investigators who find an effect get support, and investigators who don't find an effect don't get support. When times are tough it becomes extremely difficult for investigators to be objective (Taubes 1995).

The dissemination of any claim, however unlikely from the point of view of biological credibility, is facilitated by the fact that even for medical students, training in fields like toxicology, radiation biology, and statistics, leaves much to be desired. Tendencies as those described above are no doubt more or less common to most developed nations, but what distinguishes Sweden (and perhaps Denmark and Norway) from other countries is the high level of impact from environmental extremism on society. Why is this so? There are political as well as technical reasons. Among the political reasons, an important one is undoubtedly a high level of public concern for environmental protection, especially with regard to 'environmental poisons'. Another such cause is an omnipotent, centralized, and highly politicized regulatory bureaucracy combined with the lack of a balance of power between regulators, industry, and private interests. Finally, there is a general misconception that efficiency in chemicals control is proportional to the number of bans and restrictions imposed.

Technical reasons for the pursuit of a strict environmental policy in Sweden can be related (e.g.) to the impact of climatic factors of the region, implying a low rate of degradation of persistent toxic compounds, as well as a high degree of accidification with a resultant increase in mobility and bioavailability of heavy metals in Swedish soils. While working with the Swedish Environmental Protection Agency, the latter fact was used as a major reason for the present author in 1979-1981 to push through strict restrictions on the use of cadmium in Sweden (SNFS 1979, 1989; Nilsson 1990), the main content of which was incorporated into EU legislation a decade later (Directive 91/193/EEC).

With roots in the romantic era of the last century, not only Swedish intellectuals, but also prominent industrialists have a long tradition of cherishing an unspoiled nature. In a positive sense, this has no doubt promoted the progress of traditional environmental protection, as well as the introduction of stringent emission controls in industry. To justify action based on public 'concern' it has been claimed during recent years, for example by the Swedish government, that the level of risk acceptance in Sweden is particularly low (Bernson 1993). This purported oversensitivity may in a way be true for a nation that has not experienced war since Napoleonic times, and where other national disasters have been few and far between.

### *The Swedish regulatory agency*

The radical development of chemicals control that has taken place during the last decade in Sweden has been facilitated by the extraordinary regulatory powers given in 1986 to the National Swedish Chemicals Inspectorate (KEMI), previously a part of the Swedish EPA. This organization has been given a regulatory competence that approximately corresponds to that given to the Office of Pesticides and Toxic Substances of the US EPA. As in the United States, the Swedish system features a high degree of centralization, which no doubt has facilitated assertive administrative action. However, in the US many safeguards exist to ensure that the administration properly executes its obligations with respect to all interests concerned. Although providing for a balance of power, the other side of the US coin is a sluggish regulatory pace accentuated by a cumbersome bureaucracy and a litigious mood of US citizens – limitations that the Swedish regulators can avoid, though at the expense of the protection of private rights.

Unfortunately, no professional body exists in Sweden with the competence to judge agency policy and performance in a field such as chemicals control, like the Office of Technology Assessment of the US Congress, which, unfortunately, has been abolished in the US in 1995. Complaints against decisions by Swedish government agencies can be lodged at the Fiscal Court of Appeals, the highest level of appeal being the government itself. In practice this means that formally incorrect procedures may be challenged and remedied, yet an assessment is hardly ever carried out of a regulatory decision's subject matter; not to mention the evaluation of scientifically supporting material for regulatory action, or the reasons for such regulations. Thus, in contrast to many Western democracies, there is no recourse to an independent non-political court of law with respect to administrative decisions; nor does Sweden have an independent court to judge the constitutionality of proposed laws and regulations. Against this background, and given the fact that the chemical industry is small, there has been little incentive to restrain overzealous regulators. As a consequence, Sweden has introduced a number of prohibitions and regulations of chemicals that do not exist in other countries, and which more often than not reflect political expediency rather than significant levels of risk. Several of these regulations will not be found acceptable in other EU countries.

### *'Intrinsic properties' and the 'substitution doctrine'*

Much of the regulatory action taken during recent years in Sweden has been based on a regulatory tradition that focuses almost entirely on the inherent properties of chemical products, giving little regard to actual exposures. In other words, the Swedish regulatory system has mainly been based on hazard ranking. Given an initial strong emphasis on classification and labeling, this can to some extent be understood. For many chemical products the exposure upon ultimate use may be difficult to predict, and one simple risk management option is to provide adequate information to the users about potential hazards from handling the product. However, in addition to overconfidence in the impact of labeling, the serious problem concerning the preoccupation with the intrinsic properties of chemical products is that it has spilled over into Swedish chemicals control in general, and to the registration of pesticides in particular.

Current Swedish legislation states that if a hazardous chemical product can be replaced by a less hazardous alternative, such a substitution must be carried out. Used with common sense, this does not seem all that unreasonable. However, in the way the Swedish Act on Chemical Products has been interpreted, almost any chemical that fulfills certain property criteria can be subjected to a ban or to severe restriction irrespective of the actual or projected level of risk, because assessment has exclusively been based on the intrinsic properties (hazard). In addition, "a scientifically based suspicion that a chemical may cause damage is basis enough for action according to the Act" (Bernson 1993). As far as I know, no other nation takes this extremist approach in justifying regulatory action on chemicals.

However, as was already pointed out by Paracelsus (1568; Deichmann et al. 1986) in his treatise *Septem Defensiones* written during 1537-1538, any substance can elicit a toxicological response provided that the dose is sufficiently high. In order to become meaningful in the regulatory context, assessments of intrinsic properties (hazards) from exposure to chemicals should therefore not only identify potentially hazardous chemicals, but also provide a measure of risk under realistic exposure situations. In other words, a quantitative risk assessment should be made. In practically all cases where Sweden has introduced major restrictions on the import, production, or marketing of industrial chemicals and pesticides, these regulations have not been supported by quantitative risk assessment.

### *Comparative risk assessment*

The common goal in the US is to regulate any life-time cancer risk that lies above 1 in 100,000 to 1 in a 1,000,000. This means that the elimination of a factor which causes one case of cancer in a population of one million during a certain time period is believed to result in a reduction of the cancer incidence from 200,001 to 200,000 during that period. It should be remembered that the normal life-time risk for cancer in the industrialized Western world is about one in five. Although it can be debated whether the US regulatory goal makes any sense, a more realistic attitude towards cancer risks can be promoted by using comparative risk assessment. Unfortunately, except for pharmaceuticals, risk-risk comparisons are rarely considered by national regulatory agencies concerned with chemicals.

The hazards associated with pesticide use must be balanced, not only against increased food output, but also in many cases with respect to the prevention of crop contamination by significant levels of highly toxic (and carcinogenic) mycotoxins. Whereas the role of pesticide residues as a cause of human cancer was considered negligible, the inadequate attention paid by the Swedish Food Administration to the role of mycotoxins in the etiology of human cancer was underlined by the Swedish Cancer Committee (1984). Industrial chemicals, pesticides, mycotoxins, and food additives fall under different regulatory agencies – or even ministries – between which cooperation is usually less than optimal. It is, therefore, not surprising that, for regulatory purposes, comparisons are not made between risks from (e.g.) pesticide residues in food on the one hand, and risks associated with dietary factors, food additives, or toxins on the other. If solanine and chaconine were pesticide residues, potatoes would not be permitted on the market in most developed countries because of the high content of these toxic alkaloids (20-100 mg/kg), and also because these substances have not been adequately tested for long-term effects (IPCS 1993). Although exposures to man-made and natural chemicals occur by identical routes of administration and contribute to the same toxicological end points, they are, regrettably, being judged by completely different standards (Nilsson et al. 1993).

## REASSESSING CHEMICALS CONTROL IN SWEDEN FROM THE EU PERSPECTIVE

### *On the threshold of the European Union*

On July 1, 1991 Sweden applied for membership of the European Union (EU). Following negotiations starting in February 1993 and a referendum with a minimal margin of votes in favor of joining the Union on November 13, 1994, Sweden became a full member of the EU as of January 1, 1995. Finland, as well as Austria, also newcomers to the EU, found few problems in accepting the EU legislative complex on chemicals, but in Sweden public opinion forced the negotiators to press hard for exemptions, while referring to the 1963 Treaty of Rome, which stipulates a possibility for a member state to maintain stricter standards for the protection of health and environment. Several such exemptions were granted in the field of chemicals control, albeit on a temporary basis.

Harmonization of the Swedish system for Classification and Labeling has shown satisfactory progress. Certain types of tumors induced in experimental animals by non-genotoxic compounds given in very high doses have little relevance for man. Several such non-genotoxic substances were dropped from the Swedish cancer list reflecting an evaluation based on 'mode of action', contained in the 7th Amendment of April 30, 1992 to the EEC directive on labeling. The few remaining potential carcinogens and sensitizers, as well as a few other issues, will be subject to further negotiations within the EU expert group for classification and labeling.

Some of the exemptions given to Sweden – notably pesticide regulation and Swedish restrictions on chlorinated solvents – present a more formidable obstacle for integration. With respect to the Swedish regulations on phasing out certain chlorinated hydrocarbon solvents and the ban on the use of mercury in thermometers and electrical equipment, the EU has no such rules. Swedish restrictions for arsenic, asbestos, cadmium, organic tin compounds, pentachlorophenol, as well as for agents deleterious to the ozone layer, are more drastic than their corresponding EU directives. Within these areas, Sweden was granted temporary exemptions to be renegotiated after a period of four years on the basis of a technical assessment by the Commission. A similar agreement was reached on the use of the Swedish system for classification for carcinogenic agents, the use of a fourth classification category, and the Swedish rules for the classification and labeling of pesticides. Implicit in the last area are re-evaluations of a large number of pesticides banned in Sweden.

### *Chlorinated solvents*

In response to an assignment given by the government in December 1989 to identify chemicals that "are particularly harmful to the environment", KEMI and the Swedish EPA (KEMI 1990) selected methylene chloride, trichloroethylene, and tetrachloroethylene together with some other chemicals as possible candidates for far-reaching restrictions. However, no systematic approach to selection seems to have been used, evaluation of economic impact was totally inadequate, and no attempts were made to conduct a quantitative assessment in which estimated risks could be related to (e.g.) current exposures in the Swedish work environment, or to levels in the external environment. In the decree of 1991 (1991: 1289), the presence of methylene chloride, trichloroethylene, and tetrachloroethylene in consumer products was to be banned as of January 1993, and a total ban on the use of methylene chloride and trichloroethylene, also including industrial applications, was to be implemented as of 1996. However, in September 1995 an exemption was granted for 1996 with respect to two industrially important uses of trichloroethylene. During the spring of 1996 KEMI received requests from approximately 200 industries to be allowed to use trichloroethylene after 1996, evidently in response to pressure from the EU. About 90% of these petitions were rejected. For those few that were given excemptions, stiff financial charges were imposed.

Whereas the Commission could accept certain restrictions with respect to consumer use for the abovementioned solvents, in 1995 the Swedish government was notified that the Commission considers the regulations on the industrial uses of methylene chloride, trichloroethylene, and tetrachloroethylene as unjustified (Bangemann 1995). Some EU countries have filed complaints to the Commission with respect to the Swedish restrictions. The Swedish Minister of the Environment, Anna Lind, has, however, publicly declared that Sweden will not yield one inch with respect to the implementation of the regulations. In October 1996 the Commission notified the

Swedish government that it considers the Swedish restrictions to be in violation of articles 30-36 of the EU-treaty (Monti 1996). The issue will probably have to be decided by the European Court of Justice.

For pesticides, little progress has been made so far with harmonization with the EU. The application of the obsolete Swedish criteria for cancer classification to silica (quartz) would, for instance, result in classifying this material as a low potency carcinogen. Since more than 1% of sand (actually a major part) consists of quartz, sand as a product should then also be classified as a low potency carcinogen. As a consequence, every sandbox and container of sand would have to carry the label: 'A certain risk of cancer cannot be excluded after frequent exposure.' If for some reason sand was to be considered for pesticide use, it could possibly be permitted for professional applicators, but certainly not sold to the public because of its potential carcinogenic properties. Furthermore, since the regulatory goal of KEMI is to eliminate all chemicals that are not readily biodegradable (especially if they are 'carcinogenic') a total ban of sand should have to be considered.

For obvious reasons 'sand' is not classified as a carcinogen in Sweden, but better than anything else this example demonstrates that something must be wrong with the existing Swedish cancer classification criteria. In addition, when no exposure assessment is conducted, as (e.g.) required in the Council Directive on uniform principles for pesticide evaluation, regulatory action on pesticides has lost much of its rational scientific basis in Sweden.

During recent years, the KEMI has provided a special argument to justify this state of affairs: the Government decree to reduce the volume of pesticide use in Sweden by 50% during the period 1986-1990, and by another 50% until 1996. The elimination of most private uses of pesticides afforded a convenient means to help attain the first of these goals, which could, in fact, be effectuated. However, a further reduction by 50% does not seem to be compatible with the maintaining of modern agriculture practice in Sweden; moreover, the large number of pesticides that have been banned in Sweden continue to expose the public as residues in imported foods. Obviously, a 75% reduction in marketed pesticide volume does not translate into a corresponding decrease in risk. Given the extremely low average application rates in Swedish agriculture that existed already before 1986, the KEMI will find it difficult to convince the Commission that the ongoing Swedish pesticide volume reduction program provides a valid reason for the imposed far-reaching restrictions. However, the ongoing evaluation of pesticides within the EU program for re-registration of pesticides to produce a uniform list of active substances that will be permitted for use within the whole of the EU (Directive 91/414/EEC) will certainly force Sweden to revoke previous bans on a number of products.

### *The future*

Appreciating the economic importance of the European market for a country that is more dependent on export than Japan and that has a 12-13% level of unemployment, industry and a large part of the present political establishment accepts EU membership as a necessity. With respect to chemicals control policy, EU membership constitutes a sobering and restraining factor for the Swedish regulatory machinery for chemicals control. This will include the accommodation of a number of modern scientific principles related to toxicology and risk assessment. A better balance of power between regulators, private citizens, and industry will also probably be achieved. EU membership will permit Sweden to promote scientifically justified regulatory goals within the framework of international cooperation. Although assessment of hazardous substances in the EU may not always represent ultimate wisdom, the outcome will at least be competitively neutral with respect to industry and trade inside the community.

It has been very discouraging, however, that a growing part of the population favors Sweden pulling out of the Union since the country's decision to join the EU – in contrast to what is the case for Finland. With the exception of the export-industry, resistance against the EU is particularly strong among the lower social classes, especially in the northern part of Sweden, but is also prominent among personnel in the bloated Swedish public sector. Fierce EU antagonism is almost universal among the politically organized environmental movement and the previous communist party. Since these two parties are presently sympathetic to approximately one fifth of the electorate, and since the dominating Social Democratic Party and the Center Party are sharply divided about the issue of membership, the future of Sweden as a full member of the Community is full of uncertainty. This unfortunate situation is reflected by the fact that a number of prominent enemies of EU membership were recently elected as representatives to the European Parliament. Apart from serious economic consequences, canceling EU membership will accelerate an ongoing alienation of Sweden among European democracies, and an increasing part of Sweden's most successful industry will opt to move its production base outside the country.

## References

Bangemann, M. (1995) Letter from the EU Commission to Lena Hjelm-Wallen, Swedish Minister of Foreign Affairs, May 3, 1995.

Bernson, V. (1993) 'The role of science in pesticide management – An international comparison: The Swedish experience', *Regulatory Toxicology & Pharmacology* 17: 249-261.

Deichmann, W.B., D. Henschler, B. Holmstedt & G. Keil (1986) 'What is there that is not poison? A study of the Third Defense by Paracelsus', *Archives of Toxicology* 58: 207-213.

IPCS, Joint FAO/WHO Expert Committee on Food Additives (1993) *Toxicological Evaluation of Certain Food Additives and Naturally Occurring Toxicants*, Geneva: WHO, Food Additives Series No. 30.

KEMI (1990) *The task of risk reduction* ["Begransningsuppdraget"], Report to the Swedish Government from a task force, Solna: KEMI.

Monti, M. (1996) *Petition to the Swedish Minister of Foreign Affairs*, Commission of the European Communities, October 9, 1996.

Nillson, R. (1990) *Cadmium – An Analysis of the Swedish Regulatory Experience*, Report to the OECD Chemicals Group and Management Committee, January 1989, Solna: The National Swedish Chemicals Inspectorate, Report no. 6/90.

Nilsson, R., M. Tasheva & B. Jaeger (1993) 'Why different regulatory decisions when the scientific information base is similar? Part I – Human risk assessment', *Regulatory Toxicology & Pharmacology* 17: 292-332.

Paracelsus (1564) 'Septem Defensiones', in: idem, *Karntner Trilogi*, Cologne: Arnold Byrckmann Verlag.

Swedish Cancer Committee (1984) *Cancer: Causes and Prevention*, Report to the Ministry of Social Affairs from the Cancer Committee, Stockholm.

SFS (1979) *Ordinance Amending the Regulations (1973: 334) on Products Hazardous to Man and the Environment*, SFS 1979: 771.

SFS (1980) *Ordinance Amending the Regulations (1973: 334) on Products Hazardous to Man and the Environment*, SFS 1980: 84.

Taubes, G. (1995) 'Epidemiology faces its limits', *Science* 269: 164-169.

# 7

*Sheila Jasanoff*

# HARMONIZATION – THE POLITICS OF REASONING TOGETHER

> "What has been well called the long conversation of mankind may be growing so cacophonous that ordered thought of any sort, much less the turning of local forms of legal sensibility into reciprocal commentaries, mutually deepening, may become impossible."
>
> Clifford Geertz, *Local Knowledge*

## INTRODUCTION

Harmonization of technical standards is usually seen as a challenging but fundamentally objective process, requiring experts to reach a meeting of minds on the definition of 'safe' exposure levels, 'best available technology,' adequate levels of 'containment,' proper measures for personal hygiene, and so forth. I argue in this paper that standards incorporate not only 'objective' assessments of technical evidence but also collective, often tacit, cultural judgments about the appropriateness of particular social roles, power relationships, institutional forms, and styles of governance. Put differently, technical safety standards (levels of control required to protect against harm) and forms of social order (institutionalized responses to civic and political expectations) operate in any society to sustain one another. Accordingly, harmonizing standards across different cultural and political settings involves what the noted anthropologist Clifford Geertz saw as a perhaps impossible

---

In: R. Bal & W. Halffman (eds.), *The Politics of Chemical Risk*, Kluwer Academic Publishers, Dordrecht 1998: p. 173-194.

task: "The turning of local forms of legal sensibility into mutual commentaries, mutually deepening" (Geertz 1983: 234).

The first part of this paper reviews literature from the social studies of science and technology to support the point that standards are not simply technical measures but negotiated forms of social understanding. The second part looks at the specific example of quantitative risk assessment in the United States to show how formal methodologies of standard-setting are embedded in a social and cultural context. The third part suggests ways in which we might rethink the role of international expert bodies so as to encourage 'reciprocal commentary' among different conceptions of safety and order.

## THE SOCIAL CONSTRUCTION OF TECHNOLOGICAL STANDARDS

The picture of 'autonomous technology' (Winner 1977, 1986), in which the world of machines and artifacts has a life independent of the world of people, has been replaced in recent years by one that stresses the political and social dimensions of technological systems. In a suggestive historical study, Noble (1978) argued that 'numerical control,' or automated programming, was introduced into the machine tool industry partly as a method of deskilling workers and increasing managerial control on the shop floor; in this way, a seemingly neutral technological innovation reordered social relations and changed the balance of power. Winner (1986:23) provides the well-known example of Robert Moses, New York's master planner, who designed his parkways with low overpasses so as to encourage the free flow of middle-class, suburban automobile traffic while excluding busloads of poor, non-white, urban travelers. Technologies, more generally, have persuasively been described as heterogeneous systems or networks of non-human artifacts and their human (including institutional) makers, users, and regulators (Callon 1986; Bijker et al. 1987). Power is distributed across the network, and the components of the system must function harmoniously together in order for a technology to 'work.' The safe use of a machine or product depends, in this conceptualization, not only on its physical design and manufacture but also on its fit with the surrounding social context.

These works display a growing awareness of the socially constructed boundary between technology and society and prompt new questions about the nature of technological standards and the prospects for their harmonization. To what extent do *safety* standards, in particular, incorporate cultural assumptions, preferences, and practices that vary from one social setting to another? How do technological systems get standardized so as to overcome such culturally induced variations? How uniformly are standards implemented when technologies are dispersed across geographical and cultural space, and how much uniformity is desirable? Insights may be gained from a wide range of research on technology.

### *Socio-technical hybrids*

Technologies of all kinds – bicycles, lightbulbs, missiles, pesticides – acquire stable, standardized forms through social mediation (Bijker et al. 1987), in settings ranging from the protected, private spaces of industrial R&D laboratories to the highly public, often contentious contexts of regulation and litigation. In public technological controversies, 'safety' is determined through clashes among political stakeholders advancing divergent interpretations of the available data (see, for example, Nelkin 1992). Whether the issue is to site a nuclear power plant or hazardous waste facility, market a new drug or pesticide, or build a new supersonic aircraft, the advocates and opponents of new technology consistently differ in evaluating the evidence of risk, safety, and efficacy. Such controversies reveal the unavoidable 'interpretive flexibility' of scientific claims, dispelling the idea that standards can be set on the basis of 'pure' or wholly objective technical analysis. The standards adopted by policymakers are socio-technical products, developed through more or less transparent processes of negotiation and compromise. The hybrid character of standards is most visible in countries with highly participatory cultures of decisionmaking, such as the United States (Jasanoff 1986); elsewhere, the social assumptions underpinning standards are no less significant, although they may be far less open to public view (Wynne 1987).

In the domain of environmental standard-setting, the 'facts' on which experts base their judgments often fall on the boundary of 'nature' and 'society.' The very concepts that organize scientific research for use in policy – such as 'carrying capacity,' 'per capita fuelwood consumption' or 'inducing cancer' – embody prior understandings about causation and responsibility, including where human intervention ends and natural processes begin.

Where no common understanding exists, agreement on risk and safety also remains elusive. Thus, anthropologists researching environmental degradation and deforestation in the Himalayas found radical differences among experts with respect to seemingly objective facts relevant to their inquiry (Thompson et al. 1986). The 'facts' that the experts had sought to discover about the Himalayas were so contingent and socially embedded that they could not be ascertained through a universally acceptable methodology. What the experts ended up with was not a single description of reality but rather many different interpretations of uncertainty. Their conclusions were shaped by their own culturally induced perceptions of the problem and reinforced by their informants' localized experiences and locally contingent worldviews.

Testing, on which much standard-setting is based, opens up additional areas of interpretive flexibility. MacKenzie's (1990) history of American nuclear missile guidance offers relevant insights. Disputes about the 'accuracy' of intercontinental ballistic missiles (ICBMs) arose in the late 1970s, when their performance had to be assessed through tests that could not by definition exactly replicate the conditions of missile use in wartime. A perfectly dispositive test was a contradiction in terms (Collins 1985). Were tests of components equivalent to tests of the whole weapon? Could trajectories be known with sufficient accuracy in the absence of land-based tracking? Were multiple, correctable, test range firings an adequate stand-in for the one-shot firing of war? And was enough known about the earth's gravitational field to assess the operational accuracy of inertial guidance across the missile's entire trajectory?

In other words, supporters and critics of ICBMs disagreed on the second-order question of whether the tests being conducted were *sufficiently like* the expected real-world conditions to justify drawing conclusions about accuracy. Such similarity determinations must continually be made in testing any technology (Pinch 1993), and chemicals are no exception. Similar disputes have repeatedly arisen about the adequacy of animal models as a test for carcinogenicity in human beings (Jasanoff 1986; Rushefsky 1985). Are rodents sufficiently like people to serve as appropriate surrogates? Is cancer of the liver in mice a suitable diagnostic for brain, lung, or blood vessel cancers in humans? When rats and mice display different responses, which one is more similar to the likely human response, and on what basis can we answer such a question?

In the ICBM case, uncertainty about accuracy allowed the parties to argue, in turn, "for manned bombers, for the cancellation of MX and a more 'dovish' defense policy, for radio guidance and for large missile warheads!" (MacKenzie 1990:363). This controversy eventually dissipated for social rather than technical reasons – because of declining media attention and a policy change under President Reagan that shifted the weapons debate to other arenas of disagreement. As MacKenzie observed for ICBMs, a decrease in the range of policy choices often coincides with a reduction in the public perception of scientific and technical uncertainty, paving the way to agreement on standards. In environmental controversies as well, quarrels over models of natural phenomena may continue unabated until the parties can agree on a restricted set of possible responses. The lengthy battle of experts over the Storm King power plant on the Hudson River in New York provides an example. Here, years of inconclusive attempts to estimate the long-term impacts on fish populations in the river ended only when participants agreed to mitigate short-term impacts without attempting to predict and control longer-term effects (Barnthouse et al. 1984). The new framing of the problem allowed utility company and regulatory agency biologists to keep their models much closer to the observable data, and they developed mutually acceptable methods of biological monitoring over a shorter time cycle.

The forms in which standards are expressed have been shown to depend on users' and consumers' appraisals of the underlying institutional and political arrangements (Brickman et al. 1985; Wynne 1987). Such judgments are regularly built into a society's understanding of what 'safety' means and how it can be achieved in operational terms. Precise and formal regulatory controls, for example, are most characteristic of states where the level of trust in ruling institutions is relatively low. Similarly, objective, quantitative methods of policy assessment are most valued just where regulators are most vulnerable to public criticism. Thus, comparative studies of environmental policymaking reveal consistent differences between America's scientistic, numerically-grounded style of policy justification and the more qualitative, judgment-based approaches of European decisionmaking elites, who enjoy on average higher levels of trust (Brickman et al. 1985; Jasanoff 1991; Porter 1995). Quantification, as Porter (1992:47) observes, has the politically desirable effect of reducing social uncertainty and increasing trust:

> But where [the objectivity of quantification] has been applied more or less routinely, where its contexts of application as well as its methods are at least partly standardized, it can permit administrative decisions to be made quietly, discouraging public activism. In a suspicious democratic order, even truth claims depend on the appearance of objectivity in the sense of impartiality.

Through risk assessment and cost-benefit analysis, administrators can offer to the questioning, anxious citizens of modern societies the promise of impartiality, predictability, and control.

Policymakers in relatively less open and adversarial political systems may be less inclined to admit what is scientifically unknown than their more exposed American counterparts. Wynne and Mayer (1993) have argued that this is the case for British governmental experts, who deny uncertainty so as to avoid accountability; a 'greener' environmental science, according to these authors, would explicitly acknowledge the unknown. By contrast, in US regulatory science, uncertainty is both more readily accepted and more rapidly translated into the technical discourse of risk assessment (Jasanoff 1987). We will return to this point below.

Even within Europe, culturally-rooted attitudes toward state institutions are reflected in substantially different approaches to technical standards. In a comparative study of European hazardous waste management, Wynne (1987) noted that definitions of 'hazardous waste' were shaped not by any 'intrinsic natural meaning' but by the contingencies of national politics. Precise, inflexible, technical standards were adopted in the fragmented and relatively adversarial Dutch political setting, whereas Britain, with a long-established tradition of informal regulatory negotiation and institutional trust, could get by with a much less transparent system of inexplicit, ad hoc, and inconsistent rules. Wynne (1987:403) concluded: "Technical standards are socially constructed, as social languages reflecting their institutional setting." Seen in this light, the very capacity to set standards may serve as an index of social cohesion and trust. Putnam (1992) found in his classic study of Italian politics that regions with a robust civic culture and high levels of associationism were more successful in initiating policy for such contested and uncertain areas of environmental protection as strip mining, fisheries promotion, wildlife protection, and pollution control.

*Universality and contingency*

Studies of standardization have helped illuminate not only the political content of standards but also the methods by which these hybrid, socio-technical products can be made to cohere across widely dispersed geopolitical and cultural spaces. Standardization is often achieved through visual representations, such as statistical charts, questionnaires, surveys, maps, and graphic representations of risk and uncertainty. Latour (1990) terms such representations 'immutable mobiles': once fixed in form, they can be transported to distant places, carrying the same meanings wherever they are put to use. Administrative agencies with the technical capacity to create immutable mobiles become 'centers of calculation' (Latour 1990:59); such centers can gather together a wealth of information and impose on it their own compelling interpretation.

Standards 'work' because they provide valuable reassurance that risks are manageable. Scientists, policymakers, and the lay public all share an interest in reducing the range of interpretations, and hence the uncertainty, associated with hazardous phenomena. Reducing the complexity of nature to universally applicable, quantitative standards offers additional policy advantages, not least of which is the possibility of ranking various bad events according to 'objective' criteria and distributing scarce resources accordingly. For instance, in studying the catastrophic threats of ozone depletion and global warming, experts have sought to assess the detrimental properties of gases on the basis of standardized measures such as 'ozone depletion potential' (ODP) or 'global warming potential' (GWP). Yet, conflicts in 1991 between experts at the US-based World Resources Institute (WRI) and other scientists showed that the simplifying choices made in GWP calculations were not morally neutral: in particular, WRI's decision to focus on current emissions placed a higher burden on developing countries than would have been the case with a ranking based on cumulative emissions over longer time periods (Hammond, Rodenburg, and Moomaw 1991; Subak 1991). A report from India's Centre for Science and Environment stressed that all carbon releases cannot be treated as the *same* unless one adopts a reductionist view of reality (Agarwal and Narain 1991). According to the Centre's experts, WRI's methodology was morally flawed in that it disregarded the west's higher per capita contribution of greenhouse gases and placed the 'essential' agricultural emissions of the world's poor ('subsistence emissions') on a par with 'nonessential' emissions from the consumption patterns of the world's wealthy ('luxury emissions').

Standards, including many produced by non-state and supra-state actors, can be used in international trade in ways that influence the balance of wealth and power. Salter (1993) observes that standards are developed increasingly in advance of the technologies they are meant to regulate, so that they participate in shaping the actual forms of technology; and they do so, moreover, without serious political legitimation, since they represent the work of international, regional or even bilateral standards organizations rather than of democratic states. While standardizing processes open up some new opportunities for political and economic participation, the openings may be illusory, with the first and most expert players determining the gradient of the playing field for all subsequent entrants. In the arena of international environmental standards, for example, agreements about what to measure (e.g., the GWP of greenhouse gases) and how to measure it have become entrenched before divergent conceptual framings of the problem were resolved by all concerned parties. Once embedded within a network of discourse and technical practices (e.g., quantitative risk assessment, as discussed below), standards lose transparency and acquire a taken-for-granted status that resists criticism by actors who did not participate in the original standard-setting process.

Local variations in politics and practice can bring contingency back into the implementation of standards, undermining the power of 'centers of calculation' to impose strict social control. Differences in the knowledge, training, resources, and technical skills of responsible authorities, or differential supervision of implementing bodies by non-governmental organizations (NGOs), for instance, may give rise to seriously divergent regulatory practices. Variance in the institutionalization of expert knowledge within governments and in the larger political culture also creates cross-national differences in policy implementation. Manuals and protocols for the implementation of standards offer at best imperfect instruments for regularizing the behavior of human actors operating within the constraints and contingencies of widely divergent local environments. The unruliness of the real world creates discretionary space for individuals or institutions to exert their tacit knowledge and subjective moral sensibilities. Hawkins (1984:24-27) observed, for instance, that field officers enforcing water pollution standards in Britain had to negotiate variances with dischargers whose expectations of fairness came into conflict with the alleged rationality of science-based standards. Water authorities had pegged the stringency of controls to scientific assessments of the receiving waterways, hoping to achieve like quality through unlike standards; farmers and industrialists objected, saying that similar dischargers should be treated alike, with similarly stringent controls, regardless of the impact on water quality.

Even when countries claim to be complying with the *same* standard, their actual practices may well be dissimilar because of the 'interpretive flexibility' of technical standards (Bijker et al. 1987). Judgments about what constitutes adequate enforcement and compliance will inevitably reflect deep-seated normative understandings about fairness, efficiency, and the appropriate limits of governmental power (Hawkins 1984; Wynne 1987; Jasanoff 1986; Putnam 1993; Porter 1995). Tinkering, adaptation, and even outright avoidance are often the rule when incompletely negotiated and poorly understood standards are imposed on excluded or marginalized groups. A mechanical malfunction or deviation from codified practice that rings instant alarm bells in one cultural setting may be ignored in another until disaster strikes (Wynne 1988). When safety technologies malfunctioned at Union Carbide's pesticide plant in Bhopal, India, untrained and inexperienced workers relied on their sense of smell to alert them to releases of toxic, and eventually deadly, methyl isocyanate (Jasanoff 1994). In sum, technological standards offer no automatic guarantees of uniform compliance. To achieve similar levels of social welfare, standards have to be harmonized not merely at the level of testing and risk assessment but also in relation to the social context within which they are applied and implemented.

## POLITICS, CULTURE, AND RISK ASSESSMENT: THE US CASE

We noted above that quantitative risk assessment (QRA) occupies a place of unique importance in American regulatory decisionmaking, especially as a technique for controlling suspected carcinogens (Brickman et al. 1985; Jasanoff 1986; Rushefsky 1986; and, for a historical perspective, Porter 1995). Its headlong endorsement by the conservative Republican majority in the US House of Representatives in 1995, as well as support won from more moderate analysts of regulation (Breyer 1993), shows how deeply QRA influences Americans' ability to think coherently about threats from toxic substances. Even cursory comparisons with other OECD countries suggests that formal risk assessment plays a more central role in US chemical regulation than elsewhere (Jasanoff 1991; Hoberg and Harrison 1994).

The appearance of neutrality and order offers legitimation in all modern bureaucratic states, but quantitative methods of reasoning are perhaps most acutely desirable in the transparent, pluralistic, adversarial, and hence distrustful, political culture of the United States. QRA appears in this respect to be a distinctive cultural achievement, answering to particular social and political needs of the US polity. I dwell briefly below on three dimensions of this cultural role: the treatment of causation, agency, and uncertainty in QRA. Under each heading, we see that QRA, while providing a superficially impartial basis for governmental action, actually helps to control and limit potentially destabilizing political debate.

### *Causation*

In the world of regulatory risk assessment, causation generally is conceived of as a linear and mechanistic process. The classical model of carcinogen risk assessment still used by most US federal regulatory agencies views the risk of cancer as the result of individual or population exposure to single harmful agents. Of course, regulatory experts have learned over the years to add complexity to this causal picture. The recognition that cancer is a multistage process has displaced the earlier single-hit model of carcinogenesis, and modelers have tried to express the results of the new causal scheme mathematically by differentiating, among others, the initiation stage from the stage of promotion. Risk is known to be distributed over populations of diverse composition and susceptibility, exposed for variable lengths of time, and by multiple pathways. Quantitative models have grown increasingly sophisticated as they have sought to combine and manipulate all these variables. With each methodological reform, confidence rises within the regulatory community that the numbers generated by QRA are getting more reliable.

But how accurately does QRA represent the totality of what is known about the causes of cancer? A closer look immediately reveals the partial and selective character of even the most up-to-date efforts at modeling. In focusing on particular substances, for example, others are necessarily ignored. Bruce Ames and his colleagues have been arguing for many years that most industrial chemicals should be of far less concern than identical or similar substances to which exposure occurs 'naturally' through the diet (see, for example, Ames 1989). Their work has attracted an ideological following, as well as much controversy, precisely because it seeks to impose on mainstream risk assessment approaches an alternative, more comprehensive, and some would say more accurate, picture of chemically induced cancer – one that does not delegate all 'causes' to the human-made side of the human-nature boundary.

The work of Ames and his colleagues tends to exonerate many of the chemical bad actors that have occupied policymakers and social activists for 25 years. Such a refocusing of the existing policy agenda could not fail to be seen as deeply political. Moreover, complicating the idea of causation to include natural as well as non-natural carcinogens would not necessarily lead to reduced concern about exposure to industrial pollution or chemical products, as evidenced by the recent concern about 'hormone disrupters' in the environment (Colborn et al. 1996). Quantitative models often simplify the world in ways that dampen the public's perception of risk, and these understating effects, too, would have to be accommodated. The impact of multiple exposure routes and possible synergistic effects is rarely captured in routine quantitative assessments. Behavioral patterns that may aggravate risk for particular subpopulations (a well-known example is smoking among asbestos workers) are similarly downplayed or disregarded. Socio-economic factors that tend to concentrate risk from many sources for poor, minority, and disenfranchised populations are only now beginning to gain attention under pressure from the environmental justice movement. An expanded debate on causation might open up all of these issues, creating demands for reassurance that could not be met by current science or current policy. QRA helps keep such political pressures in check.

### *Agency*

A second issue that remains barely visible beneath the veil of QRA methodologies is the allocation of agency. Implicit in the use of QRA is the notion that risk originates in the inanimate world. Both regulators and the public know, of course, that this is only a simplifying assumption; yet it is an acceptable simplification because it serves modern society's need for control and social order. It is, after all, easier to manage inanimate things (and the impersonal corporations that produce them) than animate people, even when people are known to be part of the problem one wishes to control. It is this mindset that the National Rifle Association (NRA), the US gun-owners' lobby, brilliantly challenges with its well-known bumper slogan, 'Guns don't kill people, people kill people.' But a little reflection shows that the NRA's sociological insight could be generalized to most material agents that are identified as the primary risk-creators in mathematical models.

Organizational sociologists such as Perrow (1984) and Clarke (1989) have pointed out the complicated ways in which physical and human elements of technological systems interact to produce risky conditions, accidents, and disasters. The French sociologists Callon (1986) and Latour (1994) have gone even further by refashioning our understanding of the separation between animate and inanimate actors. For them, even the most humble human artifact (a door stop, a speed bump, or a bicycle) represents a physically stabilized, congealed embodiment of an entire history of social assumptions, conventions, interests, and cultural practices. One of the more remarkable achievements of human technological enterprise, in their view, is that at the end of all this activity we still have a world that seems so cleanly divided between the human and the non-human, the animate and the inanimate, the social and the mechanical.

The force of these insights is dramatically realized when technological systems fail to work, as in the wake of major disasters, and a cause must be found for the failure. The 'constructedness' of the social-technical boundary becomes most obvious at such moments. Thus, when the Challenger space shuttle exploded, the presidentially appointed Rogers Commission squarely blamed a management structure that failed to convey the engineers' concerns to the uppermost reaches of political decisionmaking (Gieryn and Figert 1990). At the same time, one Commission member, the famed physicist Richard Feynman, captured media headlines with his celebrated demonstration that the disaster had a mechanical 'cause': a crucial rocket part, a rubber o-ring, had become inelastic at the freezing temperature of water and hence had failed during a cold-weather launch. Yet in the Rogers Commission's inquiry, blame for so traumatic a national tragedy could not credibly be laid on something so mute and insignificant as a defective o-ring. *People* had to be held accountable for killing people; the management, the Commission held, should have known and acted on the defect. By contrast, prospective risk assessment – the mathematical prediction of future harm – tends to focus exclusively on the dangers of things. Little or no allowance is made for the permeability of the human and material spheres, the interchangeability of 'thing-causes' and 'people-causes' (Gieryn and Figert 1990), or the social uncertainty that flows from this sharing of the responsibility for accidents.

*Uncertainty*

A third observation about the cultural dimension of quantitative risk assessment has to do with the representation of uncertainty. It could well be argued that QRA has made the greatest strides in the past ten years in its ability to conceptualize and mathematize uncertainty (NRC 1994). Techniques are now available for capturing – often in useful and understandable forms – zones of uncertainty that previously were simplified all too often into point estimates of risk.

Uncertainty, however, is not so much a measure of the unknown as a socially constructed state of mind about what we are willing to puzzle out (Wynne 1995). To admit uncertainty in policy forums is to state, in ways that society finds acceptable, that there are certain features of the human condition that we do not know but that we have the means and will to investigate further. We have seen intriguing suggestions in the risk literature that even very similar societies, such as the nations of the industrialized west, differ considerably in the way they draw the boundaries between knowledge and uncertainty, and uncertainty and ignorance. For example, Wynne and Mayer (1993) suggest that British scientists may be particularly reluctant to admit uncertainty, let alone ignorance, in their public pronouncements on risk; the BSE (bovine spongiform encephalopathy) scare of 1996 is just one episode that lends credence to this claim (see also Irwin and Wynne 1996). The US approach, by contrast, has been to recognize many uncertainties openly but to subject them all to formal calculation through QRA. In the process of mathematization, the cultural and political origins of 'uncertainty' are erased, and numerical estimates of the unknown acquire a misleadingly objective and universal appearance.

## STANDARDIZATION AS RECIPROCAL COMMENTARY

If national safety standards and the analytic methods that produce them reflect such deep-seated cultural norms, then how should international standard-setting organizations conceive their role in attempting to harmonize national practices? A recent study of international institutions active in the area of environmental decisionmaking credited them with the ability to increase governmental concern through knowledge creation; to enhance the contractual environment for bargaining through monitoring of environmental quality and performance; and to build national capacity through provision of technical expertise (Haas et al. 1994). This model implicitly conceptualizes international institutions as instruments of policy convergence, working to bring all parties up to some common, presumably optimal and agreed upon level of safe practice. Their main contributions are to facilitate negotiation, disseminate knowledge, create transparency, and improve the condition of the weakest players, so as to compensate for radical unevenness on the playing fields of multilateral action.

One can point to an impressive roster of international organizations that conform to just this pattern of activity with respect to industrial hazard prevention. The technical harmonization efforts of the OECD and, at a regional level, the European Commission have been especially important in this regard; work products include standardized testing methods and protocols, as well as standards governing a whole range of hazardous activities, products, and substances (workplace hazards, food additives, industrial chemicals, pesticides, etc.). The role of the United Nations Environment Programme (UNEP) in fostering information exchange, as well as its proactive involvement in forging transnational 'epistemic communities' on pollution in the Mediterranean (Haas 1990) and stratospheric ozone depletion (Benedick 1991), provide additional examples. One should not underestimate the significance of these efforts, especially in terms of their ability to assist weaker, resource-poor actors. Yet, to the extent that these efforts are founded on unconscious assumptions about the objectivity of 'safety' or the value-neutrality of standards – assumptions that should no longer be taken for granted – they need to be supplemented by activities that more nearly approach the goal of 'reciprocal commentary' envisaged by Geertz.

The constructivist analysis proposed in this paper points to a potentially more dynamic role for international standard-setting agencies. Harmonization can be recognized as a fruitful site for exchange among competing views of knowledge, politics, and action – not merely as a bureaucratic procedure to facilitate convergence toward some determinate, technically calculated policy endpoint. The power of harmonization would flow importantly in this model from its capacity to reframe problems for collective solution, to extend the boundaries and parameters of relevant knowledge, and to translate experiences gained in one socio-political context to the needs and circumstances of others. Harmonization would become more explicitly a vehicle for parties with divergent views about risk to reason together.

The concept of harmonization as reciprocal commentary might be put into operation in several ways by agencies entrusted with chemical risk and safety:

*Information gathering*
Harmonizing institutions could begin to diversify the nature as well as the forms of information they collect about chemical hazards. Traditional technical inputs – toxicity data, plant design specifications, emergency response measures – could be supplemented by qualitative information, gathered and stored in unconventional formats, such as case studies or histories of prior practice. Additional types of data, too often neglected even in mature national regulatory programs, might include information about participatory procedures, monitoring and enforcement records, and feedback mechanisms. Such information would provide the social context of standards and facilitate inquiry into their success or failure.

*Effectiveness measures*
Working with a suitably expanded data base, harmonizing institutions could play a proactive role in developing criteria for cross-national comparisons of effectiveness. Such measures would necessarily require a deeper probing of the social and cultural commitments underlying divergent national approaches to risk regulation. Comparative analysis might permit programs and their effectiveness to be evaluated by criteria that are neither strictly program-specific nor solely economic and technical. One could begin to consider, for example, whether some approaches to risk management promote civic values, increase trust, and provide public information, in addition to preventing and mitigating hazards.

- *Model building*
  Harmonizing institutions could serve as a marketplace for testing and disseminating alternative models of risk management. Policy systems often fall hostage to imperfect causal models whose background assumptions (as in the case of QRA in the United States) are never questioned or reopened for review. To some degree, this state of affairs flows from the long-entrenched tendency to compartmentalize technological and social analysis in most regulatory systems, as in the separation of risk assessment from risk management. Such rigid boundary drawing can frustrate regulatory objectives. To take an especially salient example, Lipschutz (1991:40) argues that technological efforts to control air pollution in the United States fell short because they "focused almost entirely on the 'hardware' – the car – rather than on the entire web of material, structural, and ethical relations that constitute the 'Automobile'." Hajer (1995) extends this critique by showing how even a more explicitly social discourse – the discourse on sustainable development – failed to wean German policies for urban mobility from an excessive preoccupation with inflexible, large-scale technological solutions. Harmonizing bodies, as cross-cultural institutions, could seek to encourage greater creativity in policy design by bringing alternative problem framings, supported by different models of causation and agency, into productive dialogue.

- *Capacity building*
  This has long been considered one of the core functions of international institutions and should remain so. But the analytic approach I propose here implies that the 'capacity' of the makers and users of 'technical information' programs should be broadened to include a deeper understanding of institutions, culture, and history. Learning about policy performance, in particular, should focus not merely on superficial assessments of success or failure, but also on the reasons for varying outcomes, on trends and changes in trends over time, and on the systematic ways in which social and political systems respond to shocks and accidents, both big and small.

## HARMONIZATION AS A POLITICAL PROCESS

Harmonizing institutions stand, as it were, at the frontline of the clash between modernity and postmodernity. Their very existence and the increasing scope and diversity of their mandates testify to the continuing hunger of modern societies for progress toward a future of increased safety, health, material comfort, and psychological well-being. Yet in trying to meet these multiple demands, harmonizing bodies risk falling victim to the contradictions of postmodernity. Different cultural constructions of the 'same' policy problem make agreement difficult in spite of apparent similarities in national goals and aspirations; where consensus is reached, ambiguities subsequently resurface in the process of implementation; convergence among experts proves inadequate to reassure skeptical publics and command political assent.

The 1996 BSE scare in Europe provided a dramatic but typologically by no means isolated instance of the challenges of harmonization. The European Union's efforts to construct a unified, science-based standard to calm citizens confronting (ostensibly) the 'same' risk of disease from the 'same' agent fractured against the discrepant perceptions of farmers, parents, food producers, government scientists, independent scientists, public health officials, agriculture ministers, politicians facing reelection, anti-European Britons, and the Brussels bureaucracy. Quantitative analysis proved miserably inadequate for bridging these far-flung interests, as ministers wrestled week after week to agree on a single magic number – the number of cows that would have to be culled to render the beef supply adequately 'safe' for all uses. Cartoons, black humor, and bizarre role reversals seized the political stage in this latter-day *comédie humaine* (Jasanoff 1997). Butchers in the markets of Europe took over the expert's reassuring role, with official-looking signs to back up their guarantees of 'no British beef sold here.' Ministers, having vainly deferred to science in the first place, were later forced to regain credibility through personalized expressions of consumer confidence: "Beef will still be served. Myself and my family will continue to eat beef" (John Gummer, as quoted in the *Independent*, March 22, 1996:5).

National policy institutions – shored up by history, tradition, established policy discourses, and common standards of fairness and rationality – may be able to persuade most of their publics most of the time that they can deliver objective solutions to complex problems. International harmonizing bodies have few if any of these legitimating props at their disposal. As risks such as BSE proliferate and assume global proportions, harmonizing institutions can only find it more difficult to pass off as impartial expert judgment the intensely political act of mediating among competing cultural framings of risk. Standards, whether expressed in the form of numbers, work routines, protocols or practices, are likely to wear increasingly thin as they are stretched to cover worlds of perceptual divergence.

Letting the messiness of politics back into harmonization may well be more productive in many cases than leaning too hard on the supports of science. In the end, standard-setting, like politics, represents the art of the possible: how to find common ground when confronted by uncertainty and perhaps irreducible conflicts. Mutual education, even more than strict policy convergence, seems the most appropriate objective for harmonization. If culture permeates the way people reason about risk, then learning to reason together may be more productive than trying to calculate a universally valid standard of control. The former goal, more modest as well as more honest than the latter, is quite consistent with the postmodern impetus of harmonization.

## References

Agarwal, A. & S. Narain (1991) *Global Warming in an Unequal World*, New Delhi: Centre for Science and Environment.

Ames, B.N. (1989) 'What Are the Major Carcinogens in the Etiology of Human Cancer? Environmental Pollution, Natural Carcinogens, and the Causes of Human Cancer: Six Errors', in V.T. de Vita, Jr., S. Hellman, and S.A. Rosenberg, eds., *Important Advances in Oncology*, 1989, Philadelphia: Lippincott; 237-247.

Barnthouse, L.W., J. Boreman, S.W. Christensen, C.P. Goodyear, W. Van Winkle & D.S. Vaughn (1984) 'Population Biology in the Courtroom: The Hudson River Controversy', *BioScience*, 34:14-19.

Benedick, R.E. (1991) *Ozone Diplomacy*, Cambridge, MA: Harvard University Press.

Bijker, W.E., T.P. Hughes & T. Pinch (1987) *The Social Construction of Technological Systems*, Cambridge, MA: MIT Press.

Breyer, S. (1993) *Breaking the Vicious Circle: Toward Effective Risk Regulation*, Cambridge, MA: Harvard University Press.

Brickman, R., S. Jasanoff & T. Ilgen (1985) *Controlling Chemicals: The Politics of Regulation in Europe and the United States*, Ithaca, NY: Cornell University Press.

Callon, M. (1986) 'Some Elements of a Sociology of Translation: Domestication of the Scallops and the Fishermen of St. Brieuc Bay', in: J. Law, ed. *Power, Action, and Belief: A New Sociology of Knowledge?*, London: Routledge and Kegan Paul; 196-233.

Clarke, L. (1989) *Acceptable Risk? Making Decisions in a Toxic Environment*, Berkeley, CA: University of California Press.

Colborn, T., J.P. Meyers & D. Dumanoski (1996) *Our Stolen Future*, New York: Little, Brown and Company.

Collins, H.M. (1985) *Changing Order: Replication and Induction in Scientific Practice*, London: Sage Publications.

Geertz, C. (1983) *Local Knowledge*, New York: Basic Books.

Gieryn, T.F. & A.E. Figert (1990) 'Ingredients for a Theory of Science in Society: O-Rings, Ice Water, C-Clamp, Richard Feynman, And the Press', in: S.E. Cozzens & T.F. Gieryn, eds., *Theories of Science in Society*, Bloomington, IN: Indiana University Press; 67-97.

Haas, P.M. (1990) *Saving the Mediterranean*, New York: Columbia University Press.

Haas, P.M., R.O. Keohane & M. Levy, eds. (1994) *Institutions for the Earth*, Cambridge, MA: MIT Press.

Hajer, M. (1995) 'Politics on the Move: Towards the Democratic Control of the Design of Sustainable Technologies', *Knowledge and Policy* 8: 26-39.

Hammond, A.L., E. Rodenburg & W.R. Moomaw (1991) 'Calculating National Accountability for Climate Change', *Environment* 33: 11-15, 33-35.

Hoberg, G. & K. Harrison (1994) *Risk, Science and Politics: Regulating Toxic Substances in Canada and the United States*, Montreal: McGill-Queen's University Press.

Irwin, A. & B. Wynne (1996) *Misunderstanding Science?*, Cambridge: Cambridge University Press.

Jasanoff, S. (1986) *Risk Management and Political Culture*, New York: Russell Sage Foundation.

Jasanoff, S. (1987) 'Cultural Aspects of Risk Assessment in Britain and the United States', in B.B. Johnson & V.T. Covello, eds., *The Social and Cultural Construction of Risk*, New York: Reidel.

Jasanoff, S. (1991) 'American Exceptionalism and the Political Acknowledgment of Risk', *Daedalus* 119: 61-81.

Jasanoff, S. (1997) 'Civilization and madness: The great BSE scare of 1996', *Public Understanding of Science,* 6: 221-32.

Jasanoff, S., ed. (1994) *Learning from Disaster: Risk Management After Bhopal*, Philadelphia: University of Pennsylvania Press.

Latour, B. (1994) 'On Technical Mediation – Philosophy, Sociology, Genealogy', *Common Knowledge* 3: 29-64.

Laurence, D. & B. Wynne (1989) 'Transporting Waste in the European Community: A Free Market?', *Environment* 31: 12-17, 34-35.

Lipschutz, R.D. (1991) 'Wasn't the Future Wonderful? Resources, Environment, and the Emerging Myth of Global Sustainable Development', *Colorado Journal of International Environmental Law and Policy* 2: 35-54.

MacKenzie, D. (1990) *Inventing Accuracy: A Historical Sociology of Nuclear Missile Guidance*, Cambridge, MA: MIT Press.

National Research Council (1994) *Science and Judgment*, Washington, DC: National Academy Press.

Nelkin, D., ed. (1992) *Controversy*, 3rd ed., Newbury Park, CA: Sage.

Perrow, C. (1984) *Normal Accidents*, New York: Basic Books.

Pinch, T. (1993) '"Testing-One, Two, Three...Testing": Toward a Sociology of Testing,' *Science, Technology, and Human Values* 18: 25-41.

Porter, T.M. (1992) 'Objectivity as Standardization: The Rhetoric of Impersonality in Measurement, Statistics, and Cost-Benefit Analysis', in A. Megill, ed., *Rethinking Objectivity, II, Annals of Scholarship* 9: 19-59.

Porter, T.M. (1995) *Trust in Numbers: The Pursuit of Objectivity in Science and Public Life*, Princeton, NJ: Princeton University Press.

Putnam, R.D. (1992) *Making Democracy Work: Civic Traditions in Modern Italy*, Princeton, NJ: Princeton University Press.

Rushefsky, M. (1986) *Making Cancer Policy*, New York: SUNY Press.

Salter, L. (1993) 'The Housework of Capitalism', *International Journal of Political Economy* 23: 105-135.

Subak, S. (1991) 'Commentary on the Greenhouse Index', *Environment* 33: 2-3.

Thompson, M., M. Warburton & T. Hatley (1986) *Uncertainty on a Himalayan Scale*, London: Ethnographica.

Winner, L. (1977) *Autonomous Technology: Technics Out-of-Control as a Theme in Political Thought*, Cambridge, MA: MIT Press.

Winner, L. (1986) 'Do Artifacts Have Politics?', in: *The Whale and the Reactor*, Chicago: University of Chicago Press.

Wynne, B. (1987) *Risk Management and Hazardous Waste: Implementation and the Dialectics of Credibility*, Berlin: Springer Verlag.

Wynne, B. (1995) 'Public Understanding of Science', in: S. Jasanoff et al., *Handbook of Science and Technology Studies*, Thousand Oaks, CA: Sage Publications; 361-388.

Wynne, B. & S. Mayer (1993) 'How Science Fails the Environment', *New Scientist* 5 June: 33-35.

## DISCUSSIONS

### *The international arena*

Questions and comments following the presentation by *Feron*

*Rothstein*. It has been said that consensus in scientific expert committees should be reached on the basis of scientific information. However, the assessment of what is considered to be sufficient scientific information involves non-scientific considerations. The wide variation in standards as to what constitutes sufficient information in different sectors of, for example, the chemical industry suggests that this requires more examination.

*Feron*. That is a question of history. The committee itself has to decide if they can do it on the basis of the data. I would be very suspicious if you give the same basis data to two different committees and they were to come up with the same value. I trust committees much more when they have different considerations.

*Nilsson*. Feron has positive experiences with his committees, but that is because of the character of the committees: the people are selected because they are qualified. So for example, IPCS selects people for their qualities. But CODEX is completely different. Here countries' interests are represented. These people are political animals. Local administrations appoint them. There has also been a lot of pressure on the IPCS to adopt the system of government appointments.

Questions and comments following the presentation by *Van Damme*

*Bal.* Van Damme makes a plea for an independent committee which should do the assessments, free from any democratic procedures. But man-made mineral fibres have been under review by two committees, in the Netherlands and in Germany, which are both independent yet have come up with different conclusions from the same evidence. What guarantee can 'independence' give then?

*Van Damme.* The committee in Luxembourg has a rather good guarantee that it is an independent group. But my worry is that, even then, they have no control over the data, which are controlled by the industry. With respect to man-made mineral fibres, IARC has made extensive epidemiological observations, but because IARC does not have sufficient resources, the research is to a large degree financed by industry. Then we have new data, but they cannot be released because industry disagrees with the release of the data. That is a new thing we are facing now.

*Younes.* You don't need to doubt the integrity of the scientists in these two committees, because although they have looked at the same data, the reason that they came up with different conclusions was very simple: the German committee used studies where fibres were injected intraperitoneally. Whether these data can be extrapolated or not, is a matter of scientific debate. The Dutch disregarded some experiments, because they thought they were not sound. We got the two groups together and they discussed the data. That is the advantage of having an independent international group. In the end they agreed that, looking at the whole database, you cannot reach either conclusion, so what we need is more evidence, more research.

Questions and comments following the presentation by *Nilsson*

*Abraham.* I am more pessimistic on the consequences of Sweden joining the EU. In the case of drug regulation, there was always a reluctance by Sweden to adapt to international developments, but since 1 January 1995, regulators are afraid of a reduction of public interest representation.

*Nilsson.* Sweden should support its actions well, with scientific arguments, not just politically motivated ones.

*Jasanoff.* Why can we not interprete your talk as an example of the commitment a regulatory toxicologist has to the regulatory paradigm of standardisation, serving the interests of industries?

*Nilsson.* You cannot do a risk assessment without meassuring any exposure, in contrast to what Feron said before. It is not that risk assessors favour one way or the other, it is that no risk assessment is done. That is primitive, not the state of the art in 1995.

Comments and questions following the presentation by *Jasanoff*

*Millstone.* One of the consequences of the Freedom of Information Act is that the agencies are increasingly vulnerable to an infinite deconstruction. Therefore they are increasingly surrounded by expert committees.

*Abraham.* In the field of medicine, a lot of international standardisation is driven by industrial interest in harmonizing the markets. In the procedure, there is a massive bias towards industry.

*Younes.* Jasanoff said that the Red Book was a product of the political situation in 1983 (NAS 1983). But in the 1994 re-evaluation *Science and Judgement* (NRC 1994) there is no reason given for deviating from the original – except for ecological risks. Why has this not changed, when the political situation has changed?

*Jasanoff.* There have been some changes. For instance, different types of risk assessment are introduced, such as a 'quick-and-dirty' look at the data. There is also a tiered approach that has a recursive feature, which is at the heart of a non-separationist risk assessment. In addition, the committee acknowledged that science and politics are not always that easy to divide.

## General discussion

*Bijker.* It seems to me there are three groups of issues for the discussion: (1) along the line of Jasanoff: what are we talking about when we want to harmonize? (2) Along the line of Nilsson: what might happen at the national level, as a consequence of international pressure, international organisation? And (3) what can happen in the international forum?

*Jasanoff.* I feel a bit frustrated about the fact that, in efforts to reach a common language, we are always forced to strip our presentations of the underpinnings, which are the mechanisms needed to go forward to a different level of understanding.

We are discussing risk, uncertainty, and science without referring to social constructivism or whatever you want to call it, and as a result we are trying to bridge the two repertoires – the essentialist and the communitarian – without anyone being forced to come out with where they are standing, with the exception of Eric Millstone. Unless we are able to bring in constructivism, it is going to be extremely difficult to get anywhere – except on the anecdotical level – for a productive communication.

*Bijker.* We do have a vocabulary, in two ways: either we use essentialist terms, clarify differences in regulation for example by stating that the Swedish have a particular character, 'they love nature' or 'the Dutch are more interested in trade'. Then, in a controversy there can only be one answer: ask nature, and it will give the answer to what is right. So basically, there cannot be a controversy. Another way, in line with constructivism, is more fruitful. This analysis stresses that, rather than asking the essence of nature, or of science, one should study how a particular group of people adopts certain views, that there are good reasons for both the German and the Dutch committee to adopt different views. Both views can be labelled scientific.

The question is what happens in practice when, for example, different groups of different nations come together in Brussels. What process does this start?

*Halffman.* One thing that is needed is the development of a kind of sensitivity of entirely different forms of rationalities, stepping out of your own disciplinary approach. For example, there is the story that scientists will always agree eventually. But from my own research I know that some scientists do not agree; they are not in the regulatory system, and they don't want to be. As an outsider, as a social scientist, I am studying these different rationalities, and I try to understand them from the inside. So the first step is to develop more sensitivity to understanding other insights, and to accept these as rational.

*Nilsson*. What we want social scientists to help us with is not technical risk assessment. The point is more that we did not take time to explain to people who don't know. For example, I have been thinking for quite a long time about writing an elementary high-school book on toxicology. So what we need to know from social scientists is how to educate people, how to get acceptance and to know why it is that people are so concerned about a small level of industrial carcinogens, and smoke and drink at the same time, which is much more dangerous.

*Bal*. In reply to Nillson, I don't think you should expect the kind of consensus from such a book that you expect from it. Even in one discipline, there are huge differences. So raising a kind of general public understanding might even worsen the consensus, create more controversy.

As a reaction to Jasanoffs' frustration: different views in our discussions fit into each other in questions such as: what kind of harmonisation do we want? In Nilsson's talk there were three levels: Which chemicals do we ban? How do we make decisions on these chemicals? and what kind of political culture do we want? So there are more agreements on a metalevel than Jasanoff seems to presume.

*Mayer*. There is a small world created in risk assessment and this is questioned, for example by the desirability of different types of risk, different alternatives. However in the risk debate at the moment, there is no forum for this social-political debate.

*Millstone*. I have a problem with the position of Nilsson and others, originating from the group of people trained as scientists, who think that therefore, *ipso facto*, every judgement they make is scientific. During my study of toxicology I have become convinced that it is full of social assumptions that the toxicologists don't want to acknowledge. What counts as a relevant or adequate model or test, is not a purely scientific judgement. To take 50 animals per dose-group in a lifetime study as an adequate model for a heterogenous population of many millions is a social judgement, not a merely technical one. And that is been denied.

*Somers.* Harmonisation can take place at three levels in the regulatory process. On two of them, data requirements and scientific estimation, a tremendous agreement has been reached in the last twenty years. But in the third phase, decisions on risk management, you get more disagreement. For the first two phases, there exist large international networks of industrial medicine, toxicologists and international organisations.

*Stijkel.* I have studied the work of the DECOS, analyzing the starting points and criteria and comparing them with the reports (Stijkel, et al. 1996). There emerges what I call an interpretative space. But the problem is that the committee is not open to discuss this and other contributions of other sciences.

*Passchier* (referring to the Health Council committee on environmental risk assessment, of which he is the secretary).[1] Advice should not be like 'we have done this research and these are our conclusions', but more that we can only say that we have something to offer that may help. If committees were to be more modest, then the problem of different committees getting different results would not be that great, because it is clear to everybody that this is not the final word.

*Bijker.* I will try to reformulate the discussion: Let us try to get one step further than the invocation that we have to get the science right and the values right. Everybody can think about how to organize this in practice, getting the science right, for example with Feron's list of the kind of people he wants in committees, specifying not only disciplinary backgrounds, but also personal character. We can think about the kinds of affiliation committees have, and how these structures will lead to particular kinds of scientific

---

1 Editors' note: the report Passchier refers to has meanwhile been published: Health Council of the Netherlands 1996.

evidence. Thinking along those lines might get us away from the paralyzing dichotomy of science and politics.

## REFERENCES

Health Council of the Netherlands: Committee on Health-Based Recommended Exposure Limits (1996) *Toxicology-Based Recommended Exposure Limits*, Rijswijk: Health Council of the Netherlands, No. 1996/12.

National Academy of Sciences (1983) *Risk Assessment in the Federal Government: Managing the Process*, Washington, DC: National Academy Press.

National Research Council (1994) *Science and Judgment*, Washington, DC: National Academy Press.

Stijkel, A., J. van Eijndhoven & R. Bal (1996) 'Drafting Guidelines for Occupational Exposure to Chemicals: The Dutch Experience With the Assessment of Reproductive Risks', *American Journal of Industrial Medicine* 30: 705-17.

# PART III

## STANDARDIZATION

# INTRODUCTION

Standardisation of test and assessment protocols is probably the most interesting domain where harmonisation is under way. These developments offer very interesting insights into the central tensions plaguing internationalisation and science/policy relations. On the one hand, the implications of these developments for risk regulation and their specific problems are rarely fully understood by policy analysts. If the standardisation of tests and assessment protocols can be seen as a way of introducing new forms of quality control in the scientific input in decision making, several questions come to mind: why, how and where are assessment methods standardised? What is their role in decision making? And what are the problems of (international) standardisation of protocols for testing and assessment? The answers to these questions should clarify the importance of method development programs of the Commission of the European Union, of the activities of the OECD, and of various national research programs.

The development of increasingly standardised test systems also has important consequences for the position of experts in assessment procedures. Questions that can be asked in this regard are: will standardisation reduce the role of expert judgement? And would such an effect restrict the kind of health and environmental effects that can be determined by the assessment procedures?

These questions relate directly to the issue of internationalisation, since the implementation of international standardisation may offer interesting examples of the changing roles of national expert committees. But standardisation also relates to the political dimensions of the regulatory process, as well as to the boundary between risk assessment and management. In this regard the following questions are important: are standardised tests and protocols successful in limiting extensive political conflict over risk? To what extent, and in what ways, is standardisation a mechanism of exclusion?

And will increasing standardisation disturb the delicate balance between science and policy in different national contexts?

Patrick McCutcheon starts off this part with an introduction to the European Union program on environmental chemical risk regulation. He focuses on the procedure for existing substances (falling under Council Regulation 793/93), discussing the data requirements of the procedure, its priority setting, the risk assessment phase, the phase of risk reduction recommendation, as well as the relationship to the OECD and WHO programs. Standardised tests and protocols for assessment play an important role in this program. They are, according to McCutcheon, primarily intended to facilitate communication between the actors involved, as well as between different regulatory programs, and to enhance the transparency of the process.

The contribution by Alan Irwin, Elaine McCarthy, Henry Rothstein and Steve Yearley discusses the consequences of EU harmonisation and standardisation for 'regulatory science' on agrochemicals in the UK. Their research suggests that a new kind of science is emerging in which traditional boundaries – between disciplines, between research & development and (eco)toxicological testing among others – are becoming less visible. This new science, which is heavily influenced by regulatory programs, develops along different paths than the more traditional 'research science'. They discuss the characteristics of this new kind of science, suggesting five different forms in which this activity takes place, and show that these new practices are taking form in different organisational settings. They furthermore discuss the consequences this has for our view of 'science' in the regulatory process.

Peter Calow's contribution reflects and builds upon his experiences in the area of ecotoxicology testing methods, more specifically, on the standardisation of the *Daphnia* test, a key element of EU legislation. He describes the work that has to be done for the standardisation of one test, including the organisation of several workshops, the performance of round-robin tests and extensive consultation procedures. Calow perceives standardisation to be inevitable, both from a scientific and a legal standpoint. He argues that standardisation has scientific as well as political aspects, where the latter has to do, among other things, with the decision about what it is that needs to be standardised. In other words: what is most valued in nature that needs protection through standardised tests? Calow argues that in most standardisation processes such decisions are taken implicitly by scientists, and are not debated in a political arena. The challenge is, he argues, to design ways in which an informed and useful input can be made by all relevant parties.

In his contribution, Willem Halffman draws a parallel between the way trust is guaranteed amongst experts and the way trust is guaranteed between experts and non-experts. He argues that drawing this parallel can help experts to understand their status of mistrusted, about which they so often complain. He argues that trust is maintained through various 'trust devices': technical, social, or literary structures that regulate whom can be trusted and when. One of the devices of central importance in the regulatory world is standardisation. Unfortunately for those who are looking for simple solutions, he shows that standardisation and other such trust devices only have a limited capacity to restore or maintain trust. They only seem to work in rather specific contexts and can even have the opposite effect when not in correspondence to those contexts. The art of being a trusted regulatory scientist seems to be knowing when to resort to which one of the repertoires of trust devices.

# 8

*Patrick McCutcheon*

# RISK MANAGEMENT OF CHEMICAL SUBSTANCES IN THE EUROPEAN UNION

## INTRODUCTION

Control of chemical substances has developed considerably in the post-world war II period when following major developments in chemistry; initially in the area of pharmaceuticals. With the development of antibiotics, pesticides and detergents leading to major improvements to living standards, problems related to chemicals started to become apparent: Minimata disease induced by bioavailable mercury, congenital defects of Thalidomide and later a number of serious accidental releases at Seveso, Bhopal and Basel. Whereas the earliest regulatory work focused mainly on narcotics and medicines, regulation of industrial chemicals in Europe is essentially a post World War II development.

The European Union Programme on Existing Substances established by Council Regulation (EEC) 793/93 (CEC 1993a) on the evaluation and control of the risk of existing substances which was adopted by Council on 23 March 1993 and came into force on 4 June 1993 can be considered part of the third generation of chemicals legislation in the Community. Directive 67/548/EEC (CEC 1967) on the approximation of laws on classification, packaging and labelling of dangerous substances is usually considered as the basic Community legislation though it had its antecedents in the Council of Europe publication of the Yellow Book series starting in 1962 which built on earlier ILO activity during 1950-1955. Council Directive 79/831/EEC (CEC 1979), the sixth amendment to this directive introduced the distinction

---

In: R. Bal & W. Halffman (eds.), *The Politics of Chemical Risk*, Kluwer Academic Publishers, Dordrecht 1998: p. 209-230.

between new and existing chemicals with requirements to deliver a minimum premarketing dataset for new substances as part of a premarketing procedure. The Regulation provides for the delivery by industry of available data on substances produced or imported above certain quantities. This data is then used to facilitate the selection of priority lists of substances for which risk assessments will be carried out by rapporteurs in the Member States.

The substances covered by Regulation 793/93 are those which were notified under Directive 79/831/EEC as being on the market in September 1981 and were listed in the European Inventory of Existing Commercial Chemical Substances (EINECS) (CEC 1990). Council Directive 92/32/EEC (CEC 1992a), the seventh amendment to Directive 67/548/EEC, introduced the requirement to carry out risk assessments for notified new substances.

Whereas a baseset of data generated by application of standard test methods and principles of good laboratory practice (CEC 1986, 1988) and risk assessment based thereon is required for new substances according to Directive 92/32/EEC, a different approach was proposed for existing substances due to the large number of substances listed in EINECS and a need for priority setting given the resource intensive nature of risk assessment. Where the EINECS inventory lists some 100.000 substances, these represent less than 1% of the more than 10.000.000 substances for which Chemical Abstract Service (CAS) numbers exist but nevertheless overstate the number of substances of commercial significance by perhaps a factor of 5-10.

This paper outlines how the Existing Substances Regulation is being implemented, describing the successive activities and the roles of the parties involved (scheme 1), and how the programme compares with and is related to other activities on chemicals evaluation at EC and international level.

*Scheme 1*: Council Regulation (EEC) 793/93 on the evaluation and control of existing substances

*step-by-step approach*

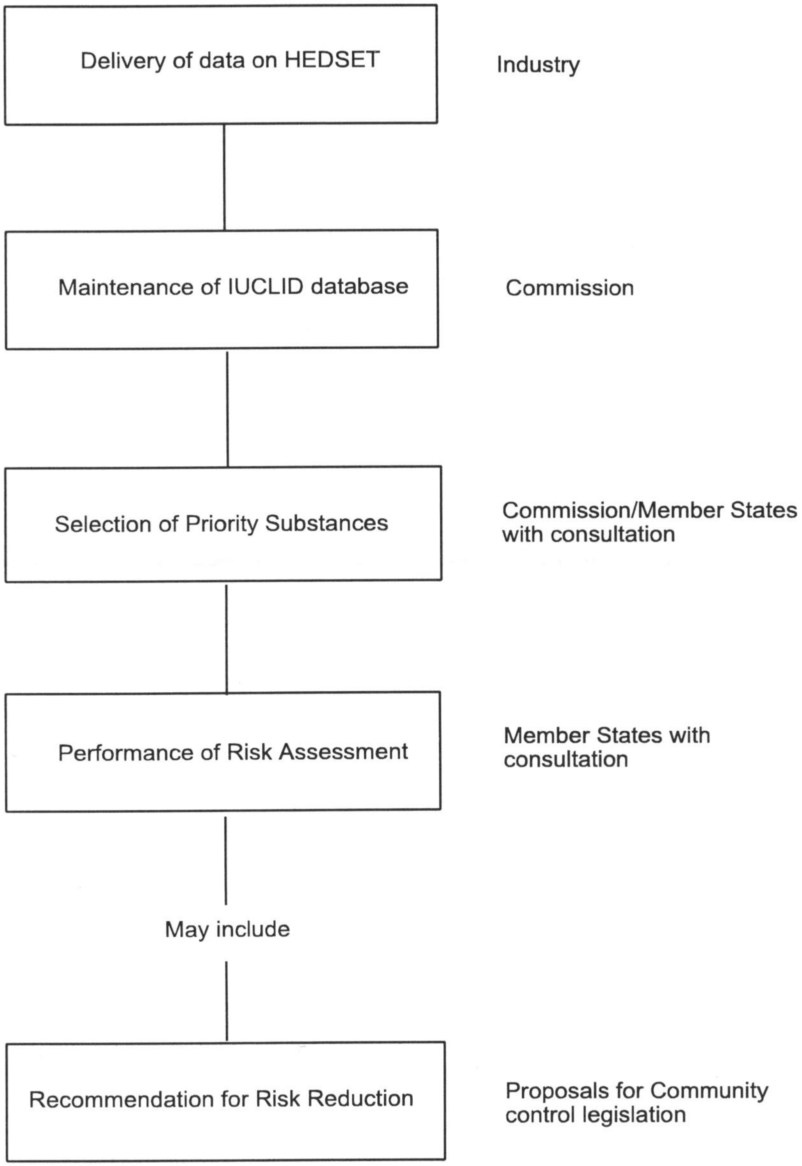

INITIAL DATA REQUIREMENTS

Recognition of the sheer number of existing substances produced or imported by individual corporate entities in excess of 10 tonnes and the resource intensive nature of the risk assessment process necessitated an approach different to that of new substances and somewhat similar to that of the active substances of plant protection products under Council Directive 91/414/EEC. Whereas a risk assessment is required for every new substance notified under Directive 92/32 and such assessments may be of a summary nature, evaluations are only required for those existing substances and pesticide active substances deemed to be of priority. The priority setting mechanism for existing substances is based on an initial delivery of available data and consideration of activity on the same substances under other programmes whereas all active substances of plant protection products require, over a 10 year period, evaluation as part of the product initial registration or re-registration process.

Regulation 793/93 distinguishes between three groups of existing substances according to the deadlines for delivery of the data:

- Data on High Production Volume (HPV) Substances listed in annex I of Regulation 793/93 had to be delivered by 4 June 1994 by all companies which produced or imported the substances in more than 1,000 tonnes per year in a defined three year period.

- Data on HPV Substances other than those listed in annex I listed in EINECS had to be delivered by 4 June 1995 by all companies which produced or imported the substances in more than 1,000 tonnes per year in the same three year period.

- Data on Low Production Volume (LPV) Substances must be delivered between 4 June 1996 – 4 June 1998 by all companies which produced or imported the substances in 10-1000 tonnes/annum in the same three year period.

The three years were defined as those preceding the adoption of the Regulation or in the year following adoption, i.e. during the period 23 March

1990 – 23 March 1994. Data on some 2500 substances was delivered during the first of these phases.

The data required in these first two phases comprised *available* information on production volumes and uses, physicochemical properties, toxicological and ecotoxicological effects as well as environmental fate as outlined in Annex III to the regulation. While these provisions provide an initial focus on high volume chemicals, a more complete data delivery may be required for lower volume substances for which there are grounds for concern. Some consideration is being given to a fourth phase delivery of some of this data for some lower volume substances.

*Data access and dissemination*

Access to all data will be, given the commercially sensitive nature of some of the data, restricted to persons *habilités aux secrets* of the Commission and the competent authorities of the Member States. Other versions excluding this sensitive data but which will still include all the scientific and technical data will also be made generally available. A more sophisticated software is more useful for searching data on existing substances as this data is being made generally available on CD-ROM whereas new substance information, like that on plant protection products is of considerable commercial value and will not be distributed beyond the regulatory authorities.

The dissemination medium foreseen is that of CD-ROM and of which two versions are available. This software, for which it is necessary to have an ORACLE licence, is essential where the user intends to exploit fully the searching permutations facilitated by the data structure. Where only basic document (dataset) retrieval or other simple queries are envisaged, this can be realised using the HEDSET software or other software which operates in a DOS environment. The Commission will also publish a simpler WINDOWS version of the non-confidential data on a CD incorporating retrieval software.

## PRIORITY SETTING

The purpose of the data delivery on existing substances is to facilitate the selection of priority substances. This will be based on an automated pre-analysis of the data and will also take into consideration both work being carried out in other fora or under other pieces of Community legislation and previous work of such programmes or legislation.

### *Ranking of existing substances for risk assessment*

The Member States have considered the use of a computerized model to rank chemicals according to relative risk comprising scores for physicochemical properties, human health and ecotoxicological effects and environmental fate, based on an analysis of the data pursuant to articles 3 and 4 of Regulation 793/93. This method, the so-called Informal Priority Setting (IPS) Methode, comprises an algorithm which selects data on about half of the endpoints covered in the initial dataset.

As data availability is variable, rules have been agreed on selection of a single result where many exist and estimated data from validated QSARs (Quantitative Structure Activity Relationships) are used to fill some data gaps. Since it is clear that a ranking produced by this or any model is certain to be based on assumptions and approximations and the relative subjectivity of weighting factors, a ranking on its own cannot constitute an adequate evaluation of risk to man and the environment and thus a model cannot be the only tool used in selection of priorities. The role of the ranking in selecting Priority Chemicals for evaluation per Regulation 793/93 is illustrated in Scheme 2.

The factors which should be considered in deriving the priority lists of existing substances from the ranking emanate from the policy outlined in article 8 of the Regulation:

- the effects of the substances on man or the environment;
- the exposure of man or the environment to the substance;
- the lack of data on the effects of the substance on man and the environment;

*Scheme 2:* Priority setting – overall scheme

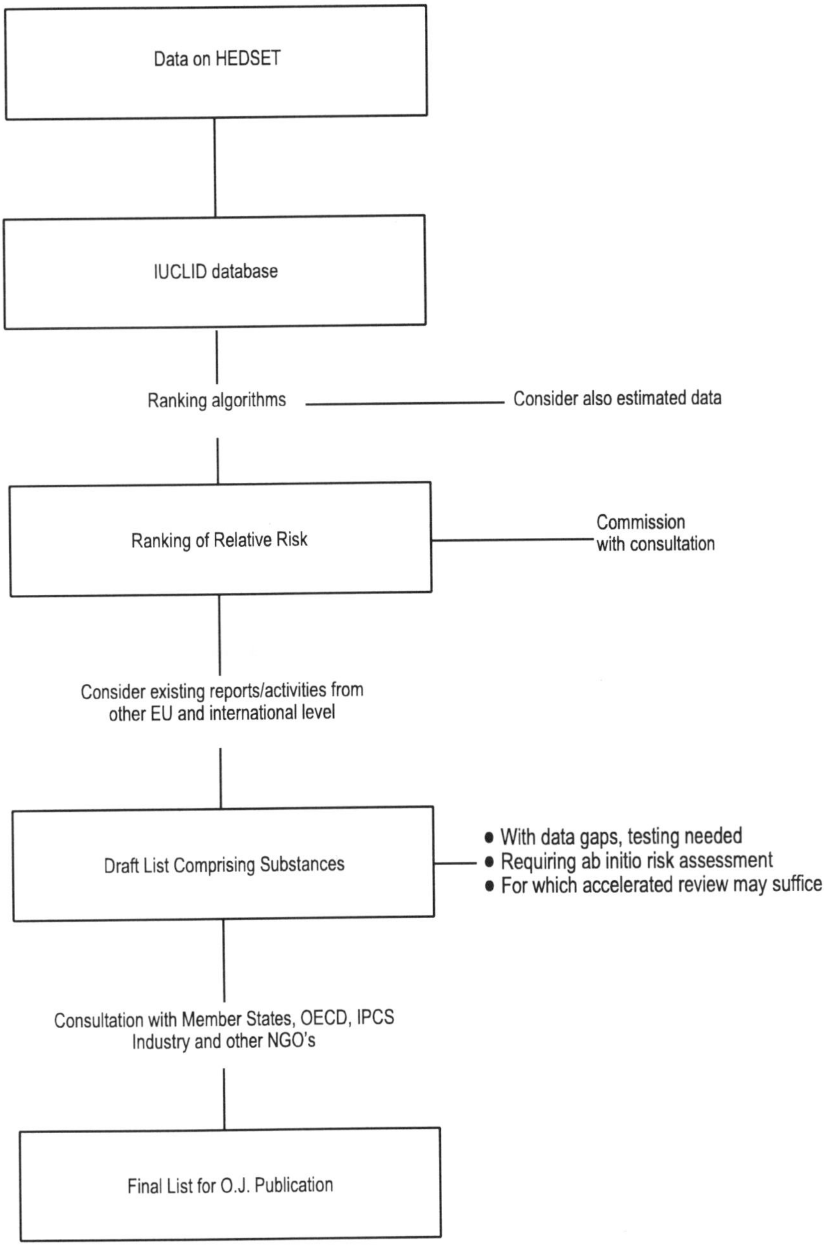

- work carried out in other international fora; and
- other Community legislation and/or programmes relating to dangerous substances.

The first two factors, the effects and the exposure, are considered by the algorithm. The lack of data on these factors is also considered, as some of the data gaps are filled with conservative default values where there are no data or QSARs. Work already carried out in international fora and under other legislative programmes and specific concerns are however not considered by the algorithm.

It has been agreed by the Member States Competent Authorities that an existing Risk Assessment report on a substance arising from work in other fora could either:

- lead to its being set-aside if that report indicates the substance is of low concern in which case the ranking is likely to be low; or
- lead to its being adopted as a candidate for a fast-track review where the report recommends risk reduction or indicates the substance is of concern.

These principles apply to reports generated pursuant to other Community legislation such as that on pesticides in the framework of Council Directive 91/414 and that on worker protection where these existing reports, although focused in their scope, may be more generally relevant. In most cases, substances which are essentially of occupational concern or used essentially as pesticides will not be considered for listing on priority lists under Regulation 793/93. The principles also apply to such international programmes as the OECD chemicals programme and the UN International Programme on Chemical Safety (IPCS), see the section on the relationship to other programmes below.

The criteria for selecting priorities for individual stages of the evaluation of existing plant protection product active substances are outlined in the recitals to Regulation 3600/92:

- health and environmental concern;
- possibility of residues in treated products;
- the importance of the preparations containing these substances; and
- manifest data gaps or conversely availability of complete data packages;

with the objective of carrying out an evaluation to determine whether or not a substance should be listed in annex I of Directive 91/414/EEC, i.e. whether or not it may be re-registered.

In considering these factors, priority lists may comprise three components:

- substances for which a preliminary analysis (using the algorithm) indicates that they are of concern (high ranking);
- substances for which few data are available and for which the ranking is high due to default values and/or acceptable QSAR estimated data;
- substances which are already the subject of a report produced in another forum indicating the substance is of concern.

Components 1 and 2 comprise substances for which a full ab-initio Risk Assessment must be carried out whereas component 3 comprises those for which an accelerated review of an existing report might be sufficient. It has been established by the Member States Competent Authorities that such an accelerated review must be in conformity with the principles and practice of risk assessment as laid down in respectively Commission Regulation 1488/94 (CEC 1994a) and the technical guidance documents; see the section on risk assessment below.

As priority setting involves the policy choices such as the number of data-poor substances to include, the derivation of the priority list will involve consultation with colleagues:

- in Member States, concerning national priorities, who may utilize product registers and other data in their consideration of priority;
- in various Commission services concerning other programmes likely to be carried out under other Community legislative action;
- in international programmes concerning current and possible future programmes;

- in Industry through the main European Chemical Industry Associations;
- in other non-governmental organisations such as labour, consumer and green organisations,

prior to formal adoption by the Member States in a voting committee which assigns each substance to a specific Member State rapporteur.

## RISK ASSESSMENT

Existing substances placed on a priority list are subject to an evaluation of risk based on Commission Regulation 1488/94 (CEC 1994b) which follows in principle that previously adopted for New Substances (Commission Directive 93/67/EEC, CEC 1993b). The Regulation is supported by more detailed *Technical Guidance Documents* which indicate how the assessment should be performed. The Guidance Documents are of a non legal status which, given the ongoing developments in the methodology of risk assessment, facilitate a more rapid review and revision than would be the case if they were formally published under legal instruments. Where separate guidance documents for new and existing substances were prepared during 1993 and 1994 respectively, a revised and amalgamated document has been developed (CEC 1996).

Given that the field of risk assessment is still developing and further revisions are likely once experience has been gathered following use of the guidance, it has been agreed that the guidance while necessary for harmonising the approach to risk assessment should not be used blindly, that it should be used with flexibility, intelligence and reasonableness. This approach of outlining principles in a piece of legislation supported by detailed guidance documents of an informal status is also followed in the Community proposal for a biocides directive (CEC 1993c).

Uncertainty with the science can only be dealt with by attempting to agree the terms for expert judgement input from both industry and regulators.

Evaluation of active substances of plant protection products is based on a set of uniform principles outlined in annex VI of directive 91/414. The basic principles of evaluation are common and involve a stepwise procedure as follows:

- Hazard Identification; identification of the (adverse) effects which a substance has the inherent capacity to cause;
- Effects Assessment; determination of the level or concentration at which the adverse effect does not result;
- Exposure Assessment; measurement or prediction of the exposure concentration at different stages of the product life-cycle for different human populations and environmental compartments; and
- Risk Characterization; estimation of the probability of the occurrence and severity of effects in a human population or environmental compartment,

noting that in drawing conclusions on the risk assessment some value judgement is involved.

Notwithstanding the common approaches, practical distinctions can be made between (1) new substances for which Annex V data is available on all toxicity and ecotoxicity endpoints required for the tonnage level of the substance and very little or no exposure information is available other than that which can be estimated, (2) existing substances where much toxicity data is available which has not been generated by Annex V tests, and exposure information may be plentiful but perhaps hard to access, and (3) plant protection active substances for which the information base is generally much larger than for many industrial chemicals.

*Evaluation, further data and testing*

Each substance selected as being of priority is formally assigned to a rapporteur in one of the competent authorities of the Member States who shall evaluate the data available in IUCLID (International Uniform Chemicals Information Database) for that substance as well as the data per annex VIIA of Commission Directive 92/32/EEC. The responsibility for delivering such data falls on those companies who submitted data on HEDSET for that substance. At this stage *all* the Annex VII data including detailed reports is required whereas the IUCLID data, while covering basically the same elements, is of a summary nature and may not be complete. Industry is required to generate any missing Annex XIIA data using Annex V tests of Directive 92/32. Risk assessment of a new substance is based on the appropriate annex VII dataset submitted with the notification dossier under the directive. Plant protection product active substances evaluated under Regulation 3600/92 are also assigned to specific rapporteurs.

For existing substances, the rapporteur shall draft a risk assessment report for consideration by the Member States and where appropriate recommend formally requesting further delivery of data and/or testing. Any further testing shall be carried out according to good laboratory practice as laid down in Directives 87/18/EEC and 86/609/EEC (CEC 1992a) and shall where possible avoid or limit use of animals. Although in principle further testing should be carried out by all companies such testing where necessary should be carried out by only one company on behalf of all. For new substances, all data should have been generated using Annex V test guidelines and GLP, whereas for plant protection product active substances, both Annex V and OECD test methods are accepted.

Whilst the rapporteur prepares a draft assessment and proposes further data delivery and testing, actual decisions are taken by a Committee of Member States which finally adopts the report which is then published; see Scheme 3. Decisions are taken by majority voting as laid down in article 148(2) of the Treaty of Rome (establishing the European Communities). The risk assessment procedure is also subject to specific deadlines. Further data and results of further testing on a priority substance must be delivered to the rapporteur within 6 and 12 months respectively of the request made by the Committee.

### *Risk assessment conclusions*

According to Regulation 1488/94 which outlines the principles of risk assessment for existing substances, risk assessment must conclude that there is:

> need for further information and/or testing (to arrive at one of the other conclusions);

*Scheme 3:* Risk assessment procedure from priority list to final assessment report

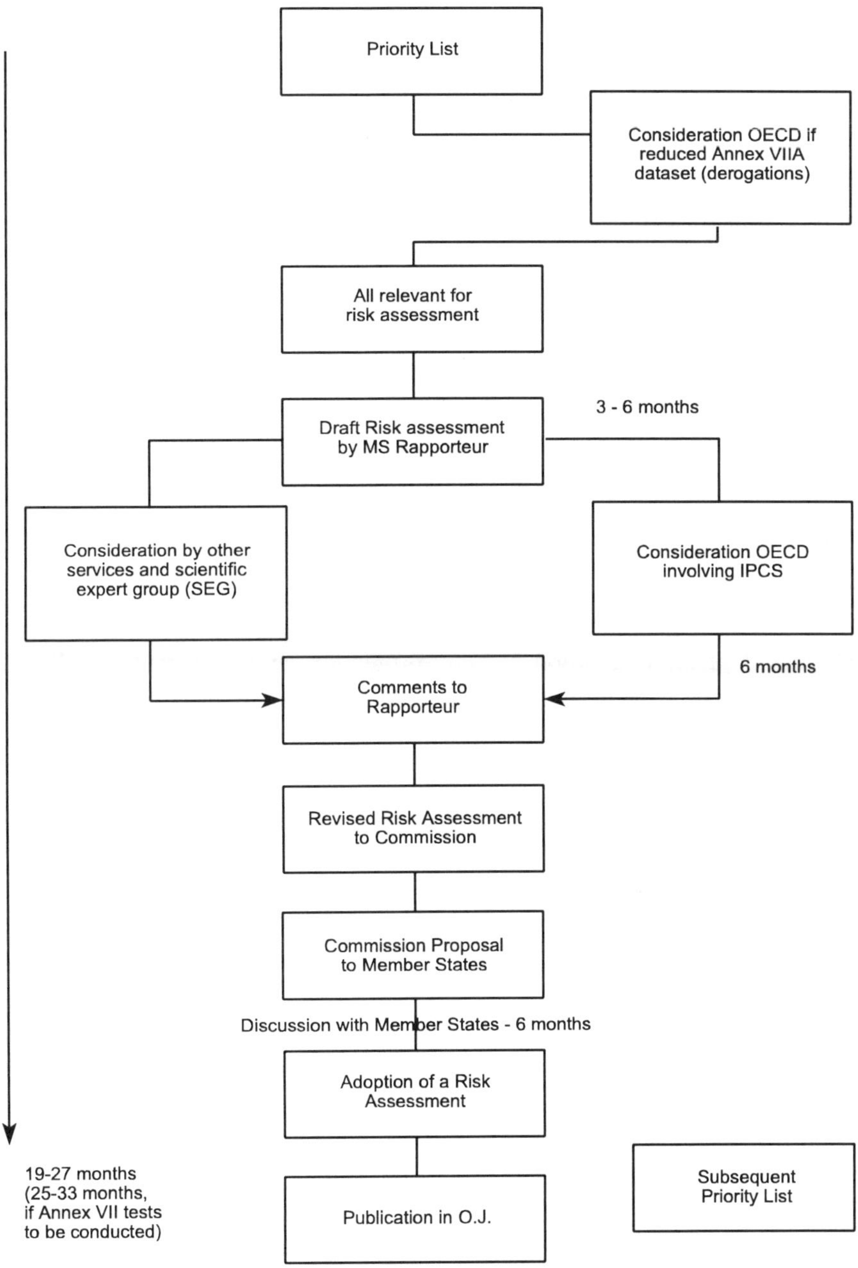

- no need for further information and/or testing and no need for further risk reduction measures; or
- need for limiting the risks and risk reduction measures are necessary in relation to one or more adverse effects on human populations and/or environmental spheres.

The risk reduction measures recommended may be taken up as the basis of proposals for Community measures in the framework of Council Directive 76/769/EEC relating to restrictions on marketing and use of certain dangerous substances and preparations and other relevant Community instruments.

In comparison, the evaluation of existing active substances under Regulation 3600/92 and Directive 91/414 conclude whether a substance is suitable for inclusion in its Annex I of the latter and thus whether or under what conditions or restrictions it may subsequently be used in re-registered products.

## RISK REDUCTION RECOMMENDATIONS

The result of the evaluation of plant protection active substances allows, or limits as the case may be, the use of that substance in product authorisations. Risk assessments of new substances accompanying notification dossiers can serve as an auto-control. As these substances are generally not used in applications where the risk would be unacceptable, these restrictions are occasionally mandatory, in other cases, assumed voluntarily. Existing substances thus remain on the market as before unless specific action is taken. Regulation 793/93 does not directly provide for risk reduction action though it may trigger it.

When the conclusion of the risk assessment of an existing substance is that the risks are not adequately managed, the rapporteur is required to propose a strategy to reduce these risks. Where the strategy considers marketing and use restrictions under Council Directive 76/769 – the essential Community instrument (CEC 1991c), which has been amended 16 times providing for specific restrictions on specific substances and preparations – an analysis of the advantages and drawbacks of the substance is also required.

Where the provisions of Regulation 793/93 are not more specific, additional guidance documents are in preparation which will assist the rapporteur in this additional analysis. Basically the guidance on the risk reduction strategy outlines the possible measures that can be taken during the life cycle of the substances to reduce the risk of exposure, the available instruments as well as the criteria, effectiveness, proportionality, monitorability and economic impact which should be considered in selecting a strategy.

Other than restrictions on marketing and use, risk reduction measures could involve redesigning processes, licencing of certain operations, emission limit values (CEC 1991a) and/or effluent monitoring as well as making available accurate information and safety training. In addition to regulatory control consideration is given to such non-traditional approaches such as voluntary agreements, information programmes, guidance and technical standards.

Where the Regulation refers to advantages and drawbacks of the substance, some such consideration might also be given to identified alternatives for which some data is available. In such a case, in stead of comparing advantages and drawbacks of a substance, alternative substances could be compared as regards their respective costs and benefits.

## RELATIONSHIP TO OTHER PROGRAMMES

This mainly concerns existing substances which require in Article 8.2 of Regulation 793/93, that priority substances shall be selected considering, inter alia, work done and programmes in other fora.

In order to avoid duplication of effort regarding future work and to go as far as possible in mutually recognizing existing work done in other fora, interaction between the Community programme and other programmes will be necessary at the various stages in the process, from defining priorities through to accepting risk assessments for those substances selected as priority (see scheme 4). This section will focus on the international programmes of the OECD and the UN. These programmes are conceptually similar to the existing substances programme of the EU and susceptible to interaction with it. Coordination is essentially and appropriately a task of interaction and demarcation between these programmes.

*Scheme 4:* Relation of Council Regulation 793/93 to international programmes on existing chemicals

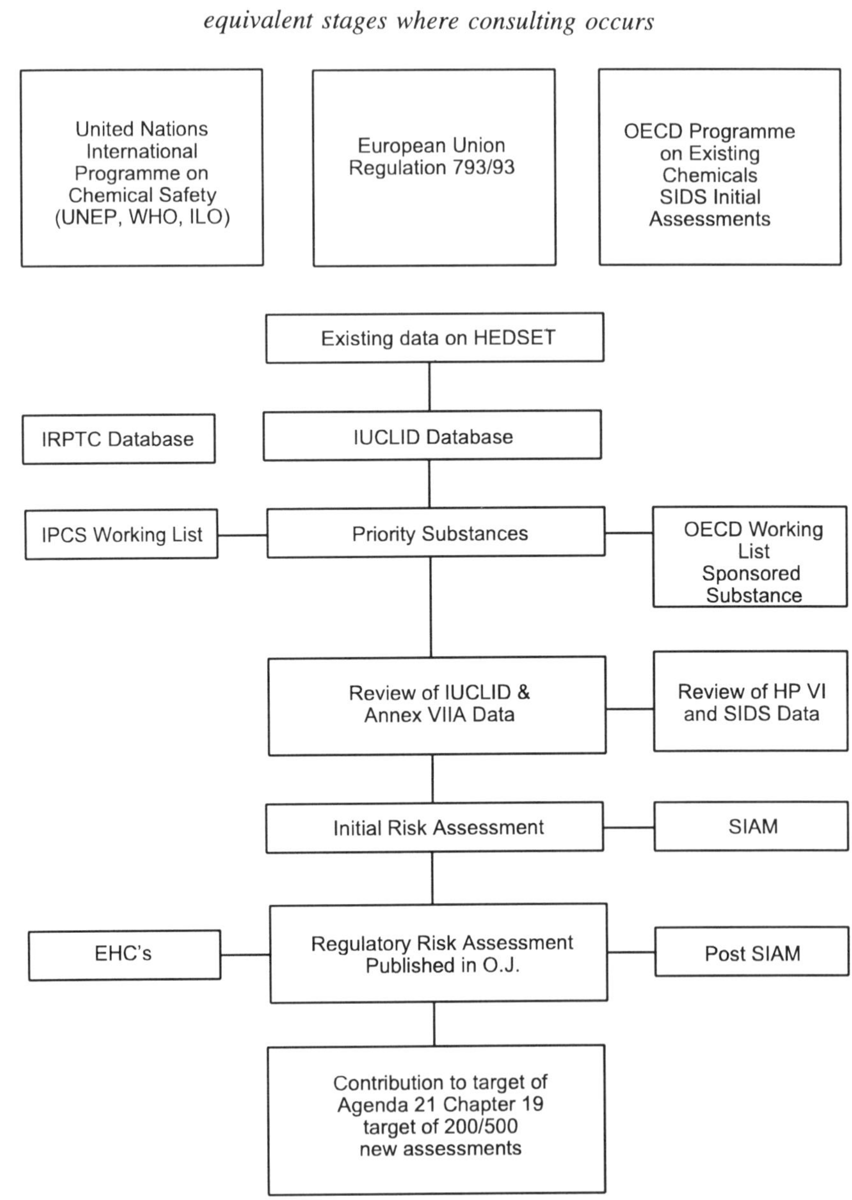

At the priority setting stage, it is necessary to consider both previous and future work carried out under other programmes. Existing reports may indicate that substances are of concern and for which a legislative risk assessment per Regulations 793/93 and 1488/94 could consist of an accelerated review and if necessary revision of an existing report to ensure:

- that the report is concerned with risk and not just hazard;
- that exposure assessment is appropriate to the EC; and
- modification in the light of data only available in IUCLID.

Effort is taken to establish that future work embarked upon in respective programmes is mutually complementary. Where such coordination is aimed at increasing the number of substances whose safety has been assessed as expressed in the objectives of UNCED's Agenda 21, chapter 19 relating to chemical safety, it has been recognised as essential that future assessments are carried out in respective programmes on the basis of very similar if not identical principles. Appropriately effort is being made to harmonise the approach laid down in the OECD SIDS manual (which is generally consistent with the EU Risk Assessment approach) and that followed by the IPCS (International Programme on Chemical Safety) in producing its Environmental Health Criteria documents, such that reports from one programme may be utilized by the other.

As such a similarity of approach exists between the EU and OECD (OECD 1987, 1991) programmes it has been agreed that Risk Assessments from EU countries carried out according to Regulation 793/93 could be presented at OECD as an EU contribution.

Having coordinated priority setting and harmonized principles and practices of risk assessment it is necessary to create a mechanism facilitating the uptake, recognition, adoption or utilization of risk assessment reports by the Community programme from these other fora. Reports at OECD from non-EU countries could only be adopted at EU level by placing them on a priority list and carrying out an accelerated review as outlined above.

The OECD Existing Chemicals Programme is now in its fifth phase for which candidate substances have been selected and for which the second EU priority list is considered as an EU contribution. It is not inconceivable that approaches in elaborating risk reduction strategies be harmonised. However, it is almost certain that decision making, which requires subjective value judgement will be taken nationally or regionally. Such harmonisation could therefore be limited to those cases where (a) there is consensus at the outset to take concerted international action; (b) it is already established that the problem is international in nature as a result of trans-frontier pollution or trade; and (c) where there is agreement on the risk assessment.

The relationship to IPCS is generally analogous to that with OECD. Existing Environmental Health Criteria (EHC) documents may have an impact on priority setting by reinforcing a ranking suggesting a substance is of concern. These IPCS Reports on substances of concern may be utilized in accelerated reviewing of priority substances. Regarding future work, IPCS will have an opportunity to comment on draft priority lists and Risk Assessments before formal adoption by the Art. 15 Committee. Published Risk Assessments will be available to IPCS as input to Environmental Health Criteria Documents, where it is interesting to note that IPCS is also considering a fast track procedure to develop assessments based on existing reports.

Existing reports generated in national programmes will be considered in drawing up priority lists in the same way as OECD and IPCS reports and may facilitate accelerated reviews of priority substances. This applies to national programmes both within and outside the EC. To the extent that non-EC national programmes are purely domestic, i.e. not presented at OECD, consultation could take place to coordinate selection of future priorities to avoid overlap.

## REFERENCES

Commission of the European Communities (1967) 'Council Directive 67/548/EEC of 16 August 1967 on the approximation of laws, regulations, and administrative provisions relating to the classification, packaging and labelling of dangerous substances', *Official Journal* EC, L196.

Commission of the European Communities (1979) 'Council Directive 79/831/EEC of 18 September 1979 amending for the sixth time Directive 67/548/EEC on the approximation of laws, regulations, and administrative provisions relating to the classification, packaging and labelling of dangerous substances', *Official Journal* EC, L259.

Commission of the European Communities (1986) 'Council Directive 87/18/EEC of 18 December 1986 on the harmonization of laws, regulations, and administrative provisions relating to the application of the principles of Good Laboratory Practice and the verification of their applications for tests on chemical substances', *Official Journal* EC, L15.

Commission of the European Communities (1988) 'Council Directive 1988/320/EEC of 8 June 1988 on the inspection and verification of Good Laboratory Practice', *Official Journal* EC, L315.

Commission of the European Communities (1990) 'Commission Communication of 15 June 1990 pursuant to article 13 of Council Directive 67/548/EEC as amended by Council Directive 79/831/EEC – EINECS (European Inventory of Existing Commercial Chemical Substances)', *Official Journal* EC, C146A.

Commission of the European Communities (1991a) 'Council Directive 76/464/EEC of 4 May 1976 on the pollution caused by certain dangerous substances discharged into the aquatic environment of the Community', *Official Journal* EC, L129.

Commission of the European Communities (1991b) 'Council Directive 91/414/EEC of 15 July 1991 concerning the placing of plant protection products on the market', *Official Journal* EC, L230.

Commission of the European Communities (1991c) 'Council Directive 76/769/EEC of 27 September 1976 on the approximation of laws, regulations, and administrative provisions of the Member States relating to the restriction on marketing and use of certain dangerous substances and preparations', *Official Journal* EC, L262.

Commission of the European Communities (1992a) 'Council Directive 92/32/EEC of 30 April 1992 amending for the seventh time Directive 67/548/EEC on the approximation of laws, regulations, and administrative provisions relating to the classification, packaging and labelling of dangerous substances', *Official Journal* EC, L154.

Commission of the European Communities (1992b) 'Commission Regulation (EEC) 3200/92 of 11 December 1992 laying down the detailed rules for the implementation of the first stage of the programme of work referred to in article 8(2) of Council Directive 91/414/EEC concerning the placing of plant protection products on the market', *Official Journal* EC, L336

Commission of the European Communities (1993a) 'Council Regulation (EEC) 793/93 of 23 March 1993 on the evaluation and control of existing substances', *Official Journal* EC, L84.

Commission of the European Communities (1993b) 'Commission Directive 93/67/EEC of 20 July1993 laying down the principles for the assessment of the risks to man and the environment of substances notified in accordance with Council Directive 67/548/EEC', *Official Journal* EC, L227.

Commission of the European Communities (1993c) *Commission proposal of 27 July 1993 for a Council Directive concerning the placing of biocidal products on the market COM (93)351 final.*

Commission of the European Communities (1994a) 'Commission Regulation (EC) 1179/94 concerning the first list of priority substances as foreseen under Council Regulation (EEC) 793/93', *Official Journal* EC, L131.

Commission of the European Communities (1994b) 'Commission Regulation (EC) 1488/94 laying down the principles for the assessment of risks to man and the environment of existing substances in accordance with Council Regulation (EEC) 793/93', *Official Journal* EC, L161.

Commission of the European Communities (1995) 'Commission Regulation (EC) 2268/94 concerning the second list of priority substances as foreseen under Council Regulation (EEC) 793/93', *Official Journal* EC, L231.

Commission of the European Communities (1996) *Technical Guidance Document on the risk assessment of new and existing substances*, in press.

Organization of Economic Cooperation and Development (1987) *Council Decision - Recommendation on the systematic investigation of existing chemicals*, C(87) 90 final adopted 26 June 1987.

Organization of Economic Cooperation and Development (1991) *Council Decision - Recommendation on the cooperative investigation and risk reduction of existing chemicals*, C(90) 163 final adopted on 31 January 1991.

# 9

*Alan Irwin, Henry Rothstein,*
*Elaine McCarthy, Steven Yearley*

## REGULATORY SCIENCE AND THE EUROPEAN CONTROL OF AGROCHEMICALS

### INTRODUCTION

Ever since *Silent Spring* (Carson 1962), the control of agrochemicals has been of central interest to the environmental movement and to consumers' organisations. Many elements within the environmental movement have pressed for substantial agricultural and regulatory reform. Meanwhile, industry and policy-makers have pursued the international harmonisation of regulatory controls – largely, of course, for economic reasons but also as part of a wider concern with the ecological and health effects of pesticides. Overall, there have been substantial changes in international regulatory regimes and in the toxicological testing required for agrochemicals.

In this paper, we consider the consequences of such changes for the kinds of scientific research carried out – both in terms of the institutional location of such research (i.e. its context) but also the form of this research (in other words, its content). The project on which this paper is based explores the extent to which new areas of regulatory science have been fostered and created. 'Regulatory science' for these purposes refers to technical activities which have grown up in response to 'external' regulatory demands. The project documents the nature and characteristics of regulatory science in the UK – its location (whether in industry, academia or public laboratories), its ethos and its mode of operation. This paper represents an early attempt to develop a sociological analysis and to propose a broad analytical framework.

---

In: R. Bal & W. Halffman (eds.), *The Politics of Chemical Risk*, Kluwer Academic Publishers, Dordrecht 1998: p. 231-250.

Of course, the agrochemical sector has not been the first (or only) area to witness the growth of regulatory science. As Bodewitz et al. (1987) have indicated, many of the sociological and institutional issues around regulation were first developed in relation to medical, and specifically pharmacological, safety. These authors point out that early regulatory activity had to do with the efficacy of treatments, that is, with preventing people being sold worthless formulations. Following this, it became apparent that "in contrast to the situation relating to efficacy tests, there is no comparable, generally acceptable methodology for testing the safety of drugs" (*ibid.:* 249).

Certainly, issues of safety and efficacy have become inseparable in the case of agrochemicals – especially within the European regulatory process. Moreover, the growth of regulatory activities has prompted many companies to consider the risks of new products alongside potential efficacy – and at an early stage in the innovation process. On that basis, the relationship between 'innovation' and 'regulation' can overlap to the extent that a practical distinction between the two may be evaporating (Irwin & Vergragt 1989).

The situation of firms and scientists conducting regulation-related research in the UK has also been affected by the changing policy context. The traditionally-closed and informal nature of the British regulatory system has been well-documented. Whilst to some it has appeared an ideal type of a consensual policy system (see Vogel 1986), to others it can be more properly characterised as a less palatable collusive system (see Millstone 1986, also Irwin and Lloyd 1992). In the specific case of the regulation of agrochemicals in het UK, a statutory regime was introduced in 1986 to replace the prior voluntary arrangements that had operated between government, manufacturers and suppliers.

However, with the strengthened position assumed by the European Union in the wake of moves towards a single market, the regulatory environment faced by UK firms has become relatively more formal and demanding. British firms are facing the task of addressing novel forms of testing, and are anticipating further changes in the light of a developing regulatory system. Meanwhile, the emergence of a European regime also raises questions of the relationship between national regulators and the European authorities: has the development of international regulatory systems served to downgrade the significance of nationally-based regimes?

The European Union's plant protection product Directive 91/414/EEC (Council of the European Communities 1991) has been designed as a two-tier approval system. Whilst Active Ingredients (AIs) will be authorised at the European level (using a rapporteur system), specific agrochemical products will be authorised at the level of Member States. Meanwhile, data requirements and evaluation guidelines will be common throughout the EU, and Member States will be expected to mutually recognise each others' approvals - subject to regional ecological variation. Quite clearly, therefore, this approval system does not deny the importance of nationally-based regulatory systems (at least not in the short, or even medium, term) but does create a possible degree of tension between national and international approval systems over which will prove to be dominant with regard to various aspects of regulation.

In this paper then, we explore regulatory scientific activity as it operates in an area of technical, economic and political complexity and, moreover, where large changes have been taking place – and are likely to continue for some time into the future as the European regime becomes established. In what follows, we have focused on these matters as they are seen from the perspective of UK-based industry. Accordingly, our account of regulatory science leads up to the point of regulatory submission – a process, as we will discuss, which remains largely invisible (and largely inaccessible) to environmentalist groups which typically can only engage in debate once regulatory clearance has been given.

## THE SOCIOLOGY OF REGULATORY SCIENCE

An initial characterisation of regulatory science has been presented by Jasanoff (1990: 76-83). Her argument is that, rather than representing a distinctive type of knowledge, regulatory science is knowledge produced in a particular institutional context. Accordingly, she points out that regulatory science differs from academic science not so much in terms of its content, but rather in terms of its context: it aims to produce knowledge for policy use under conditions of political and legal accountability, usually within tight time constraints. Typically, she argues (1990: 80), regulatory science is conducted by governmental and industrial bodies, supplemented on occasions by the "commissioning of scientific studies from highly credentialed researchers at academic institutions or from private consulting groups."

Our approach in what follows is not to impose a content/context separation but rather to consider the possible interplay between these factors within regulatory scientific activities. On the one hand, regulatory science is indeed undertaken in a wide range of institutional contexts (from contract laboratories conducting routinised animal tests to expert committees deciding on toxicological standards). On the other, it combines a variety of disciplines and specialties within its coverage – thus suggesting a divergent set of contents which cannot readily be pigeon-holed or confined to any specific technical area. Our approach overall is to view regulatory science as a hybrid area of activity in terms of both its content and context rather than simply attempting to contrast it with what may (but also may not) be a fair characterisation of contemporary 'academic science'.

Our empirical investigation is based upon an extended series of interviews with industrialists within R&D-intensive multi-national corporations with a base in the UK. We have also interviewed government officials from the relevant departments and agencies (including the Pesticides Safety Directorate, PSD), officials of the European Commission and scientists (working in university and industrial laboratories). This empirical study has so far led us to propose a five-way categorisation of conceptually-distinct but closely-related activities within regulatory science (what can be termed the 'regulatory pentangle'). The categorisation is intended to illustrate the diversity of technical and administrative activities encompassed by this concept. It also highlights the cross-institutional and disciplinary relationships, practices and knowledges that are characteristic of this domain. Outlined below are some basic features of these various regulatory scientific activities, an account of their relationships to technological innovation, and a consideration of the ways in which they appear to be distributed amongst the public and private sectors in the UK.

### *Speculative research*

In the regulatory context, speculative research is taken to embrace basic academic research on subjects which may have regulatory relevance. Some of this work may be directly concerned with agrochemicals, such as research on environmental fate, whilst other topics may have relevance across the chemicals sector, such as chemical hormone disrupters. This work is likely to be located within university or associated academic departments, but may also be undertaken in sophisticated industrial laboratories and research organisations. Our research suggests that, whilst there were some well-established links between industry and universities in this domain, there was a general problem of communication between these groups reflected in mutual uncertainties about their respective activities.

However, expectations of long-term changes in regulatory requirements have opened the door to some university/industry research initiatives. Although a major part of the rationale for such research may relate to putative regulatory developments, the research may well not have immediate applications. Industry, however, accrues some benefit from being seen publicly to support basic research whilst academic departments acquire alternative sources of funding. Such initiatives could be seen to represent low investment, high leverage opportunities for industry.

In summary then, this domain of activity is research intensive and undertaken in well resourced private laboratories and within universities. Of all the activities described in this paper, speculative research appears to be the most closely allied to conventional representations of 'academic science', albeit with sometimes commercial goals.

*Development and validation of regulatory tests*

Screening for toxic and ecological effects of agrochemicals requires the development and validation of specific and largely standardised tests. Incorporation into a regulatory regime is as much a political decision as a scientific one. This area of regulatory science therefore brings together social, bureaucratic and scientific demands. Decisions on which tests to utilise can be variously influenced by political pressures favouring environmental protection or the setting of precautionary limits, or by commercial pressures to minimise costs. The development of ecotoxicity and environmental fate tests for the new European regime, for example, has been particularly prone to scientific uncertainties and political sensitivities.

The development of new guidelines reflects the diverse institutional base for undertaking this work. Formally, the development of test requirements involves consideration of current practice amongst Member States, and *ad hoc* consultation of international organisations such as the OECD and of groups of professionals and experts. The tests are finalised in confidential inter-governmental working groups. This formal process is, however, paralleled by a more informal process contributing to the finalisation of tests.

In particular, industry can play a significant role in the development of tests by providing often-needed expertise. For example, industry took a leading role in the development of new guidelines on beneficial arthropods in order to avoid the adoption of the German system which it saw as complex and excessively cautious. Industry consequently set up the Beneficial Arthropods in Registration Testing group (BART) and the test guidelines produced are now utilised by the EU (Barrett *et al.* 1994).

This rather subtle way in which industry is active in the development of regulations could be described as 'cognitive capture' whereby established organisations can play a leading role through the *de facto* provision of expertise. At the same time, this can result in the exclusion of other actors from the regulatory process. It was generally considered by government and industry representatives, for example, that NGOs had only a limited role in this domain. Without the resources and necessary specialist expertise, NGOs were unlikely to be able to shape debate. Furthermore, without being tied into the necessary regulatory scientific networks, the access of such organisations to these informal processes was minimal.

### *Regulatory compliance testing*

Regulatory compliance testing of chemicals and products in order to obtain regulatory approval is the most rapidly expanding aspect of regulatory scientific activity. In the modern regulatory environment, regulatory strategy has to be considered throughout the innovation process so as to minimise the likelihood of costly registration failures. This approach to regulatory compliance testing (and consequently 'dossier building') is commonly termed 'process orientation' within industry.

These activities are largely conducted by industry in-house or contracted out to private laboratories (depending upon the availability of facilities and corporate strategies for maximising the use of in-house research capacity). Many regulatory scientists consider that the location of this research, including its national location, will have substantial consequences for successful registration. As will be discussed, very little of this work is carried out in public sector institutions.

A number of commercial laboratories and in-house facilities have achieved a high level of efficiency through specialisation in this field. Within thc private sector, testing has become routinised and has been subject to a considerable division of labour. Many contract laboratories have built up an extensive knowledge base on regulation and testing, often employing ex-regulatory agency staff both for their expertise and informal contacts. Our research suggests, however, that there are different strategies within industry on the use of in-house or contract laboratories.

Contract laboratories can be attractive to companies by offering well-established scientific services as well as informal knowledge and sometimes good access to regulators. However, from the perspective of agrochemical companies, opportunities to accumulate information which might aid with future development of products can be lost by contracting out research to external organisations. In some cases, therefore, it is considered that a fuller knowledge is built up by keeping such regulatory compliance work in-house.

In contrast, universities have played a relatively minor role in regulatory compliance work. The prime reason offered by industry for this has been the lack of Good Laboratory Practice certification of university laboratories (with a few exceptions in some specialised areas). This bureaucratic requirement for regulatory compliance work presents problems for universities since it involves laborious systems of record keeping and quality assurance which are expensive to institute and are sometimes perceived as 'going against the grain' of academic working practices. However, the potential for universities to be involved in this domain may also be limited by a lack of academic interest in what are often described as 'handle-turning' tests, and the lack of acknowledgement for such work within national research assessment exercises. It is also difficult for universities to compete with the economies of scale achieved by private contract laboratories.

It would appear that industry is also reluctant to use universities because of concerns over security and confidentiality, and what is seen to be a capricious academic research culture. One study as far back as the 1970s found that agrochemical manufacturers had a high opinion of their own expertise in the field of toxicology in comparison to that of government research establishments and universities (Tait 1976).

Regulatory compliance testing, therefore, is institutionally dominated by the private sector. It is largely characterised by repetitive tests, the results of which are generally kept within the private domain and assessed only within regulatory review.

### *Investigative problem solving*

Whilst there has been considerable routinisation of regulatory toxicological testing, this may not be the case if there are, or are likely to be, problems with registration. If, for example, a product appears to be harmful to a certain type of laboratory animal, this may be sufficient reason to consider that the substance would not conform to regulatory requirements and therefore to terminate its development. This responsibility to terminate development accords toxicologists a considerable importance within a company. Such a decision, at the same time, has to take into account prospective commercial gains from the marketing of the product.

However, if the result is thought to be in some way anomalous or a-typical, further investigative research may reveal a mechanism which indicates that the anomaly is irrelevant for risk assessment purposes. In such a case, regulatory approval might subsequently be secured. A decision to pursue the sometimes-costly option of further investigation will ultimately be dependent upon the expected gains from marketing the product: clearly, the greater the expected gains, the greater the incentive. Some research may be undertaken collaboratively between companies over common issues, but our interviews suggest that this has not occurred to a significant degree.

In addition to companies conducting such investigations in-house, private sector contract organisations can undertake some of this work. It may also have to be contracted out to academic experts within universities and other public institutions. From an academic viewpoint, this kind of research may make a valuable contribution to theoretical understanding – and could be seen to represent an additional source of research funding. However, it could be argued that the defensive orientation of this work implies a certain opportunism in clearing regulatory hurdles and a lack of commitment on the part of industry to the extension of knowledge *per se*.

*Regulatory submission*

The final stage of the production of regulatory science is concerned with compiling the dossier of information for regulatory review including, in the case of agrochemicals, a risk assessment. However, within the companies studied, it was clear that this stage was anticipated at an early point in the innovation process rather than being left till the product was ready for release. Certainly, companies were aware that delay (or worse) at the Regulatory Submission stage could significantly affect the eventual profitability of the product.

The process of regulatory submission has therefore become intricately entwined with the innovation process. This shift has occurred also in specific response to a past dislocation between innovation and regulatory submission which resulted in some costly registration failures. According to our interviews, whilst the voluntary arrangements that operated in the UK until 1986 were considered to be flexible and efficient, they also permitted wide discretion. This activity was traditionally accorded a low-priority by companies as it was perceived to rest upon good relations with MAFF rather than extensive and thorough presentation of scientific argumentation. The introduction of statutory regulations in 1986 and, subsequently, the new European regime have necessitated a change in corporate attitudes towards this activity.

This domain of regulatory science is particularly characterised by interdisciplinary activity. Regulatory officers in industry and officials in the regulatory agencies have to be acquainted with a diverse range of scientific disciplines, agrochemical applications, legal requirements and administrative procedures. Personnel within industry may have agency backgrounds, and will accordingly be valued for their familiarity with the regulatory process, regulatory institutions and current regulatory officials. According to our interviews, companies are acutely aware of the sometimes unpredictable nature of regulatory review and will therefore place considerable value on extensive communication with the regulatory agency for advice and guidance prior to submission. Indeed, the PSD actively encourages this kind of cooperation with companies, believing that this 'hands-on approach' best fulfils its remit.

Contract organisations may also have a role in regulatory submission, and indeed some of the larger ones make play of the fact that they employ ex-regulatory staff who are likely to maintain informal links with the agency.

Furthermore, as the workload on the PSD has increased with the introduction of statutory regulations, some dossier reviews have been contracted out to external laboratories, further tying these organisations into the regulatory network (House of Commons Agriculture Committee 1995: 46).

Of all the activities described by the 'pentangle' of regulatory scientific activities then, regulatory submission appears to be the most interdisciplinary, and to rely on accumulated tacit knowledge about both the origin and the likely reception of the dossier of evidence for regulatory approval. This is particularly facilitated by the relationships forged between companies and the regulatory agency at every stage of the regulatory process.

## *The regulatory pentangle in action*

It is important to emphasise that what has been presented so far does not represent a linear model - for different products, sectors and contexts these categories could occur in different stages. Equally, and as we have noted, the fact that, for example, Regulatory Submission is presented as the final stage does not mean that it will only be considered late in the innovation process – instead, companies must consider regulatory requirements almost from the very start of the product development process.

Therefore, this is not an attempt to reconstruct the notion of linearity which has generally been rejected within innovation research. Rather, our working assumption is that specific examples will cut across and combine categories. In methodological terms, however, the five-way model offers a heuristic or ideal-typical device in order to stimulate further empirical investigation and conceptual clarification.

This five-way conceptual and analytical categorisation has also led us to identify (or perhaps re-define) a number of wider issues. For example, it is possible to enquire about the relative significance of 'academic' and 'industrial' research within each category: at the stage of regulatory submission, industrial scientists may take precedence whilst, for speculative research, a different balance is recorded. In the remainder of this paper, we will concentrate especially on the relationship between the institutional context within which regulatory science is conducted and its cognitive (or technical) content: is it reasonable to identify any relationship between these and, if so, does this affect the technical character of regulatory science?

## THE INSTITUTIONAL CONTEXT OF REGULATORY SCIENCE

In order to summarise the institutional dimensions of our research, Table 1 sketches out the main locations of regulatory scientific activity. Whilst not pretending to be quantitatively based, the table provides an indicative and preliminary analysis of the general trends implicit in the 'regulatory pentangle'.

*Table 1*: Regulatory science in the UK

| *type of research* / *location* | Speculative Research | Development of Regulatory Tests | Regulatory Compliance Testing | Investigative Research | Regulatory Submission |
|---|---|---|---|---|---|
| R&D-Active Agro-chemical Firms | ✓ | ✓ | ✓ | ✓ | ✓ |
| Universities | ✓ | ✓ | seldom | ✓ | |
| Contract Labs./ Consultancies | sometimes | ✓ | ✓ | sometimes | ✓ |
| Government | ✓ | ✓ | | | ✓ see text |
| NGOs | | mostly lobbying | | | |

The table clearly illustrates the involvement of the agrochemical industry in all forms of regulatory scientific activity. Of course, this can be broken down further within the industrial sector, in that only the larger multinational companies have the resources to undertake the more research based activities. Companies producing generic products will generally be confined to the activities of regulatory compliance testing and submission. Furthermore, industrial involvement may also be less direct, such as through the activities of its personnel within professional bodies.

Universities tend to have a role especially within what can be defined as the most 'research-based' activities, rarely getting involved in the more 'handle turning' aspects of regulatory science. As already observed, university capacity is not readily geared to regulatory compliance testing and there appears to be a general perception within industry and universities that it could only provide a minor or specialised contribution to this activity. The lack of university involvement in regulatory compliance testing, however, raises a possibly serious problem with regard to the sometimes-expressed concerns over the dominance of industry within this area (a point to which we will return in the Discussion).

Contract laboratories and consultancies, on the other hand, are precisely focused on this aspect of regulatory science, producing the data to support approvals. In a small number of cases these organisations may have sufficient expertise to be involved in the development of test regimes through their activity within professional organisations, and may undertake commissions for more speculative or investigative research. Some organisations may also undertake regulatory submission, particularly for foreign or relatively new companies that may be unfamiliar with regulatory procedures and the regulatory agency.

Government's involvement with regulatory science has traditionally centred on the development of the regulatory regime (in this case involving especially European negotiations) and of course regulatory review. Government is also a sponsor of speculative research in the public sector through the research councils, although this may be *ad hoc* and uncoordinated with the work of regulatory officials. Furthermore, it appears to be an interesting feature of the British regulatory system that government agencies have a role in regulatory submission. This is not to suggest that they are bureaucratically involved in making submissions: companies take responsibility for this. However, they can be involved in an informal way, advising on the form, and perhaps even the content, of regulatory submissions – for example, by discussing the suitability of applications with agrochemical companies prior to review.

Finally, in this institutional overview of the sites of regulatory scientific activity, the scope for UK NGOs to participate in the regulatory science nexus has been presented as very limited in extent. Their activity has tended to be confined to lobbying around the general goals of the new regulatory regime and the resolution of certain specific regulatory issues.

Three issues arise from this discussion. Firstly, regulatory scientific activities are located in a variety of different institutional locations. Industry is, perhaps unsurprisingly, dominant – with some industrial locations undertaking the whole range of activities. Other locations, such as universities, have proved less adaptable.

Secondly, many of these activities are inter-institutional in character. Contract laboratories, for example, were perceived by one industrial representative as an extension of industrial facilities. The contracting out of review of applications for approval by the PSD to contract organisations further blurs institutional boundaries.

Finally, in the British context, the institutional networks serve to bind institutions together through regular and close personal contacts. These relationships, which emphasise trust and mutual understanding, can be seen as underpinning and fostering a cooperative and shared approach to regulatory approval. This network is reinforced by its relatively small size. There are fewer than ten R&D-active companies based in Britain, an equivalent number of larger contract laboratories and, in PSD, a high-profile government agency. This trend is reinforced by the steady flow of personnel between institutions.

At the same time, these networks can be seen as excluding wider discussion and, in particular, limiting the possibilities for 'public participation'. Much of the regulatory scientific activity is either confidential or mediated through informal contacts. This provides few opportunities for interested individuals and groups such as NGOs to examine, contribute to, or contest activities except through general lobbying. Whilst the perception of government and industry may be that such organisations have little to contribute scientifically to the process, it is common for NGOs and critics to respond that the wide range of regulatory judgements and interpretations being made necessitate wider participation and greater public oversight.

## The content of regulatory science

If regulatory science in the area of agrochemicals suggests a diversity and complexity in terms of its institutional structure, the same point can certainly be made about its intellectual and technical content. In the following section, we will discuss several of the major cognitive characteristics of regulatory science as evidenced by our empirical investigation. However, it is important to emphasise from the start that points about 'content' are largely-inseparable from the discussion of 'context' – a considerable overlap between these two elements will be observed in this section.

Perhaps the most striking characteristic of regulatory science is its interdisciplinary nature. It would appear that, within the often-immediate demands of agrochemical innovation and testing, disciplines do not reign supreme but instead are secondary to the business of problem solving and issue resolution. Regulatory science draws upon a wide range of disciplines and specialities – from botany to toxicology, from mathematics to biology. It also utilises a range of what we might term 'technical practices' – for example, routinised animal testing to the standard of Good Laboratory Practice and the presentation of scientific information within a prescribed format. Throughout its activities, regulatory science combines a complexity of technical information, a broad range of scientific practices, and a very concrete set of concerns (which, in the end, come down to the safety, efficacy and commercial viability of a chemical product).

The multidisciplinary aspect of regulatory science is closely linked to the need to operate within teams which combine various forms of expertise and operational concerns – for example, marketing and eco-toxicology, efficacy and costs of production. Regulatory scientists (whether in industry or the government agency) need to have the ability to operate within such settings and to communicate regularly with non-specialists. As in the case of PSD personnel, this requires technical skills but also a sense of the economic and commercial 'realities' of pesticide sales and production.

For these reasons also, expertise in regulatory science cannot easily be acquired by those outside the institutional patchwork described above – thus, as already noted, exclusion from technical discussions has both a cognitive and an institutional dimension which are mutually-reinforcing. This is not to deny that outsiders may have valuable knowledge and insights concerning specific technical issues (nor does it mean that they are incapable of asking appropriate questions or raising basic issues). However, discussion between regulatory scientists will often build upon such various matters as an awareness of the latest questions being discussed in Brussels or Washington DC, inside information concerning what products are in the 'pipe-line', informal talk of the difficulties being faced by various companies, a sense of the regulatory agenda and possible amendments under discussion. These discussions can be very opaque and impenetrable for those who do not inhabit this institutional nexus: thus further emphasising the relationship between institutional membership (as an 'insider') and the content of technical analysis.

However, it should also be noted that it is difficult to gauge the impact of this institutional and organisational structure upon the content of scientific work in this area since, at least in the UK context, there is no separate or 'independent' academic equivalent with which comparison might be made. As already discussed, university-based research does play a role in a number of aspects of regulatory scientific activity, but this is usually heavily dependent upon industrial funding. Other aspects of industrial regulatory scientific activity simply have no parallel within academia or hold little interest for academic scientists. We are not, therefore, dealing with an area where 'regulatory science' can be contrasted with its 'academic' equivalent – since these categories cannot be separated in any satisfactory fashion. Instead, 'academic' and 'regulatory' science inhabit the same institutional and intellectual nexus.

What should also be stressed in this discussion is that we are not simply portraying regulatory science as an *applied* area of research – although, of course, matters of practical application and implementation are very much to the fore. Instead, we are describing a field which straddles the conventional 'basic/applied' dichotomy. Regulatory science brings together activities which a traditional approach to knowledge development might categorise quite separately (for example, into distinctive disciplines and degrees of proximity to the market-place). We are therefore identifying a knowledge-production system (Gibbons et al., 1994) which largely disregards such categorisations in order to tackle a set of issues which are broad in intellectual coverage but specific in terms of application. In this, the institutional context and the cognitive content of regulatory science are highly complementary to one another.

## Discussion

In addition to developing an empirical approach to the study of regulatory science, this paper has identified a number of specific aspects of both its 'context' and its 'content'. Even at this preliminary stage in our project, it is reasonable to consider the inter-relationship between these elements

– and especially with regard to our categorisation of this field as 'hybrid' in character.

Certainly, it is possible to identify a close relationship between institutional and cognitive factors within this particular field of regulatory science. In the area of peer review, for example, the confidentiality and closed-nature of many of the processes involved means that only a limited element of external scrutiny is permitted. It is possible to suggest also that there will be a restricted scope for intellectual novelty – industrial scientists may not be especially motivated to identify whole new areas of pesticide damage or to implicate particular products either before or (especially) after release. The close relationship between scientific research and industrial funding may also represent a powerful 'conservative' influence within the field.

Of course, this limited relationship to 'basic' research may serve to restrict the intellectual energy of the field and concentrate it instead on relatively short-term questions and pressing practical concerns. This point was reinforced within our interviews by the rather vague answers typically given to questions about the significance of the international (or even British) science base – this was seen to be a matter at some distance from the everyday business of regulatory science (if scientific input was needed at any point then it could be paid for). Wider (perhaps more theoretical or basic) links to university-based research were equally viewed with some indifference. Regulatory scientists had their own networks and methods of information exchange: it was difficult again to see what general role university scientists could play within this (except on specific issues and involving particular named scientists who were seen to be highly valuable).

Whilst this portrayal suggests a somewhat worrying picture of regulatory science as disconnected from wider scientific debates due to its particular institutional structure, it is also possible to offer a contrasting picture of the area. Certainly, it would be inaccurate to portray the regulatory science studied here as either static or ossified.

Thus, regulatory scientists in the British context enjoy easy and informal relations across this institutional nexus (and especially between government, the agrochemicals industry and the key research and testing laboratories). The British Agrochemicals Association is active in terms of drawing together collective experience and sharing ideas for future development. The experience of dossier submission has caused much discussion within the whole sector as common issues are defined and considered. The government agency has been seen to offer useful feedback on 'best practice' and problems experienced by particular companies (always, of course, whilst protecting commercial confidentiality). National and international regulatory committees have brought together the major experts within the field.

On an international as well as national basis, there is a constant evaluation of different experiences and possible developments (remembering that this sector is dominated by trans-national companies and international markets). Furthermore, the high economic stakes involved in innovation and industry's awareness of its vulnerability to public criticism (with Rachel Carson herself often being invoked as a symbol of previous difficulties) have encouraged the sector to consider how to minimise future controversies – especially when perceived problems with any pesticide will reflect upon the sector as a whole. All of this suggests that agrochemical companies need to examine their products critically before release rather than face problems later on.

It is clear from our analysis that the institutional context of regulatory science affects the character of relationships and communications between regulatory scientists: not least in terms of erecting boundaries around the core of appropriately knowledgeable experts. Nevertheless, it would be premature to conclude that the impact of 'context' on 'content' must inevitably be negative. The approach we have adopted has been to study the inter-relationships between the contexts and content of regulatory science in a more even-handed (one might say symmetrical) fashion. This is all the more appropriate given the wider argument that regulatory science in the agrochemicals sector may represent just one example of an increasingly common phenomenon: the hybrid and industrially-based knowledge-production system. In our continuing research we propose to explore further these characteristics of regulatory science.

*Acknowledgments:* This research was funded by the Economic and Social Research Council (award number L323253019). The authors are also grateful for the help and assistance offered by the Science Policy Support Group within the ESRC research programme on the European Context of UK Science Policy. The authors would like to thank the industry and government representatives interviewed for this research, who for reasons of confidentiality remain anonymous. The views expressed in this paper are of course the authors' own.

## REFERENCES

Barrett, K.L., N. Grandy, E.G. Harrison, S. Hassan & P. Oomen (eds.) (1994) *Guidance document on regulatory testing procedures for pesticides with non-target arthropods*, Society of Environmental Toxicology and Chemistry – Europe.

Bodewitz, H.J.H.W, H. Buurma & G.H. de Vries (1987) 'Regulatory science and the social management of trust in medicine', in W.E. Bijker, T.P. Hughes & T. Pinch (eds.) *The Social Construction of Technological Systems*, Cambridge, MA: MIT Press: 243-259.

Carson, R. (1962) *Silent Spring*, Harmondsworth: Penguin.

Council of the European Communities (1991) 'Council Directive of 15 July 1991 concerning the placing of plant protection products on the market (91/414/EEC)', *Official Journal*, No L 230, 19.8.1991.

Gibbons, M., C. Limoges, H. Nowotny, S. Schwartzman, P. Scott & M. Trow (1994) *The New Production of Knowledge: The Dynamics of Science and Research in Contemporary Societies*, London: Sage.

House of Commons Agriculture Committee (1995) *Pesticides Safety Directorate and Veterinary Medicines Directorate*, Vol II, 391-II, London: HMSO.

Irwin, A. & P. Vergragt (1989) 'Rethinking the Relationship between Environmental Regulation and Industrial Innovation: the social negotiation of technical change', *Technology Analysis and Strategic Management* 1: 57-70.

Irwin, A. & D. Lloyd (1992) 'Pragmatism, effectiveness and institutional judgement in the British control of major accident hazards', *Technology Analysis and Strategic Management* 4: 115-32.

Jasanoff, S. (1990) *The Fifth Branch: Science Advisors as Policymakers*, Cambridge, MA: Harvard University Press.

Millstone, E. (1986) *Food Additives*, Harmondsworth: Penguin.

Tait, E. (1976) *Factors affecting the production and usage of pesticides in the UK*, unpublished PhD thesis, Cambridge University.

Vogel, D. (1986) *National Styles of Regulation: Environmental Policy in Great Britain and the United States*, Ithaca: Cornell University Press.

# 10

*Peter Calow*

# STANDARDS, SCIENCE AND THE POLITICS OF CHEMICAL RISK

## INTRODUCTION

In the EU, protecting the environment from harm from commercial chemicals has shifted over the last decade from a hazard- to a risk-based approach (Calow 1993). Regulatory instruments concerned with controlling both new and existing substances require data collection, risk assessment and the possible development of management strategies. Assessment in this procedure proceeds management.

The risk assessment in the EU (EC) legislation involves the application of scientific procedures to specify potential effects, likely exposure and hence likely harm to ecological systems. By 'scientific procedure' I mean the use of critical analysis, based upon carefully controlled observation, to further understanding of a problem. The risk management is based on the results from the assessment process, and involves using a combination of socio-political and scientific judgements to consider how much the likely harm matters and what, usually out of several options, should be done about it. By 'socio-political' I mean making judgements based upon a perception of public concerns. In general it is often considered important to separate the risk assessment, which tries to be as objective as possible by using scientific procedures, from socio-political judgements that are involved in deciding if and how to manage risks (Jasanoff 1990, Halffman & Bal, this volume).

In: R. Bal & W. Halffman (eds.), *The Politics of Chemical Risk*, Kluwer Academic Publishers, Dordrecht 1998: p. 251-263.

Yet in the development of risk-based approaches a number of management decisions ought to be made before an assessment can be carried out. Most fundamentally, a decision has to be made on what is to be managed. This is an apparently obvious requirement, but in practice it is rarely specified very precisely, leaving environmental risk assessments often somewhat vague (Calow 1994). Deciding what is to be protected and hence managed is crucial because it determines how effects and exposures are to be measured. All these issues might involve both scientific considerations – in defining 'natural' systems and their 'natural' states – and/or socio-political considerations – in defining what it is about 'nature' that society values and wants to protect from harm.

So management considerations, that involve a combination of scientific and socio-political judgements, come before (both in time *and* importance) assessments can be carried out. Moreover, the implications of these decisions 'spill over' into the assessment procedures themselves. This is not always appreciated by those involved; so that the decisions about what to measure and how to measure it are often made implicitly and may not be transparent. Moreover, given the complex, technical nature of the relationship between management targets and scientific measurements, interpretations are generally made largely by the technical community. How management decisions impinge upon risk assessment and the way this interaction is handled within the assessment procedures is illustrated below with special reference to the process of standardisation of ecotoxicity tests. An attempt is made to make explicit that which is usually implicit, and to suggest how transparency and broader involvement might be encouraged.

## To standardise itself is a management decision

Potential harmful effects from commercial chemicals are usually judged in risk assessment from the concentration-effect relationships observed in a suite of ecotoxicity tests. This is the hazard identification part of the procedure. The process of standardisation, as applied to hazard identification, has two aspects:

1 The codification of general procedures such that results are redeemable and open to scrutiny and so, if necessary, procedures can be precisely repeated. This standardisation is referred to in shorthand as good laboratory practice or GLP (OECD 1984).
2 The refinement of specific tests to ensure that results from them are repeatable and reproducible (Soares & Calow 1993a & b). Tests following the same protocol should for the same substance give results that do not differ significantly when applied by different operators, at different times. Scientific procedures can be used to identify and control sources of variability (see below) and to run ring-(round-robin) tests to assess success in standardisation (ISO 1986).

That there has to be standardisation, in both of the senses defined above, seems beyond doubt, both for the sake of scientific and legal credibility. Without it there can be no basis for sharing results, in a mutually acceptable way, within the community of scientists or more generally between the scientific and technical community and society at large. So it could be argued that the management decision to standardise is driven by both scientific and social requirements. If the same test did not give the same result in different places or at different times there would be cause for confusion that could compromise both scientific understanding and legal procedures.

On the other hand, decisions have to be made about how far standardisation should be taken; for example, in forcing the use of a few tests concerned with a few aspects of ecosystems on all aspects of ecosystems and on all ecosystems irrespective of geographical circumstances. Issues here are largely scientific: to what extent is it legitimate to extrapolate from species to species, ecosystem to ecosystem, geographic region to region? In principle, they can be decided on the basis of comparative observations on performance. But given some appreciation of the likely inadequacies in these extrapolations there are then possible decisions to make about the risks of coming to the wrong conclusion as a result of extrapolation against the benefits of convenience and costs (the expenses involved in developing new tests being nontrivial – see below), and these are not so obviously, and exclusively, scientific in content. They often colour decisions about the appropriate sizes of safety margins (uncertainty/application factors) to use in extrapolating results from laboratory to nature.

## Which tests?

Ecotoxicity tests that are currently in use in association with the risk assessment legislation have been chosen largely for historical reasons and convenience. And these are important criteria, because reliability, as evidenced by long-term use, is crucial if tests are to be used effectively in routine assessments of large numbers of substances and for legal purposes. Ecological considerations have also been involved. For example, the 'base-set' ecotoxicity requirements for new and existing substances within the EU involve 'representatives' of trophic levels – a plant (algae), plant-eating animal (*Daphnia*) and animal-eating animal (fish) – which was an attempt to introduce some ecological relevance into the testing programme. But even so the focus is still on freshwater organisms; and this is justified because it is presumed that freshwater systems are the most likely recipients of chemical contamination. Also the tests that have been developed are exclusively representative of temperate species. Now both these choices – of habitat and region – require management decisions that could either involve scientific considerations (eg. most likely fate of chemicals in the environment; most vunerable systems) and/or socio-political considerations that prioritise environments according to social values and hence dictate which representative species should be used in tests. Whether or not decisions have been, or are being, made as explicitly as this remains open to question.

## How to standardise

Variables likely to affect the performance of a test can be classified broadly into those that arise from the biological conditions of test organisms and those that arise from their surrounds (Soares & Calow 1993a & b). As far as single-species tests go, these relate in turn to which species and genetic strain within species to use, and how they are cultured and exposed to test conditions. Both these sources of variability can influence the results from tests. Some species and genetic strains are more sensitive than others, and for a particular species and genotype sensitivity can be modulated by surrounds and food supply. This has been particularly documented for the commonly used aquatic ecotoxicity test organism *Daphnia magna* (Bradley et al. 1993; Sims, Watson & Holmes 1993). Within this species genotypes can vary considerably in their sensitivity to test substances; the extent and ranking of genotype sensitivity varying with substance and the way that it is provided. Moreover, culture conditions can influence sensitivity such that for some substances the offspring of mothers fed poorly are often less sensitive than those that have been fed well. This is because poorly fed mothers often produce a fewer number of larger offspring than well fed mothers, possibly as an adaptation to deal with anticipated poor food supply for offspring.

## Management criteria for standardisation

So which species, genotypes and conditions are selected, not only for carrying out tests but also for culturing test organisms, can influence the results obtained from tests. What kinds of criteria can be used in selecting between them?

One kind of decision may well be based upon levels of protection. If, for example, the aims are to protect all (or most) species in ecosystems then the most sensitive organisms should be used in association with culture and test conditions which lead to effects at lowest concentrations of contaminants. Alternatives might be selection of test species that are representative of sensitivities within (an) ecosystem(s) (eg. Wagner & Lokke 1991) or emphasising average and median responses (Forbes & Forbes 1994). Another kind of decision is whether we want to protect ecological structure (species) or process (fluxes and cycles). The two are not necessarily tightly linked (Calow 1997). If we were interested in biodiversity it would be natural to focus on tests that address species sensitivity; but if we were interested in the yield of raw materials (eg. lumber or food (fish)) we would want to focus on process measurements. Which is chosen ought to be based on positive and transparent management decisions. However, currently possibly more as a matter of convenience than anything else (see below), tests that focus on structure rather than process are more common. Considerations about convenience and reliability of carrying tests out are nontheless important; for example, very sensitive species/genotypes might be more difficult to culture so reducing reliability (*sensu* above) of test systems. When decisions are taken on these issues there is a tendency to take worst-case scenarios

– going for most sensitivity – but the questions about convenience must also be prominent because the tests have to be workable often in a routine way. So, in conclusion, there are clearly both scientific and socio-political dimensions to all of these issues: what kind of sensitivity is needed to protect the target of interest to the extent desired? This is largely a scientific question. What are the targets and what level of protection is desirable? These questions raise issues that go beyond science and ultimately to the way society values nature and the services it obtains from ecological systems.

## How standardisation is achieved

Much of the responsibility for standardisation of ecotoxicity tests has been taken by the national and international standards organisations. In the EU, at least over the last few years, the Organisation for Economic Co-operation and Development (OECD) has played a prominent part. The philosophy is to develop systems that will allow mutual acceptance of data between bodies and nations. Within the OECD programme, the procedure for the acceptance of guidelines for protocols is by consensus, not only (formally) between representatives of member countries, National Coordinators, but (less formally) between at least some of the interested parties.

This is particularly well illustrated by the standardisation of the *Daphnia magna* reproduction study that is intended as an above base-set (level 1) test in the EU programmes (Sims et al. 1995). This test was adopted in guideline form in the early eighties, but a ring test initiated in 1985, in which two common test substances were assessed according to the standard protocol by over 30 laboratories, showed unacceptable variation between laboratories. A workshop of interested parties from regulatory, commercial and academic sectors was organised in 1989 to discuss possible sources of variability. Out of this meeting a general consensus emerged that more fully defined culture systems were desirable and that choice of genetic strain, food and culture would be important. A voluntary research programme designed to identify optimal conditions with respect to these variables was organised and results from this were received in 1991. Clear recommendations were made with regard to standardisation of genotype, medium and food and a formal updating of the OECD guideline was then initiated. But it was agreed that further work was needed to be sure that the recommendations made would lead to reduced variability across laboratories. A detailed report of the 1991 Workshop was also sent for comment to all National Coordinators of the OECD Test Guidelines Programme and to nominated national experts. In view of the importance and costs of a full ring test of the Guidelines, a pilot ring test was run in 1992 and, following another workshop to consider this in 1993, a full test with 3 test substances and involving 48 laboratories from 16 OECD member countries and the Czech Republic was initiated with reporting and discussion at a final Workshop in 1995. The overall variability between laboratories was much lower than that observed for the 1984 test and, being generally much less than a factor of 10, was deemed by the participants to be acceptable. Again results were sent out to National Coordinators and national experts before adoption by the OECD.

At all stages, then, there was a considerable amount of involvement by interested parties. In very general terms decisions between options were based upon both sensitivity and convenience. The discussions were nevertheless largely technical and it is hard to see how non-technical people could have been involved. A further important point is that the work on the standardization spanned over 10 years, involved a large number of scientists over a large number of laboratories across the world and so inevitably was very costly in time, effort and money.

## Data analysis may also matter

Conclusions are influenced by which tests are chosen and how they are carried out, but also by how the data from these are analysed. The results from both controls and treatments will be variable and so making judgements about possible differences between them is never categorical but involves statistical assessment. Important decisions have to be taken about what sorts of levels of confidence to require from analysis of data, how to do the analysis and what kind of data to use in the analyses.

As far as levels of confidence are concerned, in basic science there is usually a major concern about making false claims; of claiming differences between controls and treatments when they do not exist (ie. committing so-called type 1 errors). Significance levels here are generally set by convention at p = 0.05; ie. such that there is only a one in 20 chance of rejecting the null hypothesis when it is in fact true. In applying science, however, especially in an ecotoxicological context, it is often more important not to miss differences between a control and treatment when in fact they exist (ie. committing type 2 errors). The conventions here, in terms of chosing levels of significance, are not as clearly defined (Forbes & Forbes 1994). There are two points to note. First, levels of confidence are set by convention and are not absolute. Second, which conventions are used are context dependent. Scientists in the applied area can often be influenced by the procedures of basic science and take type 1 errors more seriously than type 2 errors. However, emphasising type 2 errors in a sense is a statistical manifestation of the precautionary principle.

There are also decisions to be made about methods of analysis. When the data are from a concentration-effect series there are at least two methods of analysis. One involves comparing each treatment with the control and each other by analysing the average response within each and the variance around it. This is the traditional method of using analysis of variance. It leads to an identification of concentrations that have no effect, not significantly different from controls, and the highest of these is defined as the 'no observed effect concentration' (NOEC). But data from the series can also be described by equations that rigorously link concentrations with effect (model fitting/regression techniques) and that can therefore be used to predict concentrations that have particular effects. Hence they can be used to predict concentrations that will have very low effects but, for mathematical reasons, never that have zero effects. This itself raises a supposed problem; ie. of chosing between techniques that seemingly give either no effect or low effect concentrations as outputs. But this problem is more psychological than substantial because strictly the NOEC is associated with a possibility of error, such that at these concentrations there might still be the probability (however low) of an effect; it is just that the model fitting technique makes this explicit. There can, nevertheless, still be differences in the sensitivity of outputs. Because a NOEC is based upon a discontinuous series of treatments there is no way of knowing how close it is to the next highest effect concentration. Clearly the problem is reduced as the interval between concentrations in the test series is reduced, but this has implications for effort and cost.

On the other hand, the regression models 'fill in the data gaps' and in principle can make more precise predictions. However, this is sensitive to the kind of model that is employed: crudely a straight-line fit between two data points is likely to lead to different predictions than either a concave-up or a concave-down curve.

Finally, even the way results are calculated can matter. The *Daphnia* study which is described above is designed to investigate *sublethal* effects on reproduction. Indeed concentrations are chosen such that they will be unlikely to cause adult mortality; to specifically investigate to what extent these lower concentrations do indeed influence reproductive performance. But even then parents do die in treatments for various reasons – eg. they may have been roughly handled or they may have been unhealthy before exposure. Adult mortality raises a problem: should offspring from adults that die during a test be ignored or not? If they are ignored effect concentrations may be overestimated by not taking account of effects on weak parents or if they are used effects on reproduction may be obscured by parental health effects! With this in mind three kinds of results can be calculated: total offspring per parents; offspring per parent per day; offspring per brood.

Apart from the decisions already noted there are also statistical issues to consider. Most statistical tests presume that in making comparisons the distributions within treatments are part of the same populations (homogenous). But the results from unhealthy parents can be so different from the rest within a treatment that they cannot be included as part of the same population. Experience from the ring test on *Daphnia* (above) showed that the statistical issues were of overriding importance and on this basis endpoints calculated in terms of total offspring produced by parents alive at the end of a test were prefered (Sims et al. 1995).

The main point of describing these somewhat technical issues is to illustrate that they can affect results and conclusions drawn from them. Moreover the rationale for chosing between options may not be exclusively or decisively technical. Not surprisingly, though, decisions on these issues are usually taken by the technical community in similar ways to those described for the tests themselves (above).

## CONCLUSIONS

There is an important sense in which, provided a problem can be defined, the scientific procedure (as defined in the introduction) can be applied to it in a way that is transparent. As has been illustrated above, judgements certainly have to be made within the scientific procedure about the way observations are made, and how they are analysed and interpreted, but these can be made explicit for discussion and debate. The main problem for environmental/ecological protection, though, is knowing what the targets are in the first place, and what it is about them, that we want to protect. Sometimes this is known precisely: particular species, habitats and ecosystems are deemed vulnerable for some reason and then, in principle, scientific effort can be put into assessing the extent of this risk and what might be done about it. But the targets are often less precise; for example, EU new and existing substances legislation is concerned with protecting the environment at large – presumably ecosystems in general, even though the current focus of its testing programmes is aquatic. There are also a number of other possible explanations for difficulties in defining targets. These are concerned with the early stage of development of the subject area, the complexity of the subject and the fact that the subjects, ecosystems, are just not as unitary in their organisation as organisms in general and the human organism in particular. Hence it will always be easier to specify the health targets for human beings than it will the well-being of ecosystems (Calow 1995).

It has been argued above that deciding what the targets are for ecotoxicology and how well they ought to be protected has both a legitimate scientific and socio-political dimension. However, it is the technical community that often predominantly takes decisions because the issues are genuinely complex; they are from complex systems and procedures and, as has been illustrated for the ring test, can involve a large number of scientists over a considerable period of time. On the other hand, decisions are frequently taken on the basis of principles that are implicit and not as clearly defined as they could be. For example, in making decision about test options most sensitive designs are very frequently favoured as a general recourse to the precautionary principle; but reliability and convenience are also of considerable prominence because of the need for pragmatism.

The challenge, therefore, given the technical nature of many of the decisions, is to enable informed and useful input from all interested parties on either side of the technical divide. This will not be easy, but two principles seem particularly important – permeability and transparency – and these are likely to influence judgements about scenarios for regulatory policy (Halfman & Bal, this volume). They should also influence the extent and form by which technical advisory bodies transmit their advice to regulators and to the public at large. For example, the Annual Report of an Advisory Committee on Hazardous Substances (to the UK Government), is written with the intent not only of informing the public on what advice has been given and what action has been taken, but also of providing general information on the nature of the decision-making processes themselves (ACHS 1995).

## References

ACHS (1995) *Fourth Annual Report 1994-1995*, London: HMSO.

Bradley, M.C., C. Naylor, P. Calow, D.J. Baird, I. Barber & A.M.V.M. Soares (1993) 'Reducing variability in *Daphnia* toxicity tests – a case for further standardization', in A.M.V.M. Soares & P. Calow, eds., *Progress in Standardization of Aquatic Toxicity Tests*, Boca Raton: Lewis Publishers; 57-70.

Calow, P. (1993) 'Hazards and risks in Europe: challenges for ecotoxicology', *Environmental Toxicology and Chemistry* 12: 1519-1520.

Calow, P. (1994) 'Ecotoxicology: What are we trying to protect?', *Environmental Toxicology & Chemistry* 13: 1549.

Calow, P. (1995) 'Ecosystem health – a critical analysis of concepts', in D.J. Rapport, D.L. Gaudet & P. Calow, eds, *Evaluating and Monitoring the Health of Large-Scale Ecosystems*, Berlin: Springer Verlag; 33-41.

Calow, P. (1997) *Controlling Environmental Risks from Chemicals: Principles and Practice*, Chichester: John Wiley & Son.

Forbes, V.E. & T.L. Forbes (1994) *Ecotoxicology in Theory and Practice*, London: Chapman & Hall.

ISO (1986) *Precision of test methods – determination of repeatability and reproducibility for a standard test method by inter-laboratory tests*, ISO 5725-1986 (E).

Jasanoff, S. (1990) *The Fifth Branch: Science Advisers as Policy Makers*, Harvard, MA: Harvard University Press.

OECD (1984) *Guidelines for Testing of Chemicals*, Paris: OECD.

Sims, I.R., S. Watson & D. Holmes (1993) 'Towards a standard *Daphnia* juvenile production test', *Environmental Toxicology and Chemistry* 12: 2053-2058.

Sims, I., P. van Dijk, J. Gamble & N. Grandy (1995) 'Final Ring Test of the *Daphnia magna* Reproduction Study'. Unpublished Final Report to the OECD Test Guideline Programme.

Soares, A.M.V.M. & P. Calow (1993a) 'Seeking standardization in ecotoxicology,' in A.M.V.M. Soares & P. Calow, eds., *Progress in Standardization of Aquatic Toxicity Tests*, Boca Raton: Lewis Publishers; 1-6.

Soares, A.M.V.M. & P. Calow, eds. (1993b) *Progress in Standardisation of Aquatic Toxicity Tests*, Boca Raton: Lewis Publishers.

Wagner, C. & H. Lokke (1991) 'Estimation of ecotoxicological protection levels from NOEC toxicity data', *Water Research* 25: 1237-1242.

# 11

*Willem Halffman*

# STANDARDIZATION AS A TRUST DEVICE

## THE PROBLEM OF MISTRUSTED EXPERTS

For many regulatory scientists, it is hard to understand why their careful and intricate risk assessments fail to resolve societal contestation over the magnitude of chemical risks. From the experts' point of view, it seems that the science of risk assessment (RA) is particularly prone to irrational responses. In spite of increasingly refined risk assessment procedures, environmental movements and consumer organizations continually question the findings of risk assessment science. Such organizations typically claim that important hazards are underestimated or ignored. On the other hand, regulated industries relentlessly insist that mitigating factors have been left out of consideration. After several decades of extensive investments in the development of risk assessment methodology, in the standardization and validation of toxicity tests, as well as in the development of assessment protocols and models, this situation has still not changed fundamentally. Nevertheless, many risk assessment experts seem to expect that their science could at least demarcate the area of political dispute. They often express the belief that further improvements in the science of risk assessment can limit societal disagreements to issues of value judgements and balancing of interests, as is shown in Sue Mayer and Gillian Clegg's contribution to this volume. Scientists then consider themselves to be the linesmen of politics – only to find their rulings questioned time and time again.

Societal debate on risk regulation frequently involves discussions about the magnitude of risks, and not just how these risks should be valued. The

In: R. Bal & W. Halffman (eds.), *The Politics of Chemical Risk*, Kluwer Academic Publishers, Dordrecht 1998: p. 265-292.

regulation of the environmental risks of pesticides provides a clear example of how regulatory decision-making can be questioned in every aspect, in spite of attempts to radically insulate the scientific issues from the political debate. In the Netherlands, the committee of authoritative experts responsible for pesticide licensing and assessment has been the object of severe criticism from the environmental movement, and even from ministeries (Reijnders et al., 1995; Projektgroep Evaluatie Toelating Bestrijdingsmiddelen, 1995). In this case, an attempt to pacify pesticide policy by relying more on the experts has failed. In other cases, policy makers seem to have lost their belief in risk assessment altogether. The European Commission's decision to set the drinking water standard for all individual pesticides at 0.1 μg/l was met with disbelief by RA experts. It went directly against the experts' standing practice to identify the precise health risks of each individual pesticide through technical refinement of testing and assessment (e.g. Royal Commission on Environmental Pollution, 1992: 126). The standard view that the best possible science will lead to a convincing basis for regulatory decisions fails to give insight into these continuing disputes over the nature and magnitude of chemical hazards. The claim that the decisions were right because they were based on the truths of science and scientific rationality is not sufficient to settle societal disagreement. Even attempts to provide better explanation to the 'lay public' do not provide a simple solution. The regulatory world is slowly becoming aware that the problem cannot be resolved by such a one-sided explanation of 'The Science' to 'The Public' (Royal Society, 1992: 135 seq.; Health Council of The Netherlands, 1995).

What might be an alternative way to understand the relation between the experts and their exacting audience of policy actors? In this paper, I suggest that it could be helpful for regulatory scientists to think of the relation between RA and its critics as a matter of *trust* rather than *truth*. Using trust as a focal point to understand the development of experimental science is a relatively new and promising approach in the social studies of science, or 'STS' (e.g. Shapin 1994, Shapin and Schaffer, 1985). The research field of STS brings together a broad range of disciplines in order to try to understand the developments of science and technology as embedded in different societal contexts. While STS has developed into a vibrant – though sometimes somewhat excentric – academic enterprise over recent decades, I will not try to catalogue its findings and debates here. An adequate overview of the key issues in the field can be found in the paper of Jasanoff in this volume (see also Jasanoff et al., 1995; Pickering, 1992). Rather, I want to show how this one approach to expertise, typical to STS, contrasts with the technical understanding of expertise common among regulatory experts. For STS, the performance and communication of research is not a sufficient condition for establishing truth. Central to an analysis of the *social* aspects of science is the attempt to understand how and when experimental practices provide arguments that are considered convincing by a community. Rather than assuming that scientific practices produce truths, this approach investigates the conditions under which scientific results are trusted.

I will start by showing how trust in toxicity testing and assessment procedures is an issue *among* regulatory scientists. Regulatory scientists use various devices to assure trust in each other's findings. I will use the standardization of toxicity tests as an example of such a device. In this analysis of regulatory practice, standardization is more than a mere technical affair, more than a matter of straightforward optimization of research practice in terms of cost efficiency or comparability of results. Without wanting to diminish the solid technical reasons for regulatory scientists to standardize toxicity tests, the paper argues that a sociological approach offers additional insights that could help us to understand how standardization 'works' or, more importantly, sometimes does not. By extending this analysis beyond the confines of regulatory science, I will suggest that the process of establishing trust *among* expert has very similar traits to the process of establishing trust *in* experts by those who are not members of the institutions of RA. Without wanting to exaggerate these parallels, I do suggest that this comparison may be useful to understand some sources of mistrust and contestation. Drawing upon ongoing research (Halffman, 1995), the analysis will focus on examples taken from non-human environmental risk assessments of chemicals in the Netherlands, the UK and the US.

## STANDARDIZATION AS A TRUST DEVICE

The standardization of environmental toxicity tests and related assessment protocols has been under way for over twenty years now. This development is more than a mere technical improvement of tests, but is closely related to the development of environmental regulation. Just a brief overview will indicate the close links between tests and the regulatory context. A landmark in test standardization was the publication of a series of protocols for acute and chronic toxicity tests with fish by the US Environmental Protection Agency in 1975 (USEPA, 1975). These tests could draw on a much older tradition of aquatic toxicity tests in US Fish and Wildlife laboratories and the UK former Water Research Centre (Hunn, 1989), as well as from the example of human toxicity tests. Nevertheless, this publication marks the recognition of the value of standardized environmental toxicity tests for routine use in environmental regulation. In subsequent years, the development of test standards quickly gained momentum. By 1977, the development of standard environmental toxicity tests was put on the agenda of the Programme on Chemicals of the OECD. This resulted in the OECD principles of Good Laboratory Practice (GLP) by 1982 and a continuing effort to develop protocols for environmental toxicity tests (Idman, 1978; OECD, 1982; OECD, s.d.). The interest of the European Union in the development of assessment protocols and standardization of environmental toxicity tests dates from the preparations for the New Chemicals Directive between 1976 and 1979 (Johnson 1978; Brickman et al., 1985: 286 seq.). Toxicity test protocols and assessment principles were further developed for the purpose of defining the classification of substances as dangerous to the environment (CEC, 1990; EEC Dir. 79/831: Annex V, Part C), as were specific EU GLP guidelines around 1986-87 (EEC, Dir. 87/18/1987). Both the EU and the OECD have continued this tradition of investing in the development of methods, often with the close involvement of national regulatory research institutes (e.g. CEC, 1980, 1984, 1993; OECD, 1991). A similar standardization process took place on the level of assessment protocols indicating how individual test results are to be integrated in one assessment. For example, the 'Uniform Principles' now provide guidance on how the results of such tests should be evaluated and assessed for pesticides, following earlier harmonized arrangements for new and old chemicals.

From this overview, it should be clear that the developmment of environmental toxicity tests and assessment protocols is a project with *regulatory* stakes. The reasons for developing tests and protocols relate to the use that actors envisage for them in the regulatory context. It is extremely unlikely that the present degree of standardization of these tests would ever have been produced for the purpose of purely academic research science. What are those specific regulatory reasons for standardization? As stated in regulatory documents or by regulatory actors, the list is diverse. A first group of reasons relates to the exchange of data. When test requirements are uniform, then duplication of testing and assessments can be minimized. In regulatory documents, this is phrased as the reduction of the cost of assessments or the abolishment of barriers to trade. Companies that operate on an international level can limit their testing effort if the same results are accepted by the regulatory agencies that accept the same test standards. Regulatory agencies do not have to repeat the assessment effort if they can rely on previous assessments (OECD, 1982: 23). Such an agenda has the political advantage of coupling minimization of industrial cost to animal protection goals. The limitation of the number of test animals used for purposes of regulatory assessment has been an important issue in the Dutch debate on dangerous substances (Malta, 1992) and is also noted at the European level (McCutcheon, this volume).

However, this objective presupposes a second set of reasons: the assessments and tests performed by regulatory scientists in one place have to be credible to regulatory scientists in other places working for other institutions or different national regulatory authorities. Techniques of quality control are supposed to guarantee the reliability of assessments to other parties. For example, the results of tests performed by commercial testing laboratories become more trustworthy to the assessors in regulatory agencies when the standardized procedures are used. Confidence in these results will increase with a guaranteed use of standard operating procedures and GLP, possibly even with a laboratory certification system. This relation of *trust* is not merely a matter of trust in laboratory results by regulatory assessors, but also a matter of trust among different regulatory agencies. As assessment methodology is standardized, assessments performed by one regulatory agency could become more trustworthy to other regulatory agencies, at least in principle. Such trust forms the basis of the distributed assessment scheme of the EU Directive on existing chemicals (McCutcheon, this volume), of the Uniform Principles for the assessment of pesticides, and of the increasing reliance of, for example, UK regulatory agencies on assessments performed by industry (UK Government/Industry Working Group, 1993). In sum, the second reason is that assessments performed by others are generally considered to be more trustworthy when assessment techniques are standardized, even in the face of conflicting interests.

Therefore, the stability of tests and assessments across contexts is an important aspect of trust among the experts. With respect to environmental toxicity testing, the development of tests, such as with *Daphnids*, is characterized by efforts to stabilize the results between different laboratories. By refining the test procedures and standardizing the equipment used, variations in the results of the same test due to laboratory ideosyncracies are gradually minimized. Whether this stability is obtained can be evaluated again by technical means, such as a 'ring test' in which the test is performed with known reference substances in different laboratories. Such a test for *Daphnia magna* has been organized by the OECD, coordinated by Professor Calow (1993, this volume). Ultimately, one could imagine fully automated environmental toxicity tests, approximating the stability of bioassays in medical research. Recent efforts to develop freeze-dried toxicity test kits seem to go in this direction. As these tests or parts of them are automated, an additional reduction of costs is implied, since labour is the most important cost factor in toxicity testing (Perez et al., 1985). Methodologically, this stability is traditionally indicated as 'reliability'.

The trust that regulatory experts have in standardized tests and protocols has another aspect. Trust in test results is not only a matter of reliability and stability of test performance, but also of the extent to which a test provides information about expected environmental effects, indicated as the 'validity' of a test. The extent to which the effects, or 'endpoints', tested by standardized toxicity tests are representative of 'real world' effects of chemicals has been a matter of contention ever since their introduction into the regulatory world. Throughout the 1980s, academic scientists and especially ecologists have continuously criticized the so-called reductionism of the tests. Allegedly, the idealized laboratory conditions of, for example, acute fish toxicity testing would not be representative of the ecological complexities of real streams (cf. Cairns, 1977, 1981, 1988; Koeman, 1982; Calow, 1993). Although this disagreement has been tenuous, here too technical solutions have been sought. The validity of single species toxicity tests has in turn been tested. Their results have been compared with the results of field studies by the USEPA or with the results of mesocosm tests, such as artificial streams by an international project supported by the European Commission (CEC, 1993). Several attempts have been made to improve the validity of environmental toxicity tests by refining the extrapolation methods (OECD, 1991).

Nevertheless, the improvement of the trustworthiness of assessments in terms of better apparatuses or procedures needs to be qualified. Environmental RA is never merely a matter of artifacts and inference rules. Regulatory experts continuously stress the importance for 'expert judgement'. No matter how stable or valid tests are, time and time again the need of expert interpretation is stated. The phrase can be found in the 1975 USEPA environmental toxicity manual and it can still be heard from regulatory experts now, 20 years later (e.g. Jager et al, 1994). There are good reasons to hold on to the margin of interpretation by experienced experts. Chemical compounds can have their ideosyncracies that are unaccounted for in the routine test procedures. The history of environmental pollution during recent decades offers a number of examples of chemicals with rather peculiar environmental effects. Some go far beyond the straight-forward environmental impacts that are part of environmental assessment procedures. Organotin compounds with pseudo-hormonal effects in shellfish are a case in point (e.g. Seager et al., 1986): only experienced experts could discover these more exotic environmental effects. However, even in routine testing, chemicals have their individual peculiarities that may require special provisions in testing protocols or interpretation of test results, for example chemicals that form hazardous metabolites or degradation products that present sollubility problems. Inversely, mitigation effects could also be ignored in overly standardized testing. In such cases, expert judgement is the only guarantee that provisions are made for the exceptional chemicals and their non-routine effects or behaviour. Even though an increasing number of effects and possible complications are now considered in formalized assessment schemes, these can never be complete.

Ultimately, trust in test results and assessments still relies on experts and their professional accreditation. This is nicely illustrated by a Dutch effort at validation of a computerized assessment tool, the Uniform System for the Evaluation of Substances (USES) program. In an effort to test the validity of the program, its results were compared with expert judgement in a prioritizing application. At a workshop, the experts were used as the measuring stick to evaluate the tool. Although results of both approaches were similar, the need for expert evaluation was confirmed. Once again, we find explicit mention of the need for expert evaluation, both of input and output of the model. The program is an expert 'decision-support system', not a fulfledged autonomous evaluator of chemical hazards (Jager et al, 1994: 2,4).

To sum up, even though the standardization of the environmental hazard of chemicals is generally presented as a technical affair, this does not imply that there are no expert judgements to be made. I have suggested that an important type of judgement concerns the balance between reliability and validity. On the one hand, trust in tests and assessments depends on guarantees of their stability in different contexts, methodologically addressed as 'reliablity'. By this criterion, a good test is a test that universally produces the same results, irrespective of the context of performance. On the other hand, trust in tests and assessments is a matter of the quality of their predictions of the effects and behaviour of chemicals in the environment, or 'validity'. A valid test is a test that predicts effects that occur in 'the real environment', inevitably involving local ideosyncracies of that environment. Requirements for valid assessments may lead to adaptations in the standard procedures to address those ideosyncracies, thereby lowering general reliability.[1] In principle, we rely on experts and their judgements to balance reliability and validity, and call the process 'risk assessment', i.e. the experts will sort out what are considered the technicalities of standardization and validation.

For these reasons, the standardization of RA methodology is more than merely a way to develop better tests and protocols in the sense of better representations of real world effects of chemicals. Standardization is also a device to increase trust among regulatory experts. Although the problem of trust in assessment has now been extended beyond a matter of technicalities of artifacts and procedures to include trust among experts, this could still be considered 'technical'; these issues seem to be unrelated to political contexts. The judgements can be made on the basis of the best possible

1 The tension between the 'general' toxicity of a chemical and its local and ideosyncratic effects in natural environments has partly been accommodated by a separation between effect and fate assessment: toxicity is a property of the chemical and is universal, fate is a matter of distribution in the environment and is therefore by definition local. However, toxicity is not a quality of a chemical alone, but of a chemical in combination with a biotic context, such as an organism, and therefore subject to local or regional variation. For these reasons, some countries stress the importance of the use of native species in environmental effect assessment. This problem is not even unique to environmental toxicology. Similar variability in effect assessment can be found with human health assessment, as the population is refined and differentiated, e.g. by sex, age, profession, or nutritional patterns.

science, be it under conditions of limited resources. I will now proceed with my analysis in an attempt to show how even these very technical questions interact with specific political contexts, following the notion of trust as the scope of analysis is widened.[2] I want to stress that my goal is not to show how noble science is contaminated by dirty politics, but rather to show that these trust devices are used differently within different political contexts.

## REGIMES OF TRUST

So far I have suggested how standardization plays a role in the maintenance of trust among regulatory experts in general. In order to make the connection with the trust of 'non-experts' in expert RA, I will extend the frame of reference and bring in the political context in which RA is set. I will call the concatenation of tools and techniques, processes of standardization and procedural guarantees that sustain trust among actors, a 'regime of trust' (parallel to Foucault, 1980: 109 seq.). For regulatory purposes, the comparison of the regime of trust of research science and of regulatory science may be informative, but a comparison of different *regulatory* regimes of trust would bring us closer to an answer to the problem of understanding the contestation of regulatory expertise. A comparison between different regulatory regimes shows different ways of organizing regulatory assessments, different ways to obtain trustworthy evaluations of chemicals, as well as different ways in which trust can be broken. Such comparisons can be made over time or between countries, but also between different regulatory regimes in the same national context. They can also involve different segments of regulatory practice.

One way to show differences in the way regimes of trust work in different regulatory contexts is by a comparison of the use of one specific trust

---

2 My analysis examines the role and stakes of standardization from the point of view of regulatory agencies and the regulatory scientists. It focuses on political rather than economic points of reference. From the point of view of multinational companies in particular, there may be entirely different stakes in the standardization of risk assessment (Abraham, 1993). However, I have chosen this focus in the light of the goals and setting of this workshop. (In response to a question by John Abraham.)

device: a comparison of the way standardized tests are actually employed by regulatory assessors in different regulatory regimes. In a comparison between the regulatory practice of assessment under the US Toxic Substances Control Act (TSCA) and the Federal Insecticide, Fungicide, and Rodenticide Act (FIFRA), I have been able to show such differences most sharply. The USEPA has invested substantially in the standardization of tests and protocols. The methodology is in many cases even more formalized than that developed in Europe or the OECD and describes test and assessment procedures in great detail (e.g. USEPA 1991). For the assessment of industrial chemicals under the TSCA, regulatory assessors rely on these standards. However, minor changes in the protocols are negotiated with companies and their laboratories for specific applications of these tests. Such changes may involve provisions for specific characteristics of chemicals, such as low solubility. When exceptional environmental behaviour of the chemical is claimed by registrants, regulators will negotiate additional testing and also negotiate the protocols to be used. This negotiation process may ultimately even result in additional testing in laboratory-scale ecosystems or 'microcosms'. Although new protocols have been developed for these tests (USEPA 1987), such tests were used before this codification. Their precise performance requires substantial additional specifications in the actual test protocol.

To regulators and companies alike, such additional provisions increase the trust in the validity of the results. Registrants can rely on their informal contacts to make sure that their test results will be considered acceptable by the regulatory assessors. The regulatory assessors will trust the test results because they have had a say in devising the test in case there was any complication. In addition, there is the limited number of regulatory toxicity laboratories and the certification programmes to back up the quality of the laboratories. According to the regulators, an acceptable balance between issues of reliability and validity has been found. Tests are considered sufficiently standard to be reliable, but there is also considerable room for negotiation to deal with the odd case.

In contrast, US pesticide assessment is far more formalized. FIFRA assessors generally do not negotiate of test protocols, and apply assessment procedures in a very strict way. Although specific questions of protocols may be answered occasionally, in general, testing rules are taken literally and assessment procedures are highly standard. The 'tiered system', in which the tests that are required for pesticides depend on previous tests, is strictly applied. In this regulatory regime, informal contact between the regulators and the assessors can easily lead to criticism from an alert environmental movement that follows pesticides much closer than the industrial chemicals regulated under the TSCA. When the strict and legalistic rules of the RA process are not followed, any of the parties can decide to go to court. In contrast to the assessment of industrial chemicals, trust in the assessment of pesticides is not in the first place a matter of negotiation and mutual adjustment of the test procedures, but a matter of strict adherence to the rules, part of which are the test protocols of toxicity assays.

One of the consequences for pesticide assessment practice is that test results that do not follow the highly standardized and formalistic patterns cannot be considered in the assessment process. Since the regime of trust is built on rules and protocols and on the scrutiny of the courts overseeing their application, other forms of knowledge are an uncertain and potentially costly gamble for all parties involved. Pond mesocosm studies are examples of attempts to use semi-field tests. Although these tests are based on protocols developed specifically for the assessment of pesticides in the US (Touart 1988, Touart and Slimak 1989), the protocols are only very general guidelines that require substantive negotiation before actual test protocols can be written. In addition, the results of these tests require a great deal of interpretation by the assessors. The use of mesocosm studies implies much more than the application of standards and rules, the trust devices normally used in this regulatory regime. The results of about thirteen expensive mesocosm tests were never used in the US, in spite of the strong conviction of the ecologists working as assessors at the EPA's Pesticide Office that these tests were of much higher validity than the standardized single-species toxicity test (based on interviews with regulators). When asked for an explanation of this situation, the regulators said they did not believe that this sort of information would survive a legal challenge. The high levels of negotiation needed to perform and use mesocosm studies did not match the high reliance on rules and standardized procedures as trust devices in this particular regulatory regime.

Pursuing the example of pesticide assessments, the consequences of these differences for the assessment process become clear. The same mesocosm test results that were left out of the assessments by the American regulators were used rather unproblematically to assess pesticide hazards in the UK. The Advisory Committee on Pesticides organizes meetings with industry scientists in which the acceptability and quality of test results are discussed. According to the regulatory assessors, the results of some of the mesocosm studies were effectively used to develop acceptable environmental concentrations. In this case, there was no possibility of legal challenges to this segment of the assessment procedures, as these proceedings are confidential and pesticide legislation does not allow for adversarial legal contestation of the decision-making. The very same tests that were seen as too high a risk in one regulatory regime were used straight-forwardly in another. When one evaluates the specific position of multi-species toxicity tests, it turns out that they are sometimes seen as producing viable results and sometimes as too weak to withstand regulatory challenges. In the international community of experts, such tests are considered to be of high validity, as close as one can get to 'real world' conditions. This is even the case for US regulators, as suggested assessment factors to be applied to micro- and mesocosm results are close to or equal to one. However, even though regulators may find these results highly trustworthy, this does not imply that they can be used in every regulatory context.

The comparison between these regulatory examples shows that the way the trust in test results is organized and guaranteed is dependent on the societal context. Regulatory scientists may have specific ideas about which data are more reliable or trustworthy, but their idea about the quality of data is not the only thing that matters. Regulators have to take the political and legal context into account. The ways in which regulators can assure their own trust in test results and assessments are constrained by the way their regime of trust is organized, which is in turn dependent upon the political, legal, and institutional conditions under which it operates. However, in this political context trust is again a crucial issue: are the experts trusted to make fair decisions or are they perceived as biased legitimators of partisan policies? In addition, whether such mistrust will have consequences for the position of the experts depends on the resources that can be mobilized against them. With these considerations, we can once more expand the context of analysis of this paper and proceed to the trust *in* the experts.

## THE ASSESSMENT OF CHEMICALS AS A MATTER OF SOCIETAL TRUST

The very idea of a division of labour between experts and political institutions depends on the assumption that the experts can be trusted with a (substantial) part of the job. However, this trust in regulatory experts is never self-evident; it has to be established and maintained. In this respect, regulatory decision-making is not different from other aspects of governmental decision making. Democracies have developed mechanisms that more or less guarantee the fairness and acceptability of government action. By constructing a specific realm for expert decision-making, the realm of 'RA', a specific set of instruments is mobilized to legitimate government action. The scientists will define what the impact of a substance will be, leaving the consequences and integration of interests to the politicians and administrators. The problem is that this distinction has no inherent foundation, in spite of positivist philosophy's attempt to devise one. The statement that the hazards of chemicals are evaluated by (the best possible) science does not by itself resolve the issues. A critical societal field of actors wants guarantees to assure that relevant information is taken into account, that evaluations take the relevant uncertainties into account, or that the experts are not too deeply involved in the culture of the parties they help regulating. A recourse to the rhetoric of 'the best possible science' for legitimation of regulatory action is not sufficient.

Just as experts use the standardization of toxicity tests and protocols as tools to assure the trustworthiness of the results, so procedural guarantees are mobilized to (re)assure the trust in experts. The way in which societies have organized this trust in experts differs widely between policy cultures. In the United States, the procedural guarantees remain dominant: membership of expert committees, the way in which data are collected for assessments, the way in which data have to be brought together to make assessments, or the value of assessment results in the ensuing balancing of interests, are all supported by legalistic guarantees. These strict rules are not always employed, as the example of the assessment of industrial chemicals indicates, but in general, the American political system provides procedural guarantees as tools to maintain the trust in expert decision-making. Just as the experts mobilize standardized and formalized testing protocols in order to trust the submitted data, so procedural guarantees are available to check the experts. When one starts to compare different regulatory regimes in the US, the additional mechanisms to sustain the trust in the experts come to the fore. The most extreme example of the mobilization of procedural guarantees is probably regulatory decision-making in the case of pesticides. In other domains of environmental policy, American regulators have developed alternative measures to increase the trust in regulatory decision-making, such as certain forms of citizen participation in the evaluation of risks (Fiorino, 1990).

British pesticide assessments, and environmental policy in general, has long been hampered by one-sided scientistic strategies for maintenance of trust. Although the British regulatory style has been characterized as informal and secretive, the legitimation of this style relies on the impartiality of professionals as the optimal way to obtain fair decisions (Wynne, 1982; Vogel, 1986; Brickman et al., 1985; Andrews, 1994). Towards the end of the eighties, a move was made towards more formal decision-making and more public accessibility of environmental information, leading some to suggest a convergence between American and British regulatory styles (Wynne, 1992). Pesticide policy can be seen as an example of this trend. After the pesticide assessment scheme became statutory in 1986, the strategy of relying on highly qualified experts in a secretive committee slowly started to change. Now, assessment documents are available that give (limited) insight into the way the evaluations have been made, whereas before one had to rely entirely on the verdict of the experts. There is also more room for discussion with other parties than just industry. The blind reliance on the professionalism of the experts that was implied in the old scheme, has therefore been supplemented with modest instruments allowing outsiders some extra assurance. Although British pesticide policy is still not exactly one of the more restrictive ones and although there is still severe criticism of assessment practice, the pesticide assessors seem to find the new, more open and responsive arrangement also more constructive (interviews; Beaumont, 1993).

Dutch pesticide assessment may well be an example of the reverse development. In 1993, pesticide assessment and licensing was mandated to a committee of three experts. The creation of this quango was motivated by the deadlock of the former corporatist decision making procedures for pesticide regulation. Under the previous arrangement, experts advised a committee mainly consisting of representatives from various ministeries. The decision-making was slow and nearly always controversial, which led to criticism of bureaucratic inertia from both industry and the environmental movement.

The slowness of decision-making contrasted sharply with the ambitious pesticide reduction goals set in the Multi-Year Crop Protection Plan of 1990 (Tweede Kamer, 1990). Part of this ambitious plan to reduce the high reliance on pesticides in Dutch agriculture was to develop a stricter licensing policy, along with more differentiated risk models. The mandate to the expert committee was based on the idea that the principles and general policy goals of pesticide assessment and licensing were clear – or would be in the very near future. The division of labour between the experts and the policy makers was not one between 'politics' and 'science', but between policy and implementation; ministeries, with the Ministery of Agriculture as *primus inter pares*, have the responsibility of developing general principles of both assessment and management. The experts have the responsibility to apply these principles in every specific case. The details of how to perform this task are rather unclear. The manual containing the assessment principles is not publicly available. The expert committee limits the information on the assessment of individual pesticide products to the legal minimum. The only basis to trust these experts is their reputation as experts.

There may be nothing wrong at all with the decision-making *per se* of the expert committee. No doubt the experts are administrating the available pesticide policies to the very best of their abilities. The tragedy is that the present arrangement leads to suspicion, not trust. The Dutch environmental movement clearly no longer trusts these experts. Environmental organizations have used their newly available legal means to challenge decision-making wherever possible. In addition, they launched an outright attack on the expert committee in the form of a 'black book'. This report goes as far as to suggest the replacement of the committee chairman (Reijnders et al., 1995). An evaluation of the functioning of the committee by a government task force also contains considerable criticism, in spite of the moderate wording that resulted from the negotiations over the text of the report (Projektgroep Evaluatie Toelating Bestrijdingsmiddelen, 1995).

In the long run, the organization of Dutch pesticide assessment and licensing will not be tenable. There are insufficient devices to guarantee trust in regulatory assessment. The only guarantees of fair decision-making presently available boil down to the argument that they are good and reliable experts. The committee claims to have strict instructions from the ministeries, but fails to provide information on how these instructions are applied. Once again, the reputation of the regulators is the only guarantee of trust. It has been precisely this reputation which has been under attack and, within the present procedures, there are no instruments to repair that trust.

Evidently, 'trust' is not the only element explaining the acceptance or contentiousness of expert decision-making. Nor is it the case that specific styles of organizing expertise inherently determine the levels of trust they arouse. For example, the present format of Dutch pesticide assessment and licensing is a format that operates without much debate in other domains of environmental policy. The assessment of new industrial chemicals, for example, is a matter of similar autonomous and 'discrete' expert committees. The same format of regulatory assessment that fails to produce a policy that is considered acceptable by actors in the regulation of pesticides passes without much contestation in the regulation of new industrial chemicals. Pesticides have traditionally drawn more attention from environmental, consumer, and labour movements. It is precisely in these more controversial policy domains that additional ways to assure trust in the experts are needed. In addition, the contentiousness of (environmental) policy domains also depends on the possibilities contesters have to mobilize resources against the institutions. These resources can be rhetorical – 'pesticides are designed to kill' – but also institutional, in the form of legal or political resources that can be mobilized against decision-making. A number of institutional arrangements oriented towards increasing trust in expert decision-making may actually increase the possibilities to challenge the decisions (by whichever party able to mobilize the resources to actually do so) and in the end lead to the suggestion that something must be wrong because the decisions are challenged so often. Trust-fostering measures can backfire by inducing more policy challenges. Experiences with science courts in American pesticide policy of the seventies are an example of this pattern: a procedure allegedly installed to make pesticide assessments more trustworthy led to polarization and deadlock in adversarial procedures (Jasanoff, 1990).

In spite of these qualifications, trust remains a central problem for regulatory policy. Every form of expert decision-making, especially in controversial policy domains, will have to foresee challenges and find acceptable ways to create and maintain the trust in the experts on which the division of labour is dependent. As in their own internal division of expert labour, trust must be earned. In this respect, the regulatory experts are no different from 'the public' they try to convince. This brings us back to the agenda of this paper:

to compare the trust *of* the experts in tests and assessments with the trust *in* experts' decision-making. I will try to show some parallels.

## TRUST OF AND TRUST IN EXPERTS: THE PARALLELS

Tensions, such as those between reliability and validity, that play a role in the trust experts have in tests and assessments have their equivalents when experts try to convince policy actors. Just as experts may try to increase the levels of standardization in an attempt to get a grip on the quality of data, so can legislators try to increase their grip on the experts by building in procedural guarantees. Experts who are perceived as being unreliable will be checked by quality control measures. Similarly, when the validity of the assessments is challenged, these same procedures may be challenged for being too inflexible or unrealistic.

On an abstract level, the structure of argumentation is very similar: a knowledge claim – an assessment of the environmental hazards of a chemical – is or is not accepted by an actor. In the one case, this actor is a regulatory scientist and the knowledge claim consists of a claim to safety based on submitted test results. In the other case, the actor involved could be an interest group and the knowledge claim is very similar: an assessment stating the hazards of a chemical. The parallel extends beyond the structure of the claim to the dynamics of trust in such knowledge claims.

As presented in the second section of this paper, regulatory assessors want guarantees of the reliability of the test results and assessments. These can be summed up in three aspects. First, the origin of the information has to be reliable. The assessor has to trust the organization and laboratory personnel that have produced the data. Similarly, it is not uncommon to find third parties questioning assessments based on a criticism of the source of the data, or simply because the source of the data is unknown. To outsiders, the regulators are also a source of knowledge claims that can or cannot be trusted. Just as assessors may want extra procedural guarantees when test results are produced by registering companies, so third parties may want extra guarantees when the assessors have close connections with the industry they regulate. This involves more than a promise to be good professionals, but as wide a range of guarantees as regulatory experts want from the sources they work with. Devices available are, for example, GLP, laboratory certification, or rules limiting career switches between regulators and regulated parties. Damaged trust is vary hard to repair here. One only needs to be reminded of commercial test laboratories caught in fraud cases.

Second, reliability is also a matter of the production of tests and assessments. Is enough information available on the precise experimental conditions? Have standard procedures been followed? It should not surprise regulators that, because much of this information may be covered by confidentiality, third parties may similarly mistrust undocumented test results. For example, an important source of mistrust in the assessments of the UK Advisory Committee on Pesticides was the lack of description of the data considered in the assessments. The more extensive reports were welcomed, even though their availability is still very limited. When it is not possible to reveal all the information and take away the source of mistrust, higher levels of trust in the experts or additional guarantees, provided by the standardization of tests, for example, are required.

Third, the trust in the actual assessment, based on test data, brings up quite similar issues. Here too, a regulatory regime that does not rely on strict and formal assessment protocols will imply a need for more integrity from the regulators. In particular, the tendency of informal assessment procedures to include negotiations with those being regulated, may not help to repair this perceived lack of integrity, even if nothing improper is going on. This is a situation that is currently confronting the Dutch expert committee on pesticides.

To continue the list, matters of trust relating to the validity of assessments, and the degree to which they correspond to relevant environmental effects are also at stake. A first issue here is whether all relevant data have been considered or – inversely – why specific data have been discarded as methodologically unsound. American legislation on both pesticides and industrial chemicals requires companies to submit all available information, in addition to the specific data required according to the regulatory status of a compound. When such requirements do not exist, the assessors may be expected to be proactive in their search for additional information, just as these assessors themselves will want guarantees from registrants that their data are complete. This issue is also at stake in the disputes over Dutch pesticide assessments.

A second aspect of validity concerns the relevance of the information that is considered in assessments. The debate on multi-species toxicity tests mentioned earlier shows that these matters are not easily resolved among the experts. Once again, it should come as no surprise that such concerns are also shared by others. Mesocoms have been supported in the past by companies such as Shell or Monsanto because they had doubts about the validity of single-species tests (and the associated assessment factors). The very idea that effects of chemicals on the non-human environment could be at all relevant has in the past been a reason to question the validity of pesticide assessment schemes. According to some, the evaluation of effects of chemicals on the terrestrial ecosystem is still underdeveloped. To the extent that the precise endpoints that require protection have not been defined in assessment procedures, such evaluations depend for the time being on trust in the experts to define them (cf. Calow, this volume).

Last, an acceptable balance of the various environmental effects is another aspect of the validity of assessments. For example, Dutch pesticide assessments have been questioned in the past because of the limited weight of bioaccumulation in the assessments. When drawing the parallel between trust of and trust in experts, this again should come as no surprise. The precise importance of bioaccumulation as a factor in risk assessments was once just as controversial in the research community.

The way these various aspects of trust are addressed in an ensemble of instruments and arrangements lead to specific regimes of trust that vary between different political contexts. These regimes imply much more than a reliance on professional accreditation of scientists or rules of good scientific practice. They also comprise principles of public accessibility of information, standardization, possibilities of legal contestation, rules on committee membership, mechanisms of participative decision-making, etc.[3] The panoply of guarantees of the reliability and validity come in different combinations and are mutually exchangeable, but only to a certain extent. The viability of different solutions depends on the context of different policy styles. For example, the degree of acceptability of reliance on experts and their professional attitude differs considerably between countries. The high degree of confidence in experts in France is not comparable with the always questionable position of experts in the US. In addition, measures that open

3 The objective of this paper was not to give a complete list of all the available measures, nor to evaluate their respective qualities, but rather to show how they have a similar trust effect.

up possibilities for legal or more adversarial contestation of RA may be productive policy innovations in countries where such measures had been lacking; in the already litigious context of US environmental regulation, they have been shown to lead to extended conflict and delegitimation of expert decision-making. There are no universal solutions.[4]

This analysis of the similarities of trust *of* and trust *in* experts needs a second important qualification. The argument that a failure of some mechanisms to foster trust in the experts will need to be replaced by other mechanisms only holds with a *ceteris paribus* clause: the level of required trust is not given or universal. It varies considerably with the specific policy domain and the degree of contestation, which is dependent on more than just issues of trust. As mentioned earlier, some issues, such as carcinogic chemicals or pesticides, receive more attention. The assessment of new chemicals follows regulatory procedures that would be entirely unacceptable for pesticides, not only because of different hazard levels involved, but also because of the controversy surrounding the chemicals involved. There are no universal problems either.

## CONCLUSION

The traditional guarantee of the trustworthiness of an expert knowledgeclaim is to say that it is produced according to solid scientific principles, as judged by the experts. Ultimately, authority of the knowledgeclaim then rests on: 'this is a trustworthy assessment, because I am the expert and you are not'. As a defence of regulatory risk assessments, this position is no longer tenable. Actors outside regulatory establishments can mobilize sufficient amounts of counter-expertise or acquire the skills and knowledge to participate in the most technical of debates. Eventually, they will question their

4 Without these two important qualifications, this analysis would boil down to an unacceptable form of 'functionalism': the idea that some social problems are universal in time and space; that the extent and nature of these problems can be defined objectively (and therefore do not vary between actors in society in any significant sense); and that the inability to address them will lead to disastrous social disruption (implying, ultimately, explanatory power for this analytic scheme).

'inferior' position as non-experts. But even if they fail to become participant experts, or refuse to do so, they will still require additional guarantees and reasons why they should trust the experts. There are no simple solutions to this problem. Making the production of regulatory assessments transparent may be reassuring when there is a suspicion of muddled interests, but it also creates possibilities to disagree with the decisions made. In addition, transparency is no guarantee of validity: a transparent clock could still tell us the wrong time. In turn, standardization may anchor parts of the assessment process in a procedural matter, but standards can also be referred to as a basis for criticism, or the adequacy of the standards can in turn be questioned. The existence of publicly available standards is still no guarantee of adequate environmental protection.

The capacity of expert authority to decide in debates on RAs has its limits. Previous efforts to expand these limits have run into unforeseen resistance, as scientific rationality was over-optimistically mobilized in regulatory conflicts. I have suggested that it could be productive for regulatory assessors not to draw too sharp a line between experts and non-experts; to think of themselves and the knowledge claims they make in the same way as the claims they have to evaluate as critical experts. They may find the reasons people have to trust the assessors very similar to the reasons the assessors have to trust test results and assessments made by others. To understand why they are mistrusted, regulatory experts should ask themselves why they mistrust other experts. To begin to build up a relationship of trust, they should ask themselves what is required for them to begin to trust other sources of expert knowledge claims. Although solutions to these matters of trust may not always be identical, this exercise may help to realize that they are at least as varied.

## EPILOGUE

The secondary agenda of this paper was to suggest ways in which a sociological analysis could be of use to an understanding of regulatory processes. I have sketched some of the patterns in regulatory processes highlighted by a social scientific analysis. In conclusion, I want to return to the issues of standardization and suggest a few specific ones in which connections with science and technology studies are possible and potentially productive.

There are three levels on which I see such possibilities concerning the role and use of standardization. For each I will suggest some preliminary conclusions from my own research and suggest interesting lines for further development.

- *The implementation of standards by risk assessors.* A more detailed analysis of the practice of regulatory assessment can clarify the role of standardized methodology in the assessment process. When standard test methodology is analyzed as a strategy and when it can be indicated what precisely the objective of these strategies is, alternative ways of obtaining such strategies could be suggested and compared. If standardized methodology is used by assessors as a way to get more grip on notifiers, then alternative resources could imply a stronger reliance on assessors' evaluations in risk management, thereby increasing the implications of their decisions for the outcome of risk management. Under what conditions will standards increase the leverage of assessors? How and why are standards accommodated to local practices? The confidentiality of the details of RA procedures makes these sorts of projects as yet very difficult for social scientists.

- *The effect of standardization on regulatory institutions.* Comparative research on different regulatory contexts can indicate circumstances qualifying the effects of the introduction of standardized methodology and RA techniques in more detail. Available research suggests that standardization may conflict with informal local assessment styles, especially in assessment practices where the boundary between RA and risk management is rather blurred. This does not necessarily lead to alterations in regulatory decision-making or forms of interest integration, but can also lead to the accommodation of standards in existing patterns of regulatory assessment. In a similar vein, the effects of standardization could be compared with other policy instruments. For example, the implementation of standard assessment methods is, among many other things, a way to attempt policy closure. An alternative path to policy closure is interest group negotiation, for example oriented towards general reduction policies (as in the Dutch Multi-Year Crop Protection Plan). Research on the Dutch system of 'convenants', fora of negotiated decision-making is beginning to show that making rules through negotiating has advantages, but also major disadvantages, especially on the level of enforcement. Comparing such patterns of advantages and disadvantages could suggest new policy mixes and priorities. For such lines of research, some basic questions need to be further investigated. To what extent does the introduction of standards alter regulatory procedures? How does this affect the position of regulatory agencies and their techniques of interest integration?

*The social context of the development of methodology.* The standardization of methods occurs in rather specific institutional formats: standardization organizations or committees. From a policy perspective, the main difficulty is to assure an independent and authorative source of test development that nevertheless follows the policy agenda. Standardizing institutions with high scientific standards that are too remote from regulatory agencies tends to suggest or develop methods that reason more from the perspective of research science than from the perspective of regulatory assessment needs. On the other hand, methods developed under close inspection from regulatory agencies may assure proper coordination with the policy agenda, but lose scientific credibility and lead to narrow and non-innovative operationalizations of environmental effects. A comparison of models for the organization of method development could indicate strong and weak points, and indicate new ways to bridge the methodological developments in research science and the needs of regulatory assessment. On a very detailed level, a study of social practices in testing laboratories could even point to social sources of variations that could in turn lead to new strategies obtaining stable standard methods.

## References

Abraham, John (1993) 'Scientific Standards and Institutional Interests: Carcinogenic Risk Assessment of Benoxaprofen in the UK and US', *Social Studies of Science* 23: 387-444.

Andrews, Clinton (1994) 'Policies to Encourage Clean Technologies' in R. Socolow, C. Andrews, F. Berkhout, V. Thomas, eds. *Industrial Ecology and Global Change* Cambridge: Cambridge University Press, 405-22.

Beaumont, Peter (1993) *Pesticides, Policies and People: A Guide to the Issues* London: The Pesticides Trust.

Brickman, Ronald, Sheila Jasanoff and Thomas Ilgen, (1985) *Controlling Chemicals: the Politics of Regulating Chemicals in Europe and the United States,* Ithaca: Cornell University Press.

Cairns, John Jr., ed. (1977) *Aquatic Microbial Communities,* New York: Garland Publishers.

Cairns, John Jr. (1981) 'Biological Monitoring, part IV: Future Needs', *Water Research* 15: 944.

Cairns, John Jr. (1988) 'Putting the Eco in Ecotoxicology', *Regulatory Toxicology and Pharmacology* 8: 226-38.

Calow, Peter, ed. (1993) *Handbook of Ecotoxicology* Oxford: Balckwell Scientific.

CEC (1980) *Principles for the Interpretation of the Results of Testing Procedures in Ecotoxicology*, Brussels: Commission of the European Communities, Symposium, Sophia-Antipolis, Valbourne, France, 30.09.80-02.10.80.

CEC (1984) *Beratender wissenschaftlicher Ausschuß für die Prüfung der Toxizität und Ökotoxizität chemischer Verbindungen, Tätigkeitsbericht 1979-83,* Brussels: Commission of the European Communities, EUR 9246 DE.

CEC (1990) *Environment and Quality of Life: Scientific Advisory Committee to Examine the Toxicity and Ecotoxicity of Chemical Compounds: Activity report 1984-88,* Brussels: Commission of the European Communities, DGV-XI.

CEC (1993) *Development and Validation of Methods for Evaluating Chronic Toxicity to Freshwater Ecosystems*, Brussels: Commission of the European Communities, DGV-XII, brochure.

Fiorino, Daniel J. (1990) 'Citizen Participation and Environmental Risk: A Survey of Institutional Mechanisms', *Science, Technology, and Human Values*: 226-43.

Foucault, Michel (1980) *Power/Knowledge: Selected Interviews and Other Writings, 1972-77,* New York: Pantheon.

Halffman, Willem (1995) 'The Boundary between ecology and toxicology: an outsider's perspective' in: Cairns, John Jr. and Barbara Niederlehner (eds.), *Biological testing at different levels of biological organization,* Boca Raton: Lewis.

Health Council of The Netherlands (1995) *Niet alle risico's zijn gelijk,* Den Haag.

Hunn, J.B. (1989) *History of Acute Toxicity Tests with Fish, 1863-87* LaCrosse, WI: US Fish & Wildlife Service, Investigations in Fish Control, vol. 98.

Idman, Mariatta (1978) 'OECD Activities: Aiming Towards Expanded International Cooperation in the Control of Toxic Chemicals', *Ambio*, 7: 263-6.

Jager, D.T. and C.J.M. Visser, eds. (1994) *Uniform System for the Evaluation of Substances (USES), version 1.0,* Bilthoven: RIVM.

Jasanoff, Sheila (1990) *The Fifth Branch: Science Advisers as Policy Makers,* Cambridge: Harvard University Press.

Jasanoff, Sheila et al., eds. (1995) *Handbook of Science and Technology Studies*, Beverly Hills: Sage.

Johnson, Stanley Patrick (1978) 'Developments in the EC for the Control of New Chemical Substances', *Ambio*, 7: 267-70.

Koeman, Jan (1982) 'Ecotoxicological Evaluation: The Eco-side of the Problem', *Ecotoxicology and Environmental Safety*: 359.

Malta, Erik Jan (1992) *Proefdier en milieu: een dreigend conflict,* Leyden: University of Leyden, thesis Biology and Society.

OECD (s.d.) *Guidelines for Testing of Chemicals,* Paris: OECD, updates.

OECD (1982) *Good Laboratory Practice in the Testing of Chemicals*, Paris: OECD.

OECD (1991) *Report of the OECD Workshop on the Extrapolation of Laboratory Aquatic Toxicity Data to the Real Environment,* Paris: OECD, Environment Directorate.

Perez, K.T. and G.E. Morrison (1985) 'Environmental Assessment from Simple Test Systems and a Microcosm: Comparison of Monetary Costs' in J. Cairns Jr., ed. *Multispecies Toxicity Testing,* New York: Pergamon Press; 89-95.

Pickering, Andy, ed. (1992) *Science as Practice and Culture*, Chicago: Chicago University Press.

Projektgroep Evaluatie Toelating Bestrijdingsmiddelen (1995) *Evaluatie van de uitvoering van het toelatingsbeleid van bestrijdingsmiddelen vanaf 1993,* Den Haag: mimeo.

Reijnders, Lucas, J. Rutteman, H. Muilerman, M.L. de Rooy (1995) *Zwartboek toelating bestrijdingsmiddelen: Aanklacht tegen het Nederlandse bestrijdingsmiddelenbeleid,* Utrecht: Stichting Natuur en Milieu, Zuidhollandse Milieufederatie.

Royal Commission on Environmental Pollution (1992) *Sixteenth report: Freshwater quality,* London: HMSO, CM 1966.

Royal Society (1992) *Risk: Analysis, Perception and Management,* London: The Royal Society.

Seager, J and S.D. Oakley (1986) *Proposed Environmental Quality Standards for Organotins in Water*, Medmenham: WRc Environment, PLC 9332 CD.

Shapin, Steven and Simon Schaffer (1985) *Leviathan and the Air Pump: Hobbes, Boyle, and the Experimental Life,* Princeton: Princeton University Press.

Shapin, Steven (1994) *A Social History of Truth: Civility and Science in Seventeenth Century England,* Chicago: University of Chicago Press.

Touart, Leslie (1988) *Hazard Evaluation: Technical Guidance Document. Aquatic Mesocosm Tests to Support Pesticide Registrations* Arlington, Va: USEPA/HED-EBB, USEPA 540/09-88-035, PB 88-172465 (micro).

Touart, Leslie W. and M. Slimak (1989) 'Mesocosm Approach for Assessing the Ecological Risk of Pesticides' in Entomological Society of America, *Miscellaneous Publications 75*: 33 seq.

Tweede Kamer (1990) *Regeringsbeslissing Meerjarenplan Gewasbeschermingsmiddelen* Tweede Kamer 1990-1991, 21677, 3-4.

U.K. Government/Industry Working Group (1993) *Risk assessment of existing substances*, London: Department of the Environment.

USEPA (1975) *Methods for Acute Toxicity Tests with Fish, Macroinvertebrates, and Amphibians,* Corvallis: USEPA-660/3-75-009.

USEPA (1987) 'Toxic Substances Control Act Test Guidelines: Proposed Rule. 40 CFR parts 796 and 797', *Federal Register*, Monday, September 28, vol.52, no.187: 36334-71.

USEPA (1991) *Methods for Measuring the Acute Toxicity of Effluents and Receiving Waters to Freshwater and Marine Organisms: Fourth Edition,* Washington DC: USEPA/ORD, USEPA/660/4-90/027.

Vogel, D. (1986) *National Styles of Regulation: Environmental Policy in Great Britain and the United States,* Ithaca: Cornell University Press.

Wynne, Brian (1982) *Rationality and Ritual: The Windscale Inquiry and Nuclear Decision-Making in Britain*, Chalfont St Giles: BSHS monograph no. 3.

Wynne, Brian (1992) 'Carving Out Science (and Politics) in the Regulatory Jungle', *Social Studies of Science* 22: 745-58.

# DISCUSSIONS

## *Standardization*

Questions and comments following the presentation by *McCutcheon*

*Heyvaert.* Does the committee have any official power to force industry, for instance, to supply more data? Is the committee accountable for its decisions, and if so, to whom?

*McCutcheon.* There is in general a lot of consultation back and forth. There is a problem with reprotox, where we don't have a standard test in the EU, and industry has systematically refused to generate data on this endpoint. If necessary, the regulatory committee can decide to force industry to generate the data, but at the same time we want to maintain the dialogue and a cooperative working relationship with industry.

*Halffman.* (1) Can you indicate why it would be wrong simply to force industry to supply all available data on all substances? (2) In which phase are non-industrial groups involved in the consultation? How do you account for different national political cultures?

*McCutcheon.* Response to (2). There are some recent discussions on where consumers and environmental groups can play a role. There is the possibilty of discussing the ranking, but there is a reluctance to introduce other actors at the political level, because of the fear that the discussion becomes rhetorical. There is also a resource problem: how to provide them with expertise? Probably any major international company has more toxicologists than the Commission, including DG XI.

Response to (1). More information would be more detailed technical information, which in comparison would not be useful for the ranking, and which we would not use for setting priorities. If there were substances that are not on the ranking lists with the current criteria and that yet would be of concern, they would manifest themselves.

*Millstone.* What checks are there that industry is actually delivering all available data, and not just a positive selection of studies, leaving out the studies that, for instance, point to carcinogenity?

*McCutcheon.* Where necessary, control measures of authorities include access to company reports. Rapporteurs are advised to carry out complementary literature searches and present and defend their report to the other member states.

## Questions and comments following the presentation by *McCarthy* and *Rothstein*

*Jasanoff.* Do we see a new kind of science emerging, and what does this mean? Can you apply 'normal criteria' for this development, for instance with new journals, new prizes, etc.? To what extent does regulatory science want to be like 'normal science'?

*Rothstein & McCarthy.* There are different aspects to the production of regulatory science which cannot be generalised under one single definition. For example, the organisation of routine mammalian toxicity tests may be very different from research investigating the relevance of positive findings in a mammalian toxicity study. Differences may occur in the location of the work, qualifications of personnel and the dissemination or publication of results.

In terms of the production of regulatory science in the UK, there is a dominance of private sector organisations, whose success will not be judged by their publication record, as has recently been the case in UK universities, but by their ability to help industry secure regulatory approval. Criteria of success in both the public and private sectors, therefore, need further examination. In general, to describe regulatory science either as distinct from, or similar to, 'normal' science is to assume that 'normal' science is itself definable. In different policy contexts regulatory science may be presented as 'normal' science or as more explicitly incorporating policy objectives. The boundaries between the two are contestable and definitions can be made opportunistically.

Questions and comments following the presentation by *Calow*

*Halffman* asks whether Calow, in his talk about protection of functions or biodiversity, was pointing to the discussion about conservation of nature or conservation of the environment.

*Calow*. Society has to make choices about what to protect. The responsibility of science is to make clear what the impacts of these decisions are on nature. Once this choice is made it is the scientist's responsibility to come up with a risk assessment procedure to implement this choice.

*Millstone* comments on *Daphnia* as Calow's favorite species, because of its sensitivity. Does it really have a uniform sensitivity, to all substances?

*Calow*. *Dahpnia* is in general more sensitive, and there are genotypes that are more sensitive than others, but not always. One tends to go for the most sensitive species in general. One wants to control the variables, to understand the system, although it is inevitably a simplification. The concern is always whether it resembles the complex system.

*Mayer*. You seem to suggest the problem is effect assessment, but I have found exposure assessment is at least as problematic.

*Calow*. Predicting environmental concentration is the easiest part of the job. You can build models that can make very precise predictions. This is easier than predicting ecological consequences. Even more difficult is the question of what we want to protect.

*Smit*. Another important question is *how* we want to protect. You very much stressed the importance of probability. In this way, science is structuring reality in a certain way, and suggesting a specific way of managing the system: when the scientist is phrasing everything in terms of probability, then he is suggesting that the management system should concentrate on – say – reducing these probabilities. So my question is, aren't there any more points where society has to come in, for instance in the way science is structuring reality, which might lead to different protection measures?

*Jasanoff.* How problematic is the role of 'function'? Are there different functions?

*Calow.* In response to Jasanoff, the different characterization of both structure and function is disputed in eco-toxicology. But my hope is to resolve these conflicts by better observations, which is the way science develops.

Questions and comments following the presentation by *Halffman*

*Abraham.* It seems to be implicit in your talk that standardization comes from regulators. But it also comes from industry, as a way to harmonize the market. An example is the HIV test, where the standardization was an industrial strategy. It is also a way to make it hard to introduce alternative products.

*Halffman.* I agree that other actors, like industry, play an important role. However, once the standards are developed by regulatory scientists and by industry, critics can also use them and confront industry with their own standards. So you don't have to be that negative about this.

*Nilsson.* Regarding deviation of tests, in the case of pesticides: Do you mean that industry can choose which test to include, that the battery of tests is negotiable?

*Halffman.* No, risk-assessors of new chemical substances in the US told me that they do not have a strong enough postion to demand certain tests and they don't see why they should not negotiate with industry on how to modify the protocol.

*Calow* (in response to Nillson). In the EU there is a base set of tests, and it is insisted upon that this should be applied. On the other hand, there are opportunities for discussing variation, and those opportunities are used by industry and by member states.

*Mayer* asks about the relation between trust in tests and public trust in a more general sense.

*Halffman*. Standardization in the regulation of pesticides in the US is a way of increasing trust. I am not sure that it is always the right way to do it, but it covers up the perceived unreliability of people making judgments within this political context.

## General discussion

*Bijker* (summarizing the main point of the papers). It seems there is need for a discussion forum, between regulatory scientists and society.

*Younes*. What can we standardize? Test methods can be standardized, but not the ways of thinking, of judgments. It is possible to give broad guidelines for risk assessment, but there has to be space for judgment, for discussion. When standardization leads to cookbook types of risk assessment, you may get the trust of non-experts or not, I don't know, but I don't see the value of that. It will straightjacket your experts. We need caution on what is standardizable and allow for consensual procedures.

*Jasanoff* (referring to similarity between processes of standardisation). Calow made the point very well, that standardization involves making choices about how to construct a macro-cosmos, resembling the real world. However, regulators too are constructing a macro-cosmos in the social-political world, expecting certain effects of their regulations.

I am quite familiar with the objections of scientists that the standardization which regulators are forcing upon them is not scientific, because the regulatory criteria are not in line with what they see in the world. For example, a mouse is not always a suitable test animal. The question then, is, are there places in standardization procedures where experts say that the representation of the physical, real world is OK, and where non-experts can challenge this judgment? Otherwise it is a rather one-sided conversation, where regulators standardizing the political world can be criticised, but experts standardizing the physical world cannot.

*Nilsson.* For a long time the tendency was towards more standardization. Now there is a contrary tendency. For example, at the conference of the National Institute of Health, in North Carolina, the National Toxicology Program was asked to introduce more flexibility, using already known data, so that you can design a more suitable test for a specific substance. You need to make a compromise between suitability and comparibility.

The question is: do you have the experts? For example, in the Philippines there are just a few experts. Maybe it is possible to help them by making clear the worst errors they can make.

*Younes.* My experience with developing countries is that they may not have the necessary infrastructure to do the risk assessment themselves. They will take over the assessement and are happy when they can apply it to their own situation. Therefore any risk assessment in the developed world has to be transparent, clear, so that people from those countries can look at assumptions.

*Calow* (in response to the question posed by Jasanoff). These questions are answered by the existing chemicals programme. There we have a base set of tests which is rather focused on specific parts of the environment.

*Bijker* (refering to the presentation by Calow and the choice between different models of protecting functions or biodiversity). I would think that this is a point you don't want to leave to scientists.

*Calow.* I agree. Science is not very good at defining how the world should be, but it can be good at describing the world. In case of change in natural systems, there is a real need for dialogue between science and the rest of society.

*Somers.* Certainly standardization is possible. But for the regulators there are two key problems: (1) the problem of extrapolation from animal results. How valid are extrapolated results to you and to society? And (2), what do you do with the high dose versus the low dose? Both questions cannot easily be answered by scientists and standardization won't help here.

*McCutcheon* (in reference to Jasanoff's comments on the first theme). EU legislation is much newer than the legislation in the US. It is interesting to note that industry is not asking for any withdrawal of this legislation.

It is true that in harmonization there is a collusion between regulators and industry, as suggested, but the reasons for the mutual interests are different. We, as regulators, are under pressure to assess the effect of chemicals. When we can use the resources in other countries, we can assess more chemicals. We can only do that by having common tests and protocols. By having agreed tests, we also limit the number of laboratory animals.

You can standardize risk assessment methodology, but not the risk management decisions, because what is an acceptable risk to one need not be acceptable to someone else.

*Sedee*. Our focus is on risk assessors. But the risk regulator has to combine different risk assessments (to health or the environment) which is quite a lot of knowledge of several aspects, with a lot of uncertainty. In order to do this, a mental simplification is needed, and therefore one needs to trust the opinion of the risk assessor. This is one of the reasons for standardization; otherwise the regulator could not do everything he has to do.

*Mayer*. There is too much focus on the technical parts of the assessment. This leads to discharging other relevant knowledge that might be important in the longer term. There is a real danger in narrowing the risk debate down to the technical issues in that it leads to denial of the real problems (for the environment and health). This may lead to a loss of political legitimacy for policy.

*Bijker*. It seems that we all have different problems. What problems do we have in common? What problems can natural scientists, social scientists, political regulators contribute to?

# PART IV

## SCENARIOS AND REFLEXIONS

# 12

*Willem Halffman & Roland Bal*

# THE POLITICS OF CHEMICAL RISK SCENARIOS FOR REGULATORY POLICY

## INTRODUCTION

In conclusion to this volume, we have made an attempt to integrate the papers in order to map different alternatives for the future development of the regulation of chemicals. Rather than drawing up long lists of all the ideas and analyses that are presented, we have tried to digest these into a set of four 'scenarios'. These scenarios are four sets of coherent choices that could guide the further development of chemical regulation. In this sense they are not to be read as predictions about the regulatory future, they are sketches of *possible* regulatory futures. As sketches, they only indicate a number of structural lines, not the flesh and bones of specific domains of regulation. Combined with an analysis of the likely developments and tensions in each of these models, they obtain a dynamic component, warranting the term 'scenarios'.

Apart from summarizing the presentations made at the workshop in a specific, somewhat unusual form, the main function of the scenarios is to create a space for discussing the future of the politics of chemical risk. The scenarios suggest that there is not *one best way* in which to organize decision making on chemical risk, but that there are many. Each scenario has its own possibilities, (dis)advantages and dynamics. In this sense they indicate that there are indeed choices to be made, possibilities to be explored.

A number of assumptions underlie the way these scenarios were constructed. Of those we are aware of, we will first present the salient ones. After that,

In: R. Bal & W. Halffman (eds.), *The Politics of Chemical Risk*, Kluwer Academic Publishers, Dordrecht 1998: p. 303-322.

we present the two main criteria that underlie our make-up of the scenarios. The criteria can be constructed as two axes, through which four scenarios can be distinguished. The two criteria are (1) assumptions about the nature of expertise, and (2) the actual organization of the boundary between risk assessment and risk management. Consequently, each of the scenarios will be briefly introduced and contrasted with each other, before expanding further into a more detailed analysis of each of them.

## OUR INTENTIONAL ASSUMPTIONS

### *Chemicals and their regulation are here to stay*

In writing up the scenarios we have assumed that the regulatory framework of chemicals is not complete. New chemicals will continue to be produced and marketed, old ones will continue to present new and unexpected problems, and the regulatory world itself will continue to develop and run into familiar and unfamiliar obstacles. This assumption runs counter to the idea that the basic tensions in the regulation of chemicals have been solved, or to the idea that the centrality of chemicals in production processes is only transitory. It assumes that even regulatory strategies that do not stress the assessment of chemicals based on their specific risk, but choose to reduce emissions in general,[1] still have to decide which chemicals to reduce and construct red, grey, black or otherwise coloured priority lists in order to do so.

Without such an assumption, developing scenarios would be pointless as the history of the regulation of chemicals would be finished.

### *A focus on the European Union*

The scenarios work from the perspective of Europe. Although they may present possible alternatives to existing national frameworks as well, the scenarios assume that the institutions of the European Union are the main

1 Examples of these are the latest North Sea Treaty, and the Dutch long-term plan for crop protection.

source of change and a central locus where tensions will appear. In spite of analyses that show that the national context remains central in chemical regulation, we assume that policy developed in the European Union will continue to influence national policies with regard to chemical regulation. Even when the importance of national influences on European decision making is taken into account, the regulatory policy of the European Union is still more than the sum of the national positions.[2]

The impact of the European Union on national chemical regulation is not only considerable with regard to the status of specific chemicals – such as in exposure standards or blacklist statuses. It is also great with regard to the way the evaluation of chemicals is supposed to be performed and organized. With respect to the evaluation of chemicals, initiatives such as the Uniform Principles or the programme on new chemicals have altered the way member countries have assessed the hazards of chemicals. In programmes such as the regulation of old chemicals, the policy of the European Union has even introduced changes in the organization of this process.

In addition, the difficulties of the European integration of chemical regulation show the differences in national styles of regulation and the variety of ways in which expertise is organized in national regulatory frameworks. The issues and conflicts in European integration are not merely a matter of different political and economic interests of national states and their representatives. In the debates, different views on the regulation of chemicals confront each other and their pros and cons are weighed. This makes a European perspective also interesting to elicit different models of chemical regulation.

### *The science/policy boundary is the backbone of regulation*

All four scenarios assume that the regulation of chemicals is only feasible if, somewhere, a boundary is drawn and maintained between science and policy. It is clear that regulatory science has assumptions and implications

---

2 Though we focus on Europe, this is not to say that the scenarios do not contain elements that might be useful for other international bodies like the OECD or the different programmes of the WHO.

that are political and that regulatory science can never be value-free. We believe that the foregoing chapters in this volume have convincingly shown that expert assessment can be successfully challenged by alternative views, even on the issues they consider firmly objective. Nevertheless, some form of institutional separation of the work of experts and that of policy makers seems to be a requirement to regulate large numbers of chemicals. Experts make choices that are value-laden and that have political dimensions, but this is most probably unavoidable. The central question is to what extent such choices should be delegated to them or how and when they should be reclaimed by political institutions.

There are several good reasons to maintain a division of labour between the domains of science and policy, of which we name just a few. First, the agenda of political institutions has only a limited capacity. Expanding this capacity implies a more than proportional expansion of the political institutions themselves. Second, experts can help to focus discussions about the political choices in chemical regulation, without necessarily themselves resolving these questions. They can steer political debate in a constructive way. Third, the decision making of political institutions has a higher cost, as conflicts over chemical regulation can escalate into political conflicts.

Conversely, regulatory decision making that is relegated to the experts alone, carries the risk of developing uncontrollable technocracies, leading to a loss of democratic control. This can further lead to a loss of the pragmatic check on negotiations, and in the end might lead to a delegitimation of regulation altogether, being perceived as inpractical, unfair or biased.

The issue addressed in the scenarios, therefore, is not whether there should be a boundary between expert institutions and policy institutions. Such a boundary is considered to be an essential part of regulation. The crucial issue concerns the attribution of responsibilities across this boundary and the organization of disputes about this attribution process.

## Underlying criteria for the scenarios

The literature contains some attempts to specify criteria which might enable analysts to classify regulatory styles or institutions. On the specific issue of environmental regulation, political science has developed parameters to typify patterns of institutionalization through comparative research. One set of parameters concerns the degree to which decision making is formalized. Environmental regulation either occurs according to strict rules, or through an informal decision making process.[3] In the former, decision making is highly protocolized and the scientific assessment of risk is highly standardized, while maintaining a strict boundary between risk assessment and risk management. In the latter no such formalization of the decision making process has been made and the boundary between risk assessment and risk managment is kept vague, or is at least mobile. A second set of parameters concerns the degree of participative democracy in a policy field, which stands against representative patterns of democracy.[4] When combined, as done by Clinton Andrews (1994), these two sets of parameters provide a tool to trace relevant parameters in different patterns of institutionalization of environmental regulation, in line with theoretical approaches of neo-institutionalist research (Jepperson & Meyer 1991).

In our construction of the scenarios we have chosen to modify these two criteria. From the foregoing chapters in this volume, two underlying criteria that can be used for the make-up of the scenarios have been distilled that are more or less in line with the ones described above. The first of these concerns assumptions about the nature of expertise. One the one hand, it can be assumed that expertise is the objective expression of the state of the art in the health and environmental sciences. Expertise, then, is a uniform and global phenomenon, which can be transferred across local contexts. On the other hand, expertise can be denied such a global status. Instead, local characteristics of expertise are stressed, and it is assumed that expertise somehow expresses contingent interests, social and political contexts, etc. Expertise, in this view, is not a global but a local (national) phenomenon, tied up to local social, cultural, and political developments and institutions.

The second criterion concerns the way the boundary between risk assessment and risk management should be organized. On the one extreme, the boundary should be very strict, meaning that any influence from risk man-

---

3 See for example Brickman et al. (1985) and Vogel (1986).

4 Older conceptualizations here indicate 'open' versus 'closed' decision making processes, but this is inaccurate since these dimensions do not consider who the process is open to.

agement on the process of risk assessment should be avoided. On the other, such a strict boundary is not deemed possible, nor desirable. Instead, the boundary should be organized in a flexible manner, allowing for a pragmatic attribution of issues.

In combination, these criteria alow for the differentiation between four paths of development for the regulation of chemical risk, which we have termed 'International experts', 'European risk consultation', 'European coordination of assessment' and 'Europe as a translator' respectively, and which can be presented in a graphical manner as follows:

| ORGANIZATION OF THE BOUNDARY | NATURE OF EXPERTISE: *Global* | NATURE OF EXPERTISE: *Local* |
|---|---|---|
| *Strict* | I International Experts | III European coordination of assessment |
| *Flexible* | II European risk consultation | IV Europe as a translator |

The first scenario, *International Experts*, starts from the assumption that the assessment of chemical risk is first and foremost a scientific issue. Since science is not linked to national social, cultural and political traditions and institutions, it is not deemed necessary that experts represent member states. The assessment of chemical risk, performed by experts working in a 'European Agency of Chemical Regulation' is strictly isolated from political issues. Important research on the toxicity or distribution of chemicals is still caried out in various national or industrial organizations, but the Agency is an important actor in setting the agenda for these institutions and in their funding.

In scenario two, chemical risk managment by the European Union is mainly thought of as a process of *consultation* between member states, supported by experts' assessments of risk. The 'European Office of Chemical Assessment' is a limited group of international experts who write risk assessment documents. An important role of the Office is to bring infomation together, stemming from various sources, national institutions among them. At several points in the risk assessment process, an exchange of views is sought and organized. Public consultative rounds are held in which country representatives, interest groups and the wider public are invited to respond. An explicit and public route of decision making is used to assure the political basis of the experts' position.

The main function of the Euorpean Union in scenario three is to *coordinate* activities of the member states. Differences between regulatory approaches are smoothed out on a step-by-step basis. The objective is harmonized risk assessment, while expertise remains distributed over the various member states. This harmonization is attempted through negotiations between experts, working in various commitees, who are not only specialists in the domain, but who also represent national institutions and views. The negotiations serve to align and integrate national differences, also in the definition of risk assessment and management. Implicitly, the negotiators accept this blurred boundary between expertise and national interests, but in the the public domain the outcomes of the negotiations are presented as strictly scientific.

In *Europe as a translator* (scenario four) differences in regulatory styles and views on risk between countries and interest groups are the starting point for European action. Levelling of these differences is, however, not a direct policy goal. Since it is recognized that the organization of the boundary between risk assessment and risk management is one of the main causes of national differences, it is also one of the central issues of the debates, rather than a given. A 'European Office of Constructive Risk Assessment' organizes the discussion between the different views and tries to elicit assumptions and find correspondences. Different risk assessments are compared, with the objective of indicating the differences in which these assessments are framed. Ways are sought to accommodate these differences. The activities of the Agency are not only directed toward the assessment of risk, but also toward the production of chemicals, since these issues are considered to be interrelated.

## The scenarios in full

### Scenario 1: International experts

*Central traits*
The expertise is centralized on the European level in a 'European Agency of Chemical Regulation'. The experts engage in informal decision making, in which expert judgement is combined with detailed and highly developed expert technology. The advantages of integrated computer modelling of effects, distribution, costs, and benefits of chemicals are combined with the judgement of the experienced experts for the idiosyncratic case: chemicals with effects not caught by the standard procedures or with unexpected impact. This requires high levels of confidence in the experts' judgements and their independence, which is shielded by confidential decision making.

Certain aspects of risk assessment are contracted out to national institutions: minor technical matters are diverted to consultants, matters that require high quality to top research institutions. Empirical data are provided by industry according to strictly standardized and harmonized guidelines. The possibility of expert judgement in the odd case in principle allows for the inclusion of non-standardized experimental results in the evaluations.

*The risk assessment/risk management boundary*
The strict boundary between risk assessment and risk management is maintained by confidential expert decision making and by the concentration of top quality expertise in one central institution.[5] The remaining margins for political decision making and interest balancing are strictly defined. The experts have a central role in the prioritizing and screening of chemical hazards. As new expert technology is developed, especially in the field of cost-benefit and comparative risk analysis, the regulation of chemicals is depoliticized and increasingly becomes a technical matter. The domain of risk assessment is expansionist: it generally encompasses a larger part of the policy process.

5 An example of such an institute is the Dutch National Institute for Public Health & the Environment.

The organization and maintenance of the boundary is an affair decided on a European level. The attribution of responsibilities across the boundary depends on the availability of expertise, but is moving in the direction of expert assessments on more and more issues of decision making.

*Dynamics and expected tensions*[6]

The concentration of decisions with a major impact in one institution raises considerable challenges to its position by organized interests. Various interest groups and national institutions try to develop means of influencing the decision making, such as lobby activities or personal networking. Such activities will be deployed by a limited range of organized interests, who have the means to organize an office near the Agency.

Interest groups develop sources of counter expertise to challenge expert decision making. In the expansionist movement of risk assessment, the experts cross political boundaries that they do not readily perceive. Because the details of decision making are not visible, there is limited possibility for constructive debate. This leads to polarization and increased political action. The decision making system lacks the flexibility to deal with these escalating controversies.

These developments lead to challenges to the independence of the Agency. In response, strict rules are developed to regulate membership and the behaviour of Agency members.[7] Professional ethics codes are eventually formalized in the regulation of affiliations with other institutions or contact with lobby groups.

Other possible reactions to these conflicts are the organization of interest integrating institutions on the European level, more external negotiation over risk assessment, or an increase in informal decision making.

---

6 Much of the dynamics discussed for each of the scenarios is extrapolated from case studies and comparative analyses taken from the political science and science and technology studies literature on the regulation of chemicals. Only at some points do we actually refer to these studies.

7 Compare the developments within the US regulatory system (Jasanoff 1990; Halffman, forthcoming).

*Advantages/disadvantages*
The expert decision making is of relatively high quality by the standards of established science. As defined by the state of the art of environmental sciences, the assessment of environmental effects is advanced. However, the questioning of the decision making leads to disagreements that block the possibilities of active environmental protection.

The possibilities of democratic control over the decision making are limited. This does not in itself lead to difficulty, as long as the Agency is able to maintain its neutral and prominent position, but leads to extra delegitimating effects when this is questioned.

*Indications of developments in this direction*
One of the examples of developments that are in line with this scenario are the talks about the formation of a European Environment Agency. These talks seem to take the US EPA as one of their examples, and one could argue that EPA has more or less followed the path of the scenario described above.

## SCENARIO 2 : EUROPEAN RISK CONSULTATION

*Central traits*
The 'European Office of Chemical Assessment' is not a fully fledged research institution, but a relatively limited group of independent experts. These experts are in constant touch with other international organizations and national research institutions, because one of their prime tasks is to collect and review data. In this sense, a concentration of experts is not the main goal, but the assessments are centralized.

At various points in the risk assessment process, intermediate assessments are circulated widely for consultation. Consultation is not only sought with country representatives, but also directly with interest groups. In hearings, focus committees, and consultation rounds in writing, the experts look for high levels of political legitimacy. The experts intentionally limit their role in deciding about uncertainties and in making judgement calls. Such decisions are refered to consultation. The experts and their evaluations are therefore very visible. The decision making process is open.

Although there is room for more informal contact in the consultation procedures, expert decision making is standardized and formal. The openness of decision making leads to possibilities for contestation of the details of the evaluation process. Strict procedures of expert decision making are developed in rcsponse to these challenges. These procedures make it harder to deal with 'exceptional' chemicals that do not fit into these procedures. For decisions about such chemicals, more weight is put on the consultation process.

*The risk assessment/risk management boundary*

The boundary between risk assessment and risk management is organized on the international level. It is flexible and mobile: when even the most technical issues in expert evaluations are contested, they are referred to the realm of risk management. In non-problematic domains, the experts develop formalized assessment tools that relieve the agenda of the political institutions (Halffman, forthcoming). This attribution process itself involves difficult manoeuvering.

*Dynamics and expected tensions*

The openness of decision making leads to several problems. First, there is substantial pressure from industry to protect the confidentiality of test data. The regulations that assure such confidentiality are under constant pressure from the consultation procedures. In controversial cases the risk assessment boundary retreats and 'confidential' information is requested in the public domain. Second, this mobility of the risk assessment/risk management boundary leads to escalating controversies. In these controversies, more and more elements of the assessment are questioned. This makes a reliance on expertise difficult to achieve policy closure. Decisions are stalled and postponed, and the political agenda is frequently overloaded. The demands on the parties involved in these debates are high: high levels of understanding of the technical aspects of chemicals are required. Prominent actors are the ones who manage to organize sufficient external expert support to participate in the debate.

Through the retreatist strategy, the experts maintain a relatively high degree of legitimacy. Pressure is oriented at the political aspects of decision making and the institutions that have responsibility for these. Depending on whether the political procedures of decision making are organized on a central or decentral level, interest group pressure will follow. Heterogeneous coalitions of such groups are likely, given the pluriform structure of the European arena. Especially slow decision making becomes an issue of criticism from broad interest group coalitions, although with contradicting motivations (Nownes 1991).

Risk management institutions try to find ways to confine these conflicts, partly in an attempt to strengthen their own position. For these purposes, they increase the pressure on the experts to come up with stricter advice. Depending on the strategy of the experts, they may either refuse or develop even more formal assessment procedures. These procedures are in turn legitimated in consultation procedures. Under high pressure, these procedures are consequently strictly applied, narrowing the space of expert judgement and leading to a number of cases of unsignalled hazards of chemicals. In case of refusal by these experts, risk management institutions will look for expert institutions that are willing to do so elsewhere, in consultancy, for example.

*Advantages/disadvantages*

The scientific decision making process is slow and difficult. The possibilities of democratic control initially construct fairly high levels of expert legitimacy. In addition, the inclusion of a wide range of actors in the consultation assures a wide variety of information and a broad range of possible effects of chemicals, but reaching a decision on their evaluation is extremely difficult. The scientific quality of decision making is variable and can deteriorate under the pressure of risk management institutions. Chemical safety can fail in the short run, but acquires more momentum in the long run because of the broader political basis that carries it (Bijker 1995a).

*Indications of developments in this direction*

The present system of setting Occupational Exposure Limits in the EU might be an example of development in the direction towards a consultative program on risk assessment, although this procedure also shares some traits with scenario 3. The same goes for the new EU programme on risk assessment and management for genetically modified organisms.

The public availability of information that is assumed in this scenario forms part of the present discussions on a European directive on disclosure of information, which, as present developments indicate, will have a similar structure to the American Freedom of Information Act of 1970.

## SCENARIO 3: EUROPEAN COORDINATION OF ASSESSMENT

*Central traits*

The expert evaluation of chemicals is a distributed process and expertise is decentralized. Countries try to hold on to their national arrangements for risk assessment and risk management because of the market advantages for their business mix and because these arrangements incorporate pacified national debates. Harmonization is striven for on a negotiated basis. Experts take a lead in this harmonization and are encouraged to do so by European institutions. A core group of European experts organizes or supports confidential and informal expert meetings. In these meetings, the negotiations revolve around a bottom-up building of expert agreement. Standardization is the codification of such agreement. However, the common basis is limited. Decision making is often *ad hoc* and codification frequently requires creative solutions. Commitment to strict standards is limited, because these restrict the manoeuvering space in future negotiations (Feron, this volume; Van Damme, this volume). However, this commitment varies with the expectations of the actors about the nature of future positions and negotiation strategies.

Expert negotiations are organized by national representation. Implicitly, it is recognized that such representation balances the fairness of evaluations and therefore acknowledges the political elements in expert decision making. But publicly, this interference is generally denied. This asymmetry is rhetorically maintained through the use of a strictly rationalistic repertoire (Bal, this volume).

The experts represented in the coordination process have close ties with national decision making institutions. This is perceived as assuring a balanced input of national views. The experts return from the negotiation with the weight of European decisions and mobilize this as a resource in national policy. The integration of interests within the European context is an important task of the experts.

*The risk assessment/risk management boundary*

The boundary is organized in a heterogeneous way. The way it is drawn in international institutions differs from varying national arrangements. On the international level, the boundary is also asymmetric. Internally, the blurred and heterogeneous nature of the boundary is recognized, which is compensated for and reflected in the representative structure of expert involvement. Externally, the boundary is presented as sharp. This asymmetry is a strategy to maintain the agreements obtained, by creating legitimacy in the national context while keeping space for manoeuvering in international negotiations.

*Dynamics and expected tensions*

The experts are continuously drawn into political positions and debates. This periodically decreases their legitimacy among expert peers, who can form competing networks and present alternative assessment procedures. This undermines the scientific legitimacy of decision making. In addition, existing expert negotiation networks develop into elites that limit the access of peers to resources. This reinforces the construction of parallel networks.

Lobby activity is intense and frequently intrudes on risk assessment. The political institutions for developing interest integration are limited (and, if they exist, they are informally organized) or oriented toward national interests only. This leads to imbalances in interest representation in expert decision making. Because of the lack of formal structures for risk management, this leads to a politicisation by under-represented interest groups and accusations of capture.

In case of controversy, the intertwinement of risk assessment and management is easily exposed.[8] This puts pressure on the rationalistic repertoire, which might make it less credible, leading in turn to delegitimation. The

8 The regulation of formaldehyde in the US provides an example (e.g. Ashford et al. 1983), as does the case of Man-made Mineral Fibres (Bal & Spit 1994; Van Damme, this volume).

most probable reaction to this is a further articulation of the rationalistic repertoire.

*Advantages/disadvantages*
A major political disadvantage is the development of circles of expert elites. These tend to develop their own networks and political resources that hamper political decision making and democratic control (Abraham 1994, Mayer, this volume). Political legitimacy is therefore low, although controversies are relatively contained. The scientific quality of evaluations is extremely variable. Chemical safety is maximized in the short run, but broad support for longer term developments is absent, and the scientific legitimation is vulnerable.

*Indications of developments in this direction*
Under the pressure of member states, many European assessment procedures in the past have been structured along these lines.

## SCENARIO 4: EUROPE AS A TRANSLATOR

*Central traits*
The 'European Office of Constructive Risk Assessment' organizes meetings with regulatory actors from varying backgrounds. It has no intention of making assessments itself, but rather facilitates discussions within Europe. Since it is recognized and accepted that assessments are embedded within national regulatory contexts, differences between member states are frequent. Through reflexive discussions, it is hoped that controversies between member states are solved, or differences are put into clearer perspective.[9] Assessment and management of chemical risk stays decentralized and standardization is lacking.

---

9 In present risk assessments it is often known that idiosyncratic factors or interests of member states leads to certain (obstructive) positions, but this knowledge always stays within the contingent repertoire. 'Europe as a translator' will build upon such knowledge in order to facilitate reflections (compare Jasanoff, this volume).

Apart from the wider political context, the frame reflection[10] focuses on differences in data sets,[11] in evaluation styles and procedures (formal/informal, etc.), in the definition of management domains, and in the operationalization of exposure measurement. This reflection process leads to new ideas for European integration in the longer run. The dominant strategy for such processes is bottom-up, with no specific preference for a priority in risk assessment or risk management.

The role of the experts in the Office is to prepare the reflection process and to suggest conclusions from it. Studies are conducted towards member states' political context of regulation and controversies within and between them. Conclusions are suggested to European institutions with a more explicit integration agenda as new and potentially promising strategies.

Since it is recognized that the assessment of chemicals and the development of new chemicals are two sides of the same coin (Rip, Schot & Misa 1995; Irwin et al., this volume), the Office develops procedures through which insights from assessments can be fed into R&D.

*The risk assessment/risk management boundary*
The national or local arrangements of the boundary are made explicit. Their alignment is not a direct policy goal, although new accommodation strategies are suggested. Expertise as such is defined in broad terms and includes both the natural and the social sciences. Since it is recognized that expertise is a local phenomenon, the Agency is reflexive upon its own interventions.

*Dynamics and expected tensions*
The reflection process enlarges (the visibility of) differences between member states, while some convergence might occur in the longer run. The process would lead to further decentralization and/or destandardization.

---

10 For the concept of 'frames' and the possibility and tensions of frame-conflicts, see Schön & Rein (1994) and Bijker (1995b).

11 For example, the stress on the use of 'native species' within environmental toxicity tests or the choices about preserving environmental functions viz. environmental structures (Calow, this volume).

There is some danger that the reflection process becomes too intellectualised, leading to a relativistic stance towards differing frames. To anticipate this, the agenda for the reflections is narrowed down (Jasanoff 1990). This might also lead to a more restricted access to the reflection process, although interest groups will concentrate their lobbying activities in the national arena. One of the main problems will be to define new criteria for the assessment of national regulatory programs.

With economic scarcity, there will be criticism because of the agency's lack of decisiveness. Criticism will also be expressed because the reflection process brings the idiosyncratic nature of member states' regulation of chemical risk into the open. These criticisms will be hard to reply to, possibly leading to a demise of the agency.[12]

*Advantages/disadvantages*

The reflexive move does not lead to energetic short-term decision making. In some occasions, it may even disrupt existing routines of efficient management. In the longer run, the output is a much higher basis for regulatory decision making with new bases for political legitimacy. Increased chemical safety is generally postponed, though new breakthroughs may be intermediate results. The scientific quality of assessment is improved through a reflection on its assumptions. However, here too, the effect on the quality of decision making is not immediate.

In general, this scenario assumes the existence and development of one or more of the other scenarios. It can be a priority for further development, but cannot take over the role of existing decision making institutions.

*Indications of developments in this direction*

Two Dutch examples are worth noting. First, the assessment of pesticide regulation by the Dutch Rathenau institute (Sterrenberg & Brandt 1996). Within this programme underlying tensions in pesticide regulation are analysed and discussed with contending parties. A second example is a recent report by the Health Council of the Netherlands, called *Not all Risks are*

12 Compare the criticisms leveled at the US Office of Technology Assessment, leading to the discontinuation of this elsewhere much celebrated organization.

*Equal*, in which it is acknowledged that risk is not only a technical, but also a social and political issue, making risk comparisons problematic (Health Council of the Netherlands 1996). A further example might be some of the work performed at the International Institute for Advanced Systems Analysis (IIASA), especially by Wynne and others (e.g. Wynne 1984), although this institute has had problems in maintaining its links to the regulatory world.

## REFERENCES

Abraham, J. (1994) 'Negotiation and Accomodation in Expert Medical Risk Assessment and Regulation: An Institutional Analysis of the Benaxoprofen Case', *Policy Sciences* 27: 53-76.

Andrews, C. (1994), 'Policies to encourage Clean Technologies', in: R. Socolow, C. Andrews, F. Berkhout, V. Thomas (eds.) *Industrial Ecology and Global Change*, Cambridge: Cambridge University Press; 405-22.

Ashford, N.A., C.W. Ryan & C.C. Caldart (1983), 'Law and Science Policy in Federal Regulation of Formaldehyde', *Science* 222: 894-900.

Bal, R. & A. Spit (1994), 'De Risicopolitiek van Man-made Mineral Fibres', *Tijdschrift voor Toegepaste Arbowetenschap* 7: 63-72.

Bijker, W. (1995a) *Democratisering van de technologische cultuur*, Maastricht.

Bijker, W. (1995b) *Of Bicycles, Bakelites and Bulbs: Toward a Theory of Technical Change*, Cambridge: MIT press.

Brickman, R., S. Jasanoff & T. Ilgen (1985) *Controling Chemicals: The Politics of Regulation in Europe and the US*, Ithaca: Cornell UP.

Gillespie, B., D. Eva & R. Johnston (1982) 'Carcinogenic Risk Assessment in the USA and UK: The Case of Aldrin/Dieldrin', in: B. Barnes & D. Edge (eds.) *Science in Context*, Milton Keynes: Open University Press; 303-35.

Halffman, W. (1995) 'The Transformation of Expertise in Two Regulatory Regimes of the EPA', forthcoming.

Health Council of the Netherlands: Committee on Risk measures and risk assessment (1995) *Not All Risks Are Equal*, The Hague: Health Council of the Netherlands, publ. No. 1995/06.

Jasanoff, S. (1990) *The Fifth Branch: Science Advisers as Policymakers*, Cambridge, MA: Harvard UP.

Jepperson, J.R. & J.W. Meyer (1991) 'The Public Order and the Construction of Formal Organizations', in: W.W. Powell & P.J. Dimaggio (eds.) *The New Institutionalism in Organizational Analysis*, Chicago/London: University of Chicago Press; 204-31.

Nownes, A.J. (1991) 'Interest Groups and the Regulation of Pesticides: Congress, Coalitions and Closure', *Policy Sciences* 24: 1-18.

Rip, A., T. Misa & J. Schot (1995) *Managing Technology in Society*, New York and London: Pinter Publishers.

Schön, D. & M. Rein (1994) *Reframing: Controversy and Reflection in Policy Design*, New York: Harper Collins.

Sterrenberg, L. & W. Brandt (1996) *Van bestrijden naar voorkomen: Een visie op duurzame gewasbescherming*, Den Haag: Rathenau Institute.

Vogel, D. (1986) *National Styles of Regulation: Environmental Policy in Great Britain and the United States*, Ithaca: Cornell UP.

Wynne, B. (1984) 'The Institutional Context of Science, Models, and Policy: The IIASA Energy Study', *Policy Sciences* 17: 277-320.

Wynne, B. (1992) 'Carving out Science (and Politics) in the Regulatory Jungle', *Social Studies of Science* 22: 745-58.

# DISCUSSIONS

*Millstone*, referring to scenario 1 ('international experts'). What is needed are both local and global types of expertise. Local experts know about the practice of chemical risk, as is shown in a study by Brian Wynne (1992b), indicating the better knowledge sheep farmers in Cumbria had about exposure data after Chernobyl. Both forms of expertise should be brought in.[1]

*Passchier* (referring to the remark that the 'social science has shown that expertise can be challenged by alternative views').[2] This implies too much polarization. Risk assessment is a combination of toxicology and other disciplines; you need different inputs. Also, reading the scenarios, I would say that a combination of the different ones is needed.

*Halffman*. Our remarks as social scientists may lead to polarization. They may look like the idea that the work of experts is not good. But on the other hand, we try to achieve agreement on the idea that different world-views are possible. For us as social scientists the problem is how to make that point clear, as was intended in the first session, on the risk assessment – risk management boundary.

Second remark: the different scenarios to a certain extent fit existing regulatory styles. For example, in the Netherlands, environmental regulation

1 After this remark, Millstone had to leave, but in a letter to the organizers of 21 December 1995, he sent some further comments, which are listed at the end of this discussion section, together with some comments by Waterton.

2 This remark has been removed from the text of the scenarios, since we believe that not only the social scientists but also most of the other participants in the workshop agree that risk assessment includes, or at least builds on political assumptions.

seems to fit in the consultation scenario, more than occupational exposure regulation, which puts more weight on the role of experts, so this fits better in scenario 1 ('international experts') or 3 ('European coordination of assessment').

*Jasanoff.* One of the questions with the scenarios is what is at stake in making this sort of classification at all. Why are we interested in the different ways we create institutions? One of the problems that came forward earlier, is the problem in Western society that, when you create a boundary between science and politics, the person on the science side no longer has to think about questions of power anymore. This is a very powerful ideology. But to label something as science can sometimes require institutional settings, again implying social issues, although this may hide issues of power. Once you consider the boundary to be permeable, you allow for the phrasing of normative questions across the boundary.

I think the scenarios are a kind of interpretive work. The typology is an invitation to all of us to think about how we want to constitute government institutions. The world could be organized in these ways. The question is how we want the world to be organized.

*McCutcheon.* As technocrat, I have more to deal with reality than try to change it. The focus on the EU in the scenarios is OK, but there is also global harmonization going on. In global harmonization of regulations, we talk about parties like the International Labour Organisation, the WHO, and the International Forum on Chemical Safety, an intergovernemental forum.

I find the scenarios rather interesting, if somewhat theoretical and abstract. The regulatory practices are generally between scenario 2 ('European risk consultation') and 3 ('European coordination of assessment'), probably closer to 3, though there are differences.

*Bijker.* I would like to come back to the question that Millstone suggested: how to integrate localized forms of knowledge in processes of globalization?

*McCutcheon.* Local forms of knowledge are about exposure information and there is no discussion of harmonizing exposure assessment, more on harmonizing test methods for effect assessment and assessment for hazard or effect classification.[3]

*Van Damme*, on the contribution of social sciences, referring to the comment made by Jasanoff: did I understand it well, that scientists may have a hidden agenda and that that is the reason why social sciences should come in?

*Bijker*. There is no accussation of conspirancy in the natural sciences intended here. Sociology of science has tried to show that scientific knowledge and experiments are basically human work. You can understand them in terms of groups of people trying to make sense of experiments, negotiating among each other. This has enormous implications: it is a group of people making scientific knowledge, rather than Nature dictating it. Then other things come in, like values and disciplinary perspectives, normally not discussed in the Popperian ideology of science, and thereby giving science a divine, church-like character, which in my view prevents the democratisation of science.

*Van Damme*. OK, because otherwise my remark would be that social scientists may have a hidden agenda as well. An expert committee, as independent as possible, may agree that a social dimension is missing. However, this aspect may be introduced at the wrong place, introducing, in fact, the hidden agenda of experts from industry. Therefore, I maintain to my earlier remark that we should communicate with different other disciplines, but under the condition that we share the same objectives.

*Bijker*. I oppose the vocabulary of the hidden agenda. You will not understand what is happening by means of this. I think it is begging the question to say that we have to agree on objectives and then everything will work

---

3 Editors' note: this remark implies that the question of how to think about local and global types of expertise is already answered by the scenarios. More specifically, it can only be a problem in those scenarios in which local knowledge about exposure is relevant for the assessment of risk, which is presumably only the case in the fourth scenario ('Europe as a translator'). For the other scenarios, it is only relevant concerning the assessment of exposure. This could then of course be seen as a disadvantage of these other scenarios.

smoothly. The definition of the problem needs discussion now, and need not be confined to one arena, scientific, political or whatever. These terms have different meanings in different worlds.

*Smit.* I think these are useful scenarios, even when they are out of touch with the reality of regulation at the moment. This was also the idea behind the Shell scenarios: make challenging scenarios, encouraging thoughts about alternative futures. I appreciate this. However, I was puzzled by the meaning of the horizontal axis: the 'nature of expertise'. The difference between scenarios 1 ('International experts') and 3 ('European coordination of assessment') on the one hand and between 2 ('European risk consultation') and 4 ('Europe as translator') on the other seems not just to be a difference in technical expertise. It has more to do with pluriform vs. uniform regulation, or autonomy of regions on the one hand and a central organisation on the other. An alternative might be that there is more of a difference in the problem definition: a centralized vs. a local definition.

*Piney.* The trouble with scenarios of a globalized/harmonized world is that it is no longer clear where the numbers come from. That will blind people, and make them believe in the numbers like a kind of religion.

*Birrer.* The nature of expertise is in the scenarios referred to as local vs. global. But what is not in the scenarios – or only barely – is the form of decision making. For me, the choice between the different scenarios would very much depend on the checks and balances provided. For example, in the EU where, at the moment, there is little control, this has the implication in my opion that it is better to regulate chemical risk at a local level. Or we should think of how the EU can work in a more ideal way.

*Sedee.* I would choose scenario 3 ('European coordination of assessment'), with two restrictions: in the scenario it is stated that the assessment is confidential and not standardized. But in the EU going so far, it is standardized and not confidential, at least in the risk assessment phase of the existing chemicals programme. So, maybe it is better to use a third axis with confidential/non-confidential and standardization. Then it is easier to understand what is going on in the EU.

Scenario 3 is closest to what is going on at the moment. The movement is to take power *away* from Brussels; not give them more money, but less. In the comming years, risk assessment will be decentralized, not done in Brussels.

*Bal.* Translated in terms of scenarios, you are saying that it is agreed that assessments are done within the member states, on a local level, then negotiated between member states and NGO's and then presented as the result of a scientific debate, then followed by a political debate. That kind of system would fit in the third scenario, maybe apart from the confidentiality.

As to the remark made by Smit, I think you are right in pointing at the problem definition, but I think this is included in the scenarios. The consequence of defining expertise as a local phenomenon would imply that the risk assessment would also have to be done on a local level. Scenario 4 ('Europe as translator') builds precisely on that, whereas in scenario 2 ('European risk consultation') the different local assessments are negotiated on an international level.

*Halffman* (in reaction to the checks and balances point of Birrer). We know that there is a problem there, we have to think about it. But if you take openess-closedness of information and standardized-informal as the second axis, you come very close to what has been proposed for the comparison of environmental controls on technology (see the opening remarks of the paragraph on the criteria for the scenarios).

In reaction to Sedee's point: If the assessments are open and they are standardized, that would be more like scenario 2 ('European risk consultation'), which stresses open consultation procedures. Crucial for scenario 3 ('European coordination of assessment') is that the experts suggest that politics can be kept outside, and that their decisions should be and can be defended as scientific decisions, but in the interim there can be negotiation over politics. This is the crucial mechanism; it implies secrecy, implies limited standardization, because too much standardization would mean less room for negotiation.

Scenario 2 looks for feedback, so something has to come back; it is more than communicating assessments and decisions made by the experts.

*Vogelezang* (on the issue of decentralization). In the case of pesticides, perhaps this is different from other chemicals, there clearly is a tendency towards more centralization. Pesticides are – in legislatory terms – *products* and I think that product regulation is centralized by definition. If the instrument is national and centralized, it does not fit into local situations. That is one of the problems: how to change the instrument, so that it fits into local situations.

*Smit*. An intermediate situation could be to have local arrangements, coordinated to some extent to other local situations, not central regulation. You can compare this with the currency in different countries: it is local and there is coordination.

*Heyvaert*. Processes of globalization and localization can run parallel. Science becomes more global, but regulation follows slowly, and that is cumbersome. Therefore, I suggest using Europe more as a coordinator of knowledge, leaving regulatory work more to the local level, for efficiency reasons, but also because they can experiment with different kinds of regulations. That also leads to new knowledge, to alternative forms.

The problem is that we are talking about products: it means that industry is more interested in uniform regulation than in local arrangements.

*Jasanoff*. Three observations from the US context may be relevant to the discussion here: (1) In the early eighties there was a discussion of splitting risk assessment from risk management, and whether to centralize it. Everybody understood that this was a highly politically motivated proposition, because the power balance between experts and lay input changes radically when you have a centralized bureau. The National Academy (1983) decided that this was the wrong way to go, that risk assessment ought to be close to policy formation. Different agencies should do different assessments for health, environment, food and drugs. The idea that in Europe assessements should be centralized and regulation left to the member states, to some degree runs against the thinking in the US at that time.

(2) About checks and balances: formal systems of control make it very difficult to cash in on theoretically available systems of checks and balances. In the US, the theoretical possibilities of control are the most developed of the industrial world, but it is by no means the case that a person in the street

can make use of these kinds of power. So, checks and balances should not be discussed as formal mechanisms, and the more one makes one's decision making more technocratic, the more it becomes clear that people don't have access to the kind of information they need to challenge these decisions. So more informal systems, with space for dialogue, may offer more real opportunities for changing people's minds, although they don't look like offering checks and balances.

(3) In the last 3 to 4 years, the public has turned away from the risk-based regulation paradigm. People are asking for control over risks, for them not to be shipped home to states or localities. Many states have comparative risk excersises. One subaspect of this is that they say: 'we don't believe the formal risk assessment, we want a more common sense, a more local knowledge-based set of approaches, and we don't want to be controlled by methodology from Washington.' Heralds of this movement in California say: 'we don't care about risk, just hazard'. If a substance is shown to be reprotoxic or carcinogenic, then exposure should be brought back as far as possible.

There is a much more full scale rejection of methods and procedures, which people feel have become so opaque that, despite all oportunities of public influence, people don't feel attached to it anymore. People felt that they had no ownership of technical assessment. Discussions became so detailed and technical that there seemed to be no more relation with safety.

In the Californian case of comparitive risk assessment, there was a subcommittee on environmental equity. This meant that a new and different kind of people came in: 'non-experts'.

Followed by a discussion between *Van Damme* and *Bal*, in which Van Damme stresses the importance of independent scientific, uniform health-based values for occupational exposure. The worst case for workers is when scientists do not agree, because then the worst exposure limit will be taken. But Bal points to the DG V-experience (the Directorate General of the EU responsible for setting occupational exposure limits), where it is possible to get independent health-based standards, but impossible to implement them in the local contexts. This would suggest that, in order to be productive, risk assessment should be in touch with local institutions.

*Stijkel.* 'Think global, act local', that was once a slogan of the environmental movement. I think you can develop international health-based standards and then make local feasibility standards. This would lead to the construction Mark Piney suggested: two independent lists. Then, locally you would not have an expert group, but a group with labour and industry.

*Bijker.* In conclusion, I think the global-local knowledge discussion is a central point. Science and putting down numbers has become equal to global power, global truth. We have argued for the need to take in other groups, considering the local dimension. This is more than a theoretical discussion; it is also an empirical observation. Also in Europe, science is criticized and questioned about whether it is enough to ritually invoke the methods of science. There is a need to supplement them with other kinds of knowledge and local practice.

*Millstone* (excerpt taken from his letter to the organizers of 21 December 1995). While I understand your focus on the European Union, and accept that it is important, I am especcially anxious about the implications of the Urugay GATT Treaty and the relocation of regulatory powers to the World Trade Organization, and to bodies such as the IPCS of the WHO. The problem there has to do with the almost lack of transparancy, and the complete absense of any mechanisms for democratic accountability. Those problems arise in EU institutions, too, but are even more acute at the global level.

The distinction between, and the relations between, science and politics is clearly a crucial issue. While it is important to retain the boundary between science and politics it is also important to continue to explore the extent to which nominally 'scientific' issues contain concealed within them political assumptions and judgements. As Sheila Jasanoff and others have shown, it is in transparent and accountable systems such as those in the USA in which the regulators are (at least sometimes) compelled to identify and defend their non-scientific assumptions and judgements, and where they are under some pressure to show that those judgements are made in a consistent fashion.

Concerning scenario 1 ('International experts') one could argue that in practice it seems unrealistic to think that global experts can be entirely decoupled from their national or local institutions, unless and until the EU sets up its own centrally located and controlled scientific institutions. Scenario 2 ('European risk consultation') looks rather like a situation towards which some Commission officials think we are moving. The limitation here has to do with the lack of formal channels for many NGOs, consumer and trade union groups. The problem arises because consultation procedures are failing. Scenario 3 ('European coordination of assessment') is perhaps the one preferred by some members of the current British [1995] government. They pay lip service to European integration, but in practice they also want subsidiarity and localised or national autonomy. Whatever this might be, it would not be harmonization; and trade disputes could easily arise.

*Waterton* (exerpt from a letter to the editors, January 1996)
I think my main feeling about the scenarios was that they were pre-emptive and boxed the debate in the workshop in too much. Perhaps also a little too model-like in a way that was a little artificial?

## References

National Academy of Sciences (1983) *Risk Assessment in the Federal Government: Managing the Process*, Washington, DC: National Academy Press.

Wynne, B. (1992) 'Sheep Farming After Chernobyl: A Case Study in Communicating Scientific Information', in: B. Lewenstein (ed.) *When Science Meets the Public*, Washington: AAAS, Committee on Public Understanding of Science and Technology; 43-67.

# 13

*Willem Halffman & Roland Bal*

## POSTSCRIPT:
## NOTES ON THE WORKSHOP AS AN EXPERIMENT

### THE GOAL OF COMMUNICATION

This workshop had two goals. The first was to understand the patterns of integration between science and policy making in the area of chemical hazard regulation, in the light of the relation between European and national regulatory agencies. The second was to create a dialogue between social scientists who study these regulatory systems and natural scientists, administrators and representatives from interest groups, usually also with a background in the natural sciences, who are involved in regulation. We have presented our conclusions with respect to the first goal in the previous chapter, where we have tried to summarise and integrate the various views and processes signalled by the participants of this workshop in the form of scenarios: different courses that the European regulation of chemical hazards could take and the typical dynamics that could be expected in each of them. In this chapter we focus on the process rather than the product: on the goal of creating communication between social and natural scientists. We find it important to make available our experiences in this respect, since we find them at least as valuable as the substantive results. We hope these experiences can be used by others who seek to organise similar projects. In this respect, the things we did not plan and foresee are probably the most interesting and we will try to scrutinise these here.

In: R. Bal & W. Halffman (eds.), *The Politics of Chemical Risk*, Kluwer Academic Publishers, Dordrecht 1998: p. 333-344.

## THE PLANNING

We wanted to trigger a debate between natural and social scientists in order to mobilise a broader scope of interdisciplinary experiences to devise regulatory futures. While people in the 'regulatory world' have ample opportunities to meet and exchange views (although somewhat familiar with the phenomenon, it was a surprise to us to see in how many different forums some of the people we invited do meet), policy analysts and social scientists interact relatively little with this community. In spite of an impressive body of research on risk regulation, only a relatively small portion of social science research is fed back into the regulatory world. This is unfortunate, first because the widely differing forms of integration and distinction of science and policy, as well as issues of internationalisation and standardisation have been central topics for the researchers in science and technology studies (STS). We believe that the 'regulatory community' concerned with chemical risk might benefit from at least some of these contributions. Conversely, there is a clear need for the STS community to confront itself with practitioners of all sorts, to get more grasp on the practicalities of chemical risk regulation.

Organising such feed back is not self-evident, since the tools and insights of social scientists do not enter into a previously empty discursive space. The social science approach to risk differs considerably from the presently dominant one of the natural scientists in some crucial aspects. As we noted in the genaral introduction, this can be illustrated sharply with a recent report of the British Royal Society, *Risk: Analysis, Perception and Management*. The first section of the report is entirely devoted to quantitative approaches that interpret risk analysis as a purely scientific problem; the second section points to the close interconnection between culture, policy and risk and the impossibility of a 'purely scientific' approach (Royal Society 1992, Levidow 1994; cf. Health Council of the Netherlands 1995). Our idea was to try and get beyond this gap, to combine the advantages of first-hand, practical experience and detailed technical knowledge with the power of social scientists' reflexive contributions. Evidently, nobody expected this to be achievable within the setting of one two-day workshop, but nevertheless, this was the context in which we envisaged a role for the project.

The debate really started a year before the actual workshop took place. We worked from a ten page starting document that was sent out to the first set of participants we had in mind. The document specified the themes and goals of the workshop, as well as our ideas on the format. In particular by seriously considering the feedback from people familiar with the regulatory world, we could make sure the project retained maximum relevance for all parties involved. That is where our attempt at a dialogue started, in these contacts about what the workshop should be about. In the process, we gathered more participants, which continued throughout 1995. Unfortunately, those participants that came on board later were less involved in the construction of the workshop, which became manifest during the deliberations at the workshop itself.

Evidently, we expected communication difficulties, which we assumed would be caused mainly by the use of different frames of reference by the social and the natural scientists. We decided to send out a reader containing some ten basic texts from both the regulation of chemicals and reflections upon these regulatory systems (Haigh 1992, McCutcheon 1994, Brickman et al. 1985, Jasanoff 1987 and 1993, Hood et al. 1992, Zielhuis et al. 1991, Nilsson et al. 1993, Gillespie et al. 1982, Cairns 1986, Soares & Calow 1993, Wynne & Mayer 1993). We thought it important to keep a close grip on the programme in order to keep the project on its intended track, (e.g.) by asking speakers to talk on specific subjects. We limited the time for presentations as far as possible in order to have time for longer discussions. To facilitate this, we sent out abstracts or full texts of all talks to the participants beforehand. We planned much time for informal gatherings in order to maximise informal contacts. We aimed at the possibility that both parties would at least develop an understanding for each other's view. The presentation of the conclusions to the workshop in the form of four different scenarios, we believed, would accommodate the wide variety of these views, while still providing a maximum of analytic clarity.

## WHAT HAPPENED

The workshop had a difficult start. The first presentations on the risk assessment – risk management boundary brought out the diametrical positions. On the one hand, regulatory scientists, such as toxicologists Victor Feron and Robert Nilsson, felt the need to defend regulatory assessment procedures as being scientific and therefore independent of political influencing. Science and scientific independence were defended from this side as an important guarantee of just and reasonable decision making. Critical accounts from policy analysts, such as former Head of Science of Greenpeace UK, Sue Mayer, on the other hand, insisted on the 'politics' in the 'science' of risk management. The position taken from this side was that scientific independence, and the split between risk assessment and risk management, is a myth. Based on empirical examples, these accounts show how decisions of a political nature are taken by regulatory scientists, under the heading of risk assessment, rather than risk management. In this view, the myth does not serve to increase the independence of the regulators, but rather covers up the biases in regulatory assessment procedures towards allowing higher risk levels.

The indication of the mixing of politics and science was perceived as an outright attempt to delegitimise the conscientious and meticulous work of the regulatory scientists. We were half-way into the first morning, and the opposition that we had based the set-up of the workshop on, was laid bare. This was the tension that we were trying to overcome, but it took quite a bit of informal debate to get beyond the polarising confrontation of this first phase of the discussions. Nevertheless, at least it made clear what the problem was that we wanted to address.

By the next morning, when we turned to the more detailed, and perhaps more concrete matters of standardisation of chemical evaluation, some cracks seemed to have appeared in the natural scientists' defensive shield. Professor Peter Calow presented his account of the development of standardised toxicity tests to indicate where exactly he saw the decisions in his practice as a scientific expert that are 'actually' political. The main issue he identified was the choice between the environmental endpoints that chemical regulation should protect. More precisely, he signalled the need for a political choice between the assessment of the environmental impact of chemicals in terms of protection of species or in terms of protection of the ecosystem, i.e. the choice between protecting environmental *structures* or *functions*. When the evaluation of such potentially contrasting goals of environmental assessment is left to the experts, they will have to make political choices. The risk assessment processes, normally portrayed as pure science, then, according to Calow, can no longer be portrayed as such. As a regulatory scientist,

Calow wanted a clear mandate indicating the goals of chemical regulation, in order to deploy his own specific skills and expertise to achieve these goals.

The presentation of Peter Calow marked the changed atmosphere of the discussions and the growing appreciation of each other's position. However, even when one accepts that there may be some issues in regulatory science that are 'really' political, the consequences of this point are far from clear. Should one attempt to further 'purify' the scientific and the political? Or should the mix of science and politics be considered unavoidable? During the debates, two crucial and related issues in the organisation of risk assessment processes were identified and recognised by most of the participants. First, the tension between the difficulty of dividing 'science' from 'politics' on the one hand and the need, somehow, to organise such a divide for the purposes of policy making on the other. There was general agreement that substantial parts of the decision making process over the hazards of chemicals need to be delegated to the experts, the theme of discussion being how substantial this part should be and how this process should be organised. Some argued that if only the process of risk assessment were to be 'transparent', that is, observable and controllable, there would be no problem. A particularly clarifying intervention in this debate was made by Sheila Jasanoff. She argued that the model of a sharp split between 'risk assessment' and 'risk management' was a very specific product of a very specific (American) political situation of the early eighties, not necessarily a universal solution to all regulatory tensions. Furthermore, Jasanoff contested the corollary notion of 'transparency' of the risk assessment, since a transparent mountain of regulatory red tape may not necessarily mean accessible, understandable, and meaningful regulation of chemicals.

The second issue identified concerned the tension between local and translocal knowledge, an issue put firmly on the agenda by Erik Millstone, using very concrete and adequate examples. Even if we could agree on what constitutes 'science' and what constitutes 'politics' in a specific area, which knowledge should be included in the 'science' side of the devide? Especially the attempts to harmonise risk assessment procedures on an international level seem to run the risk of ignoring important *local* variations, which could radically alter levels of risk *locally*. Local knowledge about specific conditions of exposure or specific forms of natural environment could alter the parameters of the evaluations in such ways that an international assessment may obscure major local hazards. To be able to include such local knowledge under pressure of unifying markets, harmonised regulation, and multinational companies, new and creative forms of risk regulation seem to be required.

At this point in the discussion, we thought these two classic points of the Science and Technology Studies work on risk regulation would provide the input for a debate on the four 'possible future' scenarios we had prepared. However, proceeding so quickly to this primary goal of the workshop encountered some resistance. Most participants insisted upon exploring the differences and resemblances in positions more profoundly. Wiebe Bijker, our extremely agile chairman, proposed a very useful way to do this: take a quick inventary of what participants considered to be the most important problems of risk regulation. This indeed showed an extremely wide variety of priorities. Concerns ranged from the difficulty of proceeding with harmonisation, a problem especially for international regulators; over how to get rid of the politics in expertise, which mostly concerned regulatory scientists; to how to assure a fair balance of positions in the risk assessment process, especially aired by policy analysts; and how to avoid a gridlock of reflexive loops of analysis, a central problem for some of the science studies people present (see further below).

In the end, the tone of the discussions was clearly dominated by the attempts to communicate across interdisciplinary boundaries and between diametrically opposed conceptions of risk. The attempts to discover each other's frame of thinking, differing problem definitions and especially differing strategies to convince each other were quite fascinating. Unless they were interculturally misunderstood acts of politeness, we registered a clear will to continue the debate, some of which clearly happened during the preparation of the Proceedings.

## ANALYSIS

We want to make explicit a number of processes that occurred during the workshop. Some of these we noticed as organisers, some were pointed out to us by participants, in particular in later communications with Sue Mayer,

Erik Milstone, our chairman Wiebe Bijker, and Claire Waterton. Four of these will be discussed below.

*What is the problem?*

As indicated, the bottleneck we expected in the communication process was the use of different discursive repertoires by the participants. What became clear during the workshop was the difference in what the participants saw as the most salient problems of current regulatory practices. Participants shared a loosely defined interest in the problems we put on the agenda, but had quite different priorities. When asked what they saw as their most important problem, the range turned out to be remarkably wide. Here is a list, summarising these problems.

1 *Legitimacy*. How can we assure the legitimacy of the regulatory process? How do we organise 'regulatory science' in a way that is trusted, and accountable to public control?
2 *Shared definitions*. How do we reach agreement on the definition of regulatory problems and objectives?
3 *Communication*. How do we communicate uncertainties to legislators? How do we communicate science to the public?
4 *Participation*. How do we organise public participation in regulatory decision making? How do we open the black box of regulatory science to allow this?
5 *Other knowledge*. How do we prevent regulatory systems from locking in to specific forms of knowledge? How can we bring in other disciplines or 'lay' forms of knowledge that have been ignored?
6 *Conflict*. How do we make productive use of regulatory conflict?
7 *Reflexive paralysis*. How do we prevent a meaningful reflection on regulatory practice from turning into generalised doubt and paralysis that keeps us from actual change?
8 *Access to knowledge*. How do we make sure that even actors with less power get access to knowledge? How do we overcome inequalities in availability of expertise?
9 *The RA/RM boundary*. How convincing is this boundary? How do we organise the division of labour between experts and policy makers?

10 *The burden of proof.* Who should prove whether specific chemical risks are within acceptable limits? Should we prove reasonable safety or prove reasonable absence of risk?
11 *The local and the global.* How do we integrate local variabilities in risks? How do we organise the balancing between these and between local and global risk perceptions and definitions?

Although there are clear relations between them, the definition of what 'the' problem of regulation is shows considerable variability. Note also that the 'we' that is standard in these problem definitions is not always the same. Some problems, such as communication, are very much a problem of those who are at the core of the regulatory process. The 'we' who want access to knowledge or want their knowledge included as valid in evaluations, is clearly a different 'we'. The confrontation of these different problem definitions made clear that a large part of the difficult communication does not just consist of 'speaking a different language' but on having different problems altogether. For some policy analysts, this has been the reason to shift the attention of endeavours such as this one to engineering a shared definition of the problem (Hischemöller & Hoppe 1996). We more or less overlooked this in the preparations to the workshop. Organisers of similar endeavors might want to start with a discussion of the way participants define their problems. However, as shown below, differing problem definitions are only one set of bottle-necks.

### *Communication*

We very much based our workshop on the idea that the communication between social scientists and natural scientists (in regulatory positions) would be a good thing. Maybe we even had an idyllic secret phantasy of some sort of agreement or consensus that could be reached through this. However, some participants indicated that they saw no need for further communication. They were disappointed by the lack of response from 'the other side'. When one looks at the list of prominent problems participants presented, then communication corresponds to only a limited range of these. Those who interpret the problems of regulation as a matter of power or unequal access to knowledge, may find that communication can lead to co-optation and compromising. For example, some NGO's which have attempted communicating with, and even participating in the regulatory process, have found themselves ending up in the labyrinth of technical debates on chemical risks, having made compromises that they did not wish to make and that were not accepted by their constituencies (e.g. Van Damme, this volume). Likewise, some people who arc in the regulatory arena might be willing to communicicate, but not to open up positions that had some time been reached only with difficulty.

Furhtermore, it became clear to us during the workshop that whatever consensus we were able to forge in the very limited setting we had created, would probably not survive once people returned to their everyday jobs. The very goal of obtaining a communication process between the 'two cultures of risk assessment' (Jasanoff 1993) may have been a project that was biased by our own academic ethos.

### *Bridge builders*

We had two clear-cut groups in mind. We managed to get the divide between these groups into the open in an early phase of the workshop, maybe even more harshly than we wanted. What we overlooked was the importance of participants with multiple memberships in the construction of the dialogue. We discovered some of our natural scientists had social science experience, that some of our regulators could illustrate points of the policy analysts with more authority than they had, and that some of the social scientists could very convincingly mobilise examples of natural science. We have already mentioned the importance of Erik Milstone's interventions with examples of experimental practices that require decisions that reach beyond science. Also important were regulatory examples of Dr. Somers, a well respected and highly experienced regulator, indicating the limitations of unidirectional risk communication to manage regulatory controversies.

Participants with multiple memberships can enjoy respect in the different constituencies. In addition, their understanding of conceptualisations, problem definitions, and sensitivities allows them to build bridges across gaps that others would not even notice. For a project like this one, never leave home without them!

### *Scenarios*

We chose to work with scenarios to allow for different views and accommodate different expectancies of where the future of European chemical hazard regulation lies. We thought that this would help the debate because no point of view would have to be squeezed out, no artificial New Speech consensus language would have to be invented. Scenario building is normally a long and difficult negotiation process, used increasingly to mobilise knowledge in changing organisations (Becker 1994). We went through an iterative process, while writing and re-writing the proposal, receiving the abstracts, then drafts of the papers. We even modified the scenarios we had prepared beforehand during the workshop, based on the debates.

But the participants of the workshop did not make the scenarios themselves. *We* presented them at the end as an account of the debate and the different positions, leaving participants too little opportunity to participate in the construction of the scenarios. We kept too much of a grip on the process. It is difficult to see how more participation in the construction of scenarios could have been fitted into two days, given the gap in communication that we started from. Nevertheless, it would be worth finding more space for such participation while using scenarios as a workshop tool. We still believe we have covered most of the positions presented during the workshop, but we also know some of the participants still do not agree with us.

## CONCLUSION

In spite of the difficult and persistent differences in frames of reference, we found this workshop an extremely useful social experiment. Talking back to the communities we study under the pressure-cooker conditions of a workshop allowed us to appreciate the variety of problems in chemical regulation and to proceed with solutions for the problems we see from the analyst's perspective. One could call this action research; we also see it as a way of 'doing politics'. It is not only a way to learn more about regulation, it is also an attempt to re-formulate findings of Science and Technology Studies (STS) into messages understandable and viable outside our little circles. Call it STS extension work too, if you want. In any case, we would like to see more of such workshops happening and invite you to share experiences with us.

## REFERENCES

Becker, H.A. (1994) *Werken met scenario's: Minigids voor strategic learning*, Amsterdam: Thesis Publishers.

Brickman, R., S. Jasanoff and T. Ilgen (1985) *Controlling Chemicals: The Politics of Regulating Chemicals in Europe and the United States*, Ithaca: Cornell UP.

Cairns, John Jr. (1986) 'What is Meant by Validation of Predictions Based on Laboratory Toxicity Tests?', *Hydrobiologia* 137: 271-78.

Gillespie, B., D. Eva & R. Johnston (1982) 'Carcinogenic Risk Assessment in the USA and UK: the case of Aldrin/Dieldrin', in: B. Barnes & D. Edge (eds.) *Science in Context: Readings in the Sociology of Science*, Milton Keynes: Open University Press; 303-335.

Haigh, R. (1992) 'The European Community Programme on Health and Hygiene at Work', *Annals of Occupational Hygiene* 36: 675-680.

Health Council of The Netherlands, Committee on Risk measures and risk assessment (1995), *Not All Risks are Equal*, Den Haag: Health Council of the Netherlands, publication no. 1995/6.

Hischemöller, M. & R. Hoppe (1996) 'Coping with Intractable Controversies: The Case for Problem Structuring in Policy Design and Analysis', *Knowledge and Policy* 8: 40-60.

Hood, C.C., D.K.C. Jones, N.F. Pidgeon, B.A. Turner, R. Gibson (1992) 'Risk Management', in: Royal Society, *Risk: Assessment, Perception, and Management*, London: Royal Society; 135-92.

Jasanoff, S. (1987) 'Contested Boundaries in Policy-Relevant Science', *Social Studies of Science* 17: 195-230.

Jasanoff, S. (1990) *The Fifth Branch: Science Advisers as Policy Makers*, Cambridge, MA: Harvard UP.

Jasanoff, S. (1993) 'Bridging the Two Cultures of Risk Analysis', *Risk Analysis* 13: 123-129.

Levidow, L. (1994) 'De-Reifying Risk', *Science As Culture* 4: 440-56.

McCutcheon, P. (1994) 'Implications of Council Regulation 793/93 on the Evaluation and Control of existing Substances', *Annali dell'Instituto Superiore de la Sanita* 30: 367-72.

Nilsson, R., M. Tasheva & B. Jaeger (1993) 'Why Different Regulatory Decisions When the Scientific Information Base is Similar? – Human Risk Assessment', *Regulatory Toxicology & Pharmacology* 17: 292-332.

Royal Society (1992) *Risk: Analysis, Perception and Management*, London: Royal Society.

Soares, A.M.V.M. & P. Calow (1993) 'Seeking Standardization in Ecotoxicology', in: J. Cairns Jr. (ed.) *Progress in Standardization of Aquatic Toxicity Tests*, Boca Raton: Lewis Publishers/CRC; 1-6.

Wynne, B. & S. Mayer (1993) 'How Science Fails the Environment', *New Scientist* 138, June 5: 33-35.

Zielhuis, R.L., P.C. Noordam, C.L. Maas, J.J. Kolk & H.P.A. Illing (1991) 'Harmonization of Criteria Documents for Standard Setting in Occupational Health: A Report of a Workshop', *Regulatory Toxicology and Pharmacology* 13: 241-62.

# CONTRIBUTORS

*Roland Bal* studied Health Sciences at the University of Maastricht before becoming a research assistant at the Leyden Institute for Law & Public Policy. He is now a consultant on issues at the interface between science and policy. His research includes standard setting for occupational chemicals and the societal responses to risk in the changing welfare states of Western Europe. He has published several articles and reports on this research, as well as on wider themes in the study of science and technology. His thesis on occupational standard setting will be published in 1998.

*Peter Calow* is professor of Zoology and former director of the Institute of Environmental Sciences and Technology at the University of Sheffield. He is chairman of the UK Government Advisory Committee on Hazardous Susbtances and member of the EC Scientific Advisory Committee on Toxicity and Ecotoxicity. He has published over 150 articles in international journals and more than 10 books, including *Rivers Handbook*, volumes 1 and 2 (1992/4, editor with Petts) and *Handbook of Ecotoxicology*, volumes 1 and 2 (1993/94). He is the founding editor of *British Ecological Society's Functional Ecology* and *Integrated Environmental Management*.

*Karel van Damme* is a doctor of medicine and holds certificates in occupational medicine and hygiene and radiation protection. He is president of the Belgian Fund for Occupational Disease, a medical labour inspector for the Belgian Ministry of Employment and Labour, fellow at the Centre for Human Genetics of the University of Leuven, and fellow at the Department of Epidemiology and Community Medicine of the University of Antwerp. He served as a Research Officer at the European Trade Union

Technical Bureau for Health and Safety (1990-1995), and as such served on several advisory committees of the European Commission on both occupational and environmental health. He published numerous articles, reports and book chapters on occupational health and politics as well as on the social, ethical and scientific problems related to the application of genetic screening and monitoring of workers.

*Vic Feron* (toxicologist/toxicologic pathologist) is senior research fellow in the Toxicology Division of the TNO Nutrition and Food Research Institute, Zeist, The Netherlands. He holds a part-time professorship in Biological Toxicology at the Research Institute of Toxicology (RITOX) of Utrecht University. He is chairman of the Dutch Expert Committee on Occupational Standards (DECOS), a committee of the Health Council of The Netherlands. He is also a member of the Scientific Expert Group on Occupational Exposure Limits, Health and Safety Directorate, European Community, Luxembourg.

*Gillian Glegg* obtained her doctorate in marine chemistry in 1988, after which she worked for five years on the scientific aspects of environmental pollution with Greenpeace UK. She now lectures and researches at the University of Plymouth on marine science, pollution and policy.

*Willem Halffman* is a sociologist lecturing at the Department of Science and Technology Dynamics and a consultant on issues at the interface between science and policy. He is currently finishing a Ph.D. thesis on the integration of scientific knowledge in the regulatory control of environmental hazards of chemicals. This project compares the development of the involvement of ecologists and toxicologists in regulatory assessment in The Netherlands, the UK, and the US, over a period of several decades.

*Alan Irwin* is a Reader in Sociology in the Department of Human Sciences, Brunel University. His research interests are in the study of science and its publics, regulatory science and environmental sociology. Among his publications, he is author of *Citizen Science: a study of people, expertise and sustainable development* (Routledge, 1995) and co-editor (with Brian Wynne) of *Misunderstanding Science?* (Cambridge University Press, 1996).

*Sheila Jasanoff* is professor of Science Policy and Law and the founding chair of the Department of Science and Technology Studies at Cornell University. Her primary research interests are in the areas of risk management and environmental regulation, interactions between science, technology and the law, and the implications of social studies of science for science and technology policy. Her publications on these topics include *Controlling Chemicals: The Politics of Regulation in Europe and the United States* (1985; with R. Brickman and T. Ilgen), *The Fifth Branch: Science Advisers as Policymakers* (1990), and *Science at the Bar: Law, Science, and Technology in America* (Harvard University Press, 1995). She is a Fellow of the American Association for the Advancement of Science and recipient (1992) of the Distinguished Achievement Award of the Society for Risk Analysis. She has served on numerous advisory committees and panels of the National Science Foundation, the National Academy of Sciences, and the Institute of Medicine.

*Sue Mayer* has degrees in Veterinary Science and Pharmacology from the University of Bristol. After working in veterinary practice she returned to Bristol and gained a Ph.D. in cell biology/immunology in 1987 following which she lectured on Veterinary Therapeutics and Toxicology at Bristol Vet School. In 1990, she joined Greenpeace UK as a biologist, becoming Head of Science in 1991. In 1994/5 she spent a 14 month sabbatical at the Centre for the Study of Environmental Change, Lancaster University, working with Brian Wynne and Robin Grove-Withe. She left Greenpeace in September 1995 and is now an independent researcher/consultant with a special interest in the regulation of the risks of genetic engineering.

*Elaine McCarthy* was a researcher at the University of York at the time of writing. In addition to the papers which have emerged from this research, she has published (with Steven Yearley) in *Environmental Politics*. She is now working in the IT industry.

*Patrick McCutcheon* studied organic chemistry at University College, Cork, and legal studies at the Dublin Institute of Technology. Before joining the European Commission, he worked briefly in the aluminium industry in Sundsvall, Sweden, as a pharmaceutical representative, and as a forensic scientist for the Irish Department of Justice. He was the (founding) editor of *Irish Chemical News*, the official journal of the Institute of Chemistry of Ireland from 1984-1988 and represented the institute in various activities of the Federation of European Chemical Societies. From 1987 to 1993 he worked at the Commissions' Joint Research Centre in Ispra on the development of information systems on environmental chemicals and pharmaceutical products. From 1993 until recently he was the secretary for the regulatory committee of the EU existing substances programme on the evaluation and control of high volume existing substances and also for international activities at the OECD and UN level on chemical regulations. In the latter context he was the Commission's principal negotiator on the OECD discussions on lead, which culminated in the 1996 Ministerial Declaration, the UNEP/IFCS discussion on Persistent Organic Pollutants and the 19th UNEP Governing Council which adopted the suite of decisions 19/13 in February 1997. Since April 1997 he has assumed responsibility for chemical issues in International Water Conventions (OSPACOM, HELCOM, Rhine Commission and North Sea Conference). He is vice chair of the OECD Steering Group on Existing Chemicals and the OECD Advisory Group on Risk Management.

*Robert Nillson* has a background in biochemistry and radiation biology, and for four years acted as a sole technical advisor to the plaintiffs in the civil action against the producer of Thalidomide in Sweden. He was head of the Toxicology Division of the Swedish EPA from 1979 to 1984. He served as an advisor to the ministries of environment in Iran and India, and in various capacities as an expert to the OECD, the WHO and the IPCS. More recently he has initiated and coordinated several research projects supported by the Swedish authorities, the Commission of the European Communities as well as by the US chemical industry. Since 1986 he has been adjunct professor of molecular toxicology and risk assessment at Stockholm University, and European representative at the Council of the US-based International Society for Regulatory Toxicology and Pharmacology. He has published various articles in international journals, as well as several book chapters, both on issues in toxicology and on risk assessment and management.

*Mark Piney* has worked as an occupational hygienist for 17 years, first at Aston University Health and Safety Unit and then attached to Birmingham University Institute of Occupational Health. His long term interest in the history, philosophy and politics of science came together when he started research for his Ph.D., *The development of chemical exposure limits for the workplace*, which he was awarded in 1990. Since 1989 he has worked as a Specialist Inspector in occupational hygiene for the Health and Safety Executive. He is a Visiting Research Fellow at Aston University. His research is directed at the social, historical and philosophical aspects of standard setting for occupational chemicals.

*Henry Rothstein* is currently a Research Officer at the London School of Economics, undertaking research on UK risk regimes. At the time of writing he was a Research Fellow at the Centre for Research into Innovation, Culture and Technology (CRICT), Brunel University. His D.Phil. research at the Science Policy Research Unit (SPRU), Sussex University, was on food chemical safety policy in the UK and EU, with special reference to food contact plastics.

*Steve Yearley* has been professor of sociology at Queen's University of Belfast and the University of Ulster and a visiting professor at Cornell University; he currently holds the Chair in Sociology at the University of York. His research interests centre on the sociology of scientific knowledge and on the sociology of environmentalism. Recent publications include *Sociology, Environmentalism, Globalization* (Sage 1996) and *The Green Case* (Routledge 1992).

# WORKSHOP PARTICIPANTS

*John Abraham,* University of Reading, United Kingdom

*Roland Bal,* Maastricht, Netherlands

*Wiebe Bijker (chair),* University of Maastricht, Netherlands

*Frans Birrer,* University of Leiden, Netherlands

*Pieter van Broekhuizen,* University of Amsterdam, Netherlands

*Peter Calow,* University of Sheffield, United Kingdom

*Karel van Damme,* Universities of Antwerp and Leuven, Belgium

*Victor Feron,* TNO Nutrition and Food Research Institute, Zeist, Netherlands

*Willem Halffman,* University of Amsterdam, Netherlands

*Veerle Heyvaert,* European Institute, Florence, Italy

*Sheila Jasanoff,* Cornell University, United States of America

*Patricia Koundakjian,* Health & Safety Executive, United Kingdom

*Georg Krücken,* Bielefeld University, Germany

*Sue Mayer,* Litton Buxton Derbyshire, United Kingdom

*Elaine McCarthey,* University of York, United Kingdom

*Patrick McCutcheon,* European Union, Directorate General for the Environment (DG XI)

*Eric Millstone,* University of Sussex, United Kingdom

*Robert Nillson,* University of Stockholm, Sweden

*Flip Noordam,* Ministry of Social Affairs and Employment, The Hague, Netherlands

*Wim Passchier*, Health Council of the Netherlands, The Hague, Netherlands

*Mark Piney,* Health and Safety Unit, Aston University, United Kingdom

*Henry Rothstein,* London School of Economics, United Kingdom

*Aad Sedee,* Ministry of Public Health, Housing and the Environment, The Hague, Netherlands

*Wim Smit,* University of Twente, Enschede, Netherlands

*Arjan Spit (minutes),* RIGO, Amsterdam, Netherlands

*Emanuel Somers,* WHO International Forum on Chemical Safety, Geneva, Switzerland

*Anne Stijkel,* University of Utrecht, Netherlands

*Liesbeth Vogelezang,* University of Amsterdam, Netherlands

*Claire Waterton,* Centre for the Study of Environmental Change, Lancaster University, United Kingdom

*M. Younes,* WHO International Program on Chemical Safety, Geneva, Switzerland

# ABBREVIATIONS

| | |
|---|---|
| ACGIH | American Conference of Governmental Industrial Hygienists |
| ACHS | Advisory Committee on Hazardous Substances (UK) |
| AI | Active Ingredient |
| AIHA | American Industrial Hygiene Association |
| AFARP | as far as is reasonably practicable |
| ASA | American Standards Association |
| BATNEEC | Best Available Technology Not Entailing Excessive Cost |
| CEC | Commission of the European Communities |
| CEFIC | Conseil Européen des Fédérations de l'Industrie ChImique |
| CMR | Carcinogens, Mutagens and substances toxic to Reproduction |
| DECOS | Dutch Expert Committee on Occupational Standards |
| DFG | Deutsche Forschungsgemeinschaft |
| DoE | Department of the Environment (UK) |
| EC | European Commission |
| ECETOC | European Chemical Industry Ecology & Toxicology Centre |
| EINECS | European Inventory of Existing Commercial Chemical Substances |
| ENDS | Environmental Data Service Ltd. (UK) |
| EPA | Environmental Protection Agency (USA) |
| ETUC | European Trade Union Confederation |
| EU | European Union |
| FI | Factory Inspectorate (UK) |
| FIFRA | Federal Insecticide, Fungicide, and Rodenticide Act (USA) |
| GLP | Good Laboratory Practice |
| HBEL | Health Based Exposure Limit |
| HBL/Z | Health Based Limit or Zone |
| HBROEL | Health Based Recommended Occupational Exposure Limit |
| HMIP | Her Majesty's Inspectorate of Pollution (UK) |
| HPV | High Production Volume |

| | |
|---|---|
| HSE | Health & Safety Executive (UK) |
| IARC | International Agency for Research on Cancer |
| IEH | Institute of Environment and Health (UK) |
| IH | Industrial Hygiene |
| IFCS | International Forum on Chemical Safety |
| ILO | International Labour Organization |
| IPCS | International Programme on Chemical Safety |
| IT | Industrial Toxicology |
| IUCLID | International Uniform Chemicals Information Database |
| KEMI | KemikalieInspektionen (Sweden) |
| LOAEL | Low Observed Adverse Effect Level |
| MAC | Maximum Acceptable Concentration (USA) or Maximum Accepted Concentration (Netherlands) |
| MEL | Maximum Exposure Limit (UK) |
| MMMF | Man Made Mineral Fibres |
| MSAE | Ministry of Social Affairs and Employment (Netherlands) |
| NAS | National Academy of Sciences (USA) |
| NIOSH | National Institute for Occupational Safety and Health (USA) |
| NOAEL | No Observed Adverse Effect Level |
| NOEC | No Observed Effect Concentration |
| NRA | National Rivers Authority (UK) |
| NRC | National Research Council (USA) |
| NSC | National Safety Council (USA) |
| OECD | Organization for Economic Co-operation and Development |
| OEL | Occupational Exposure Limit |
| OSHA | Occupational Safety and Health Administration (USA) |
| PEL | Permissible Exposure Limit |
| PHS | Public Health Service (USA) |
| ppm | parts per million |
| QRA | Quantitative Risk Assessment |
| QSAR | Quantitative Structure Activity Relationship |
| RA | Risk Assessment |
| REL | Recommended Exposure Limit (set by NIOSH) |
| RIVM | Rijksinstituut voor Volksgezondheid en Milieuhygiëne (Netherlands) |
| RM | Risk Management |
| RPEL | Reasonably Practicable Exposure Level |

| | |
|---|---|
| SEG | Scientific Expert Group (of Directorate General V of the European Commission) |
| SETAC | Society of Environmental Toxicology and Chemistry |
| SCOEL | Scientific Committee for Occupational Exposure Limits (former SEG) |
| STS | Science and Technology Studies |
| TLV | Threshold Limit Value (set by the ACGIH) |
| TSCA | Toxic Substances Control Act (USA) |
| TWA | Time Weighted Average |
| UNICE | Union of Industrial and Employers' Confederations of Europe |
| USEPA | United States Environmental Protection Agency |
| WHO | World Health Organization |
| WRC | Water Research Centre (UK) |

# INDEX